Today's Nursing Leader

Managing, Succeeding, Excelling

Edited by:

Marilyn Klainberg, EdD, RN
School of Nursing
Adelphi University
Garden City, New York

Kathleen M. Dirschel, PhD, RN
St. John's Riverside Hospital
Cochran School of Nursing
Yonkers, New York

JONES AND BARTLETT PUBLISHERS
Sudbury, Massachusetts
BOSTON   TORONTO   LONDON   SINGAPORE

World Headquarters
Jones and Bartlett Publishers
40 Tall Pine Drive
Sudbury, MA 01776
978-443-5000
info@jbpub.com
www.jbpub.com

Jones and Bartlett Publishers Canada
6339 Ormindale Way
Mississauga, Ontario L5V 1J2
Canada

Jones and Bartlett Publishers International
Barb House, Barb Mews
London W6 7PA
United Kingdom

Jones and Bartlett's books and products are available through most bookstores and online booksellers. To contact Jones and Bartlett Publishers directly, call 800-832-0034, fax 978-443-8000, or visit our website www.jbpub.com.

Substantial discounts on bulk quantities of Jones and Bartlett's publications are available to corporations, professional associations, and other qualified organizations. For details and specific discount information, contact the special sales department at Jones and Bartlett via the above contact information or send an email to specialsales@jbpub.com.

The authors, editor, and publisher have made every effort to provide accurate information. However, they are not responsible for errors, omissions, or for any outcomes related to the use of the contents of this book and take no responsibility for the use of the products and procedures described. Treatments and side effects described in this book may not be applicable to all people; likewise, some people may require a dose or experience a side effect that is not described herein. Drugs and medical devices are discussed that may have limited availability controlled by the Food and Drug Administration (FDA) for use only in a research study or clinical trial. Research, clinical practice, and government regulations often change the accepted standard in this field. When consideration is being given to use of any drug in the clinical setting, the health care provider or reader is responsible for determining FDA status of the drug, reading the package insert, and reviewing prescribing information for the most up-to-date recommendations on dose, precautions, and contraindications, and determining the appropriate usage for the product. This is especially important in the case of drugs that are new or seldom used.

Production Credits
Publisher: Kevin Sullivan
Acquisitions Editor: Emily Ekle
Acquisitions Editor: Amy Sibley
Associate Editor: Patricia Donnelly
Editorial Assistant: Rachel Shuster
Associate Production Editor: Katie Spiegel
Marketing Manager: Rebecca Wasley
V.P., Manufacturing and Inventory Control: Therese Connell
Composition: Auburn Associates, Inc.
Cover Design: Timothy Dziewit
Cover Image: © Jaroslav Machacek/ShutterStock, Inc.
Printing and Binding: Malloy, Inc.
Cover Printing: Malloy, Inc.

Library of Congress Cataloging-in-Publication Data
Today's nursing leader : managing, succeeding, excelling / [edited by] Marilyn Klainberg and Kathleen M. Dirschel.
   p. ; cm.
   Includes bibliographical references and index.
   ISBN-13: 978-0-7637-5596-6
   ISBN-10: 0-7637-5596-6
   1. Nursing services—Administration. 2. Leadership. I. Klainberg, Marilyn B. II. Dirschel, Kathleen M.
   [DNLM: 1. Nurse Administrators. 2. Leadership. 3. Nursing, Supervisory. WY 105 T633 2010]
   RT89.T63 2010
   362.17′3068—dc22
                                                                        2009002216

6048

Printed in the United States of America
13 12 11 10 09   10 9 8 7 6 5 4 3 2 1

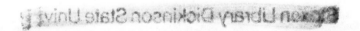

To family and friends who sustained and put up with me during the preparation and writing of this book, especially my husband Bernie, who is the love of my life; my children and their spouses, Dennis and Dana, Danielle and Mark, Gregory and Jenny, Joshua and Shelly; and especially to my grandchildren, who are my life and who will be delighted to see their names in print: Adam, Emma, Sydney, Jacob, Sofia, Simon, Samantha, Max, Shayna, and Sari.

—Marilyn Klainberg

For my husband George. You are more than the wind beneath my wings. You are my wings. For my children and their families: Mark and wife, Tricia; Nicholas, Jacqueline, and Grace Kathleen; Kristen; Michael, Agustina, and new baby-to-be; John; Brian, fiancée Christi, and Brianna. You are all the loves of my life.

—Kathleen M. Dirschel

Table of Contents

Introduction

This book is intended to help prepare the new nurse or nursing student to enter the nursing profession. It contains important components to help the new nurse achieve success. To be successful, you must know some specific and nonspecific information about how to manage your new role as a nurse and leader, as well as the history of the profession and how nursing evolved into the profession it is today. This knowledge is intended to help the new nurse understand the role of the leaders and managers with whom they will be working.

Understanding how a profession emerges and the impact of the profession on society is important in understanding health policy, delegation, management and legal issues, and how to affect these by making changes if necessary. Knowledge of these issues is important so that you can assume your role in leadership positions.

Porter-O'Grady and Malloch describe the role of a leader: "The leader is a primary facilitator of the journey to a new way of working. The leader's role is to keep people on the journey and help them understand what that means to them" (Porter-O'Grady & Malloch, 2007, p. 26). This is an important consideration to how you approach the content of this book. Nurse leaders need to be open to new ideas and able to communicate these ideas. Nurse leaders value professional growth by becoming lifelong learners and being open to change.

Charisma, creativity, and good ideas are only a portion of the role of the leader. Leaders must be able to communicate their ideas and embrace the notions of others. This goes beyond the technical ability to manage and meet the needs of the organization where you are employed. A good leader regards peers, subordinates, and those to whom they report in a just, fair, honest, and understanding manner (Porter-O'Grady & Malloch, 2007). Without this ability, a leader may not be able to go forward. People will put obstacles in your way to successful leadership. Part of the leadership role, then, is successfully working with others as a team as well as working with individuals, subordinates, and other leaders. Leaders must collaborate, coordinate, listen, be open to new ideas, and acknowledge and realize when they are wrong or have made an error. As you read and explore the ideas presented in this book, be open to them and try to incorporate these notions and strategies into your new experiences as a professional nurse.

The intent of this book is to present undergraduate nursing students with valuable reference information that is also readable. We have provided sources for students to review and hope that this book encourages you to seek further information about topics of interest to you. Because no book such as this that contains so many diverse subjects can contain all the information you will need, if we spark an interest in you to search for more in-depth information, we have accomplished what we intended.

Thank you to Rachel Shuster and Katie Spiegel of Jones and Bartlett, who put up with a great many questions from these authors! Special thanks to Jones and Bartlett for helping us realize our dream of creating a book for students that we believe will enhance their careers.

Thank you to Marie Anker, Polly Bednash, Sue Buchholtz, Tara A. Cortes, Jeanette Ives Erickson, Theodora T. Grauer, Jacqueline Rose Hott, Dawn F. Kilts, Marilyn H. Oermann, and Claire Shulman for their memoirs, which help to mentor students in their careers. To the book contributors, all specialists in their field, we thank you and appreciate your hard work and participation in this project.

Reference

Porter-O'Grady, T., & Malloch, K. (2007). *Quantum leadership: A resource for health care innovation* (2nd ed.). Sudbury, MA: Jones and Bartlett.

Contributors

Marie Anker, MS, RN
Assistant Vice President for Nursing
New York City Health and Hospitals Corporation
  (HHC)

Veronica Arikian, PhD, RN
Assistant Professor, College of Nursing
SUNY HSCB

Barbara Stevens Barnum, PhD, RN, FAAN
Consultant

Polly Bednash, PhD, RN, FAAN
Executive Director, American Association of
  Colleges of Nursing

Sue Buchholtz, EdD, RN, NP
Department of Ambulatory Surgery
North Shore University Hospital

Patrick R. Coonan, EdD, RN, CNAA
Dean, School of Nursing
Adelphi University

Tara A. Cortes, PhD, RN
President and CEO
Lighthouse International

Christine Coughlin, EdD, RN
School of Nursing
Adelphi University

Patricia Eckardt, MBA, RN
School of Nursing
Adelphi University

Jeanette Ives Erickson, MS, RN, FAAN
SVP for Patient Care/Chief Nurse
Massachusetts General Hospital

Bonnie Ewing, PhD, RN
Assistant Professor, School of Nursing
Adelphi University

Theodora T. Grauer, PhD, RN
Dean, School of Health Professions
Long Island University, C.W. Post

Marie Hayden-Miles, PhD, RN
Dean, School of Health Sciences
Farmingdale State College

Mary T. Hickey, EdD, NP
Assistant Professor, School of Nursing
Adelphi University

Stephen Paul Holzemer, PhD, RN
Associate Professor, School of Nursing
Adelphi University

Jacqueline Rose Hott, PhD, RN, CS, FAAN
Former Dean, School of Nursing
Adelphi University

David M. Keepnews, PhD, JD, RN, FAAN
Associate Professor, School of Nursing
Adelphi University

Dawn F. Kilts, MA, ABD-PhD
Dean, School of Nursing
Long Island University, Brooklyn

Sharon R. Kowalchuk, MA, BSN, RN
Staff Development, Westchester County
    Medical Center

Deborah Ambrosio Mawhirter, MS, RN
Clinical Professor, School of Nursing
Adelphi University

Marilyn H. Oermann, PhD, RN, FAAN, ANEF
Professor & Adult/Geriatric Health Chair
The University of North Carolina at Chapel Hill

Jerelyn Peixoto Weiss, RN, FNP, JD
Healthcare Consultant

Claire Shulman, BS, RN
Former Borough President of Queens, New York

Unit One

Genesis and Development of Professional Nursing as a Leadership Role

Chapter 1

Experiential Drivers of Leadership

Kathleen M.
Dirschel

OUTLINE

PURPOSE

The purposes of this chapter are fourfold:

- to understand the leadership role in nursing
- to understand the management role in nursing
- to analyze the nursing leadership role in implementing mission, vision, and strategic planning
- to identify components of an organizational assessment

3

The Leadership Role

Leadership in nursing is a goal, vision, and expectation for all professional nurses in any form of practice. Leadership has numerous definitions, but the key inherent components of all definitions are vision, communication, ability to encourage and develop people, and ability to bring about innovative change. Bringing about change in healthcare institutions that is lasting and measurable and that results in improved practices and outcomes is daunting and exciting.

A goal of this book is to help the reader grasp opportunities for leadership. Companions to this awareness are an understanding of the characteristics and skills of a nurse leader and a better understanding of the environment in which nursing leadership most often occurs. The leadership role is often tied to and inclusive of the management role. Although there are some similarities, there are also considerable differences in the practices of leader and manager. Some views on these differences are addressed in this chapter.

It is most common to think of nursing leaders with such titles as *vice president*, *director*, *president*, *chair*, *administrator*, or *dean*. Other titles such as *manager*, *nurse practitioner*, *educator*, *clinical specialist*, and *doctor* (of nursing practice, of nursing science, of education, of philosophy) also imply leadership or managerial responsibilities and authority. In all cases, with the preceding titles, a significant educational background goes along with the roles. The educational components of nursing leadership are presented later.

In the final analysis, all forms of nursing leadership must result in excellent patient care and patient outcomes. All forms of nursing leadership must also result in an environment that supports and encourages evidence-based nursing practice, essential for the practice of nursing at the cutting edge of recognized standards. To achieve these two outcomes the nurse leader must also provide for and support the growth of the scarce resource of the "bedside nurse."

The clinically practicing nurse fully implements and represents to the public and professional colleagues nursing as a practice profession. The nurse leader in the institution is the force behind clinical practice in the nursing role. Nurse leaders bring the vision for growth and the power to create the environment needed to preserve and develop the profession. The nurse leader is the visionary and the catalyst who brings power to nursing practice and creates an environment in which innovation and ideas about nursing practice can flourish. The nurse leader must create and orchestrate an environment that supports and encourages excellence in nursing and scholarly, caring practice. The nurse leader has the interesting challenge of creating and maintaining openness in a multidimensional, complex healthcare delivery system and enriching the practice field of nursing for the benefit of the institution.

There is a bridge between leadership and patient care outcomes: the nurse clinicians who are at the bedside and who do not necessarily hold any of the titles listed earlier or, indeed, any title other than *nurse*. That said, it is essential that organizational structures in which nurse–patient encounters occur and where nurses practice are supportive and encouraging of nurses' professional roles. When the environment allows nursing practice to flourish, excellent patient outcomes (in particular) and other nurse-driven outcomes (in general) can be achieved. Nurses, a scarce resource, can stay at the same institution because it is professionally supportive, and they can continue their work while meeting and exceeding standards of practice.

The institutions in which nursing is practiced are generally organizationally and structurally complex and always evolving. For the nurse leader at the highest level to influence all aspects of such an organization—not just the nursing sector—so that nursing can flourish is a role, responsibility, and challenge of enormous magnitude and opportunity.

Nursing leadership at the highest level occurs primarily in healthcare delivery systems and in educational institutions. The nursing roles in these environments, although related, are significantly different. However, both must operate to support the growth and development of nursing, as well as its other constituencies. The nursing leaders in both environments essentially have the same challenges and opportunities to move the profession forward and, indeed, move nursing as it is expressed in their institutions to exceed expectations and be so situated and energized to move standards of practice to the cutting edge.

Shaping and energizing the nursing component of any complex, dynamic system involve extraordinary knowledge and capabilities of nursing and the ways it is practiced in the environment. Accordingly, nursing is based on its underpinning theory and research that directs evidence-based practice. Such recognized behaviors move nursing to be a recognized partner in delivery of care.

The nursing leader also energizes the dynamics of the other personnel groupings and the vision, mission, structure, and resources of the broader institution. Doing so creates an open, more fluid system throughout the healthcare organization where individuals' resources and roles can work together with greater understanding and cooperation. When this level of communication is reached, sharing between roles, growth, and innovation occur in all sectors so that seamless care can be achieved.

Technology infrastructure, human resource development, operational definitions of quality, and measurements of achievement are key tools for the nurse leader to use to implement the organization's vision. What will be achieved is a cutting-edge standard of nursing practice that is a universal model. The nurse leader can use education, benchmarked practices, and analysis of data of outcomes from nursing practice as resources to achieve the vision and model for practice standards of excellence. The model must be flexible and sensitive enough to be responsive to evidence-based research, thus maintaining its positive energy forces and remaining strong enough to achieve the goals of the institution despite conflicting and competitive forces.

The Nursing Leader in a Senior Position

The potential for nursing leadership to serve at the highest level of responsibility in the healthcare delivery system, specifically the level of the chief executive officer, should be included in the vision of the nurse as leader. In the CEO position, the nurse transcends the traditional nursing role to one with multidimensional, multidisciplinary, and multisystem characteristics. The leader exercises effective power to achieve quality, cost efficiency, and access to services across all sectors and operational divisions.

Nursing leadership at the uppermost level can and must have the power and the ability to create an environment that stimulates the practice of nursing to the highest levels of evidence-based practice. Providing effective nursing leadership at this level to achieve evidence-based practice that exceeds expectation is arguably a most complex and challenging practice to which nursing can aspire and achieve. The educational pathways open to those aspiring to be nurses are quite varied. Chapter 3 reviews the educational pathways and concomitant experiential credentialing to achieve leadership abilities.

Ultimately, the top administrative position is the one with greatest opportunity to influence change and reinforce excellence in services across the entire system, whether it is a healthcare delivery system or an education system. The top administrative position is also situated to be the catalyst for developing relationships with the system's customer organizations and populations, and inherently shapes and analyzes the resources so as to be fully responsive to customer needs.

Wherever the nurse leader is in the organizational structure, the power to generate change and influence should be as broad and multidimensional as possible. The education to support this power must provide a framework for vision, planning, and action to ultimately achieve an organization that is true to its mission and socially responsible to its constituents in all aspects of its operation. Yet the leader must also avoid creating a culture that is over-managed and underled.

Mission and Vision as Forces of Leadership

The components of practice that become the driver for the nurse leader at any level are strategic planning and strategic management. These components position the organization in an infrastructure that is characteristically flexible and responsive to the demands of the customers of the system. Organizational infrastructure that consists of mission, vision, and values documents exhibits commitment and belief, which in turn are drivers for nurse leaders in all realms of practice as they evolve from a role at the bedside to a role in the boardroom.

The Mission Statement as It Relates to Nursing Leadership

Early on, nurse leaders must address their organization's mission statement, vision, and values. The ethical beliefs of the organization and its goals can provide direction and strategies to achieve these stated commitments. The mission statement states the institution's reason for being. It is usually a brief but enduring and broadly defined statement of the purposes of the institution. It is simple, despite the complexities encountered in carrying it out. Mission statements sometimes also state something about the scope and quality of the institution's services and the actions of the workforce to achieve those goals. In healthcare institutions, the mission states a goal of achieving a level and breadth of health care and the institution's way of achieving that goal, such as by employing educated, ethical, and committed healthcare professionals.

Mission statements can be refined as consumers and mergers change the structure and purpose of the organization (Swayne, Duncan, & Ginter, 2006). As the nurse leader begins to set his or her operational style and direction, the mission, vision, values, and codes of ethics are among the most important structural components that can be used to describe the distinctive nature of the organization.

Community is usually mentioned in the mission statement. If not in the mission statement, then elsewhere in the operating materials will be a description of the geographic and demographic profiles of the individuals, families, and groups to be served. The scope and breadth of the services further explain the goal statement. The phrases that address this could refer to the inpatient, outpatient, treatment approaches, and scope of services offered.

Mission statements are short and relatively simple statements of the working heart of the organization. An example of a written and succinct mission statement is "The mission of California Cardiac Care Center is to eliminate coronary artery disease in the state through research, prevention and education programs, and healthcare treatments."

The nurse executive utilizes the stated mission of the organization and leads the processes of interpretation and implementation in his or her areas of responsibility. The diverse areas under the nursing leader's responsibility and authority will respond and organize resources in a variety of ways to meet the expectations. Clearly stated, understood, and supported mission statements are the first step toward innovation in health care. The staff develops ways to carry out the mission through innovation, knowledge of their profession, and loyalty to the institution and its mission. The role of the senior leader is to generate creativity in carrying out the mission while respecting and enhancing the traditions and expectations of the institution.

As a profession, nursing can, should, and must have a greater say in how professional nursing practice in an organization reflects the organization's mission. Formal standards of practice, including expected outcomes as related to various nursing areas, will provide the evidence that demonstrates how nurses creatively and professionally innovate nursing practice to carry out the institutional mission.

The Vision Statement as It Relates to Nursing Leadership

As the nursing practice of the institution clearly demonstrates how the mission is brought alive to all constituents and the nurse leader generates the energy to carry it out, the vision of the organization must then be considered. The vision is a picture of what the future of excellence in healthcare delivery will look like in the arenas in which the institution competes. It is a statement of commitment and hope of what is to be achieved; it is a "will be" statement. For example, the hospital "will be the leading trauma center" and "We will deliver innovative technologies." Some visions suggest continuous actions, such as customizing care according to patient needs and values.

Vision statements should have the effects of empowering employees and being inspirational; they should be a basis on which decisions about the future directions of the organization are made. Although the vision looks to the future, the statements also honor and acknowledge past achievements, because the vision comes from the organization's history. Vision statements guide the organization in a direction where staff can reach their potential.

Strategic Planning as a Function of Nursing Leadership

The governing board sets mission and vision statements, and changes to them are relatively infrequent. However, in a dynamic environment some shifts may occur that require a reevaluation and reconsideration of the focus of both statements. Such a reevaluation would also focus on the strategies in place to achieve organizational goals. Examples of such shifts would be institutional mergers or additions and deletions of services.

Current strategies and possible alternatives are identified not only by the mission and by goals, but also by the performance of the institution regarding finances, operations, customer satisfaction and growth of the customer base, innovations and learning that occurred compared to a prior year, recognized benchmarks, and any changes in the environment. Operationally, healthcare institutions also strive for and measure success at meeting the standards of care using guidelines that are safe, effective, patient centered, timely, efficient, and equitable (Institute of Medicine, 2004).

When such an analysis translates to action goals and is prioritized, an improvement agenda and eventual strategic plan to achieve the new goals are established. Strategic planning is a process conducted at the level of the board and senior leadership. It is a decision-making and documentation process that results in a plan of action based on three components: situational analysis, strategy formulation, and strategy implementation. In some cases, a SWOT (strengths, weaknesses, opportunities, threats) analysis enhances the information used in the planning process (Swayne, Duncan, & Ginter, 2006). Any institutional strategic planning is of all services across the enterprise.

Characteristics of strategic planning in healthcare systems include the following:

- Guides members of the organization to see its future in terms of operations, relationships, and innovation
- Develops procedures and operations to optimize future outcomes, thereby establishing organizational focus
- Decreases costs and expands resources to serve community needs and interests
- Adds efficient and effective services and programs in such areas as primary care, rehabilitation, hospice care, and home care
- Establishes fruitful relationships with patients, intermediaries, other stakeholders, and potential competitors

The strategic plan is a planning and marketing document that defines the institution's responses to its internal and external environments in the present and in the near future. It involves resource allocation and is proactive and market oriented. Environmental assessments are a key aspect of the plan.

The internal and external environment assessments should be factual and quantitative. They should address changes in such topics as attitudes toward the organization and the services it provides, and beliefs about its ethics, values, commitment, quality of care, and the use of technology to achieve its goals.

Demographic information about the communities served, including health trends and economic and diversity profiles, supports planning. Patient surveys, complaint analyses, and direct interviews with consumers of care, insurers, and payers provide insight into what is expected and future trends that can affect the organization. Data about trends in clinical practice including attitudes of patients and clinicians about new services and modes of delivery; trends in physician and nurse availability; trends in attitudes of current employees, physicians, and volunteers; and roles of other provider organizations must be collected.

Once the strategic assessments and planning are completed, managers must manage the strategic momentum and the changes that will occur. Those in leadership roles set the direction and mobilize the energy for the changes. Managers have the key role of evaluating the organization's success and learning more about what works. New information received by the managers may result in adjustments in the plan and the process of implementation.

Leadership Strategies

The mission, vision, and strategic planning statements play a key role in producing change by helping the leadership direct, align, and inspire action. For example, without a clear vision statement, any transformational efforts can easily weaken, be confusing, and be incompatible with efforts to change current practices that do not address these principal documents of operation.

The mission and especially the vision set the stage for nursing leadership agendas for innovative change, especially because they guide decision making. Leaders and managers need to focus on communication skills and dissemination of information approaches and must create short-term wins, performance improvement goals, and rewards and recognition systems.

With mission and vision shared by staff and senior leadership, changes produce improved quality performance, increased customer satisfaction, ease of communication between employees to reduce extra work and time spent on notifications, financial savings, increased customer base, and reinforcement of promotion criteria.

Nursing leaders work with broad institutional teams and more local nursing teams to process changes for the diverse nursing staff to meet and exceed the goals of carrying out the mission and implementing the vision. They do so by establishing strategic direction and motivating and inspiring nurses to create energy and reduce barriers, and they produce extremely useful change. An effective leader invites a variety of individuals with different backgrounds and perspectives to provide input to the process.

The leadership must recognize that the arenas of change will be technological and educational, and some restructuring and increased quality monitoring and management must take place. Accordingly, any changes that occur will have upheaval and disruption as counterforces, and the management staff needs to be prepared for and skilled in maintaining order and predictability while monitoring implementation and overseeing delegation of responsibility.

Complacency can be a negative force against change. Leadership actions that create a sense of urgency, set higher standards for practice and day-to-day interactions, and increase the amount of internal performance feedback enhance energy and commitment to change. The leaders and managers can encourage, reward honest feedback in meetings, and develop an environment in which staff is able and willing to confront problems.

The complexities of healthcare institutions and the diversity of backgrounds and positions of nursing staff may move the nursing leader to embrace bolder approaches to change. For example, after examining work goals of divisions and departments and comparing them to benchmarks of like areas, the leader communicates that he or she expects the staff to improve their output so that they are first or second when compared with others within 24 months. With that expectation, the leader must provide support for the training necessary and the help of the managers to simplify some activities so that staff can reach higher response rates to patient outcomes that support the stated mission and vision.

Setting productivity expectations at higher levels for qualitative outcomes is a further expression of a bolder approach to implementing change. Creating expectations of improved customer satisfaction and setting and enforcing high standards for quality evidence-based patient care set an expected achievement level that supports the mission and the placement of the organization at the forefront of the healthcare industry of choice.

To maintain and improve the perception of the institution as a desirable place to work, such goals as higher staff retention ratios, less absenteeism, and staff education and practice achievements balanced by rewards and recognition must be set. Throughout the change process, leaders must stress the importance of communication and continuously roll out information on current and future growth opportunities and the rewards and benefits that are tied to them.

commitments. Accordingly, managers are prepared to manage by their education, their experience, and the arrangement by the leadership that there is sufficient time to work with the staff. Managers frequently come from the ranks of clinical staff and possibly may confuse their previous clinical, patient care-oriented roles with managing and overseeing staff clinicians. In positions where nurse managers also hold clinical responsibilities, the potential for role confusion and lack of job satisfaction is high. Nurse managers who spend an inordinate amount of time on staffing are not able to perform the management functions as well as should be expected.

Managing through supervision, guiding the staff to high achievement, helping staff feel a sense of satisfaction from their work effort, and encouraging advanced education and certification to facilitate delivery of quality care should be prominent in the nurse manager role. The goal of the supervision role is to bring about nursing practice, consistent with evidence-based standards, and carried out with as little variation as possible.

Management Strategies

Managers are key players in the change process. The overall role of the manager is to direct, coordinate, and reinforce expectations of the work of others. Implementation of the goals and visions as set by leadership become the focus at the managerial level. It is managers' responsibility to facilitate achieving the goals in a stable and rational environment. Managers focus on short-term goals that include cost effectiveness and staff retention and satisfaction.

Managers are empowered to hold staff and others accountable for meeting objectives and

Management Roles and Behaviors

Successful managers use specific skills to facilitate the implementation of change. Changes in the healthcare environment are always fluid and occur in an environment that is diverse, chaotic or almost so, complex, and demanding. Managers can grow into great managers that create success—individually, in their teams, and for their organizations. Box 1–1 gives one nurse leader's perspective on how to be an effective manager.

Box 1–1 Being a Contemporary Nurse Leader

Jeanette Ives Erickson

Who I am as a nurse leader was defined early in my life. I grew up in Portland, Maine, surrounded by an extended family of first-generation Italian immigrants. We lived over a grocery store owned and operated by my great-grandparents. I was blessed with a strong family system where the values of hard work and putting people first were well known and engrained into us.

My first mentors were family members who shared invaluable lessons that have carried me throughout my nursing career. My mother taught me how to solve problems, my uncle taught me the value of participatory management long before there was a name for it, and my aunts taught me a lot about business. My father, who traveled extensively, helped me understand that work needed to be balanced with family. And all of them taught me that you can create your own destiny, and that success takes vision, courage, perseverance, and hard work.

Despite our humble socioeconomic status, my parents instilled in me a belief that I could do anything I put my mind to. Going to college was important, but money was not readily available; I knew I would have to work hard both to secure scholarships and funds for the remaining costs. So, at age 16 I started my first job, working in a grocery store. I have worked ever since and working has become an integral part of who I am.

During my senior year in high school, I decided I wanted to go to nursing school, and our next door neighbor, Mrs. Alice Haskell—

a nurse—took an active interest and helped me with my applications. She also introduced me to Sr. Mary E. Consuela White, RN, head of the Mercy Hospital School of Nursing and director of Nursing at Mercy Hospital in Portland, Maine. From my initial interview, Sr. Consuela became a role model, and because of her, I decided to attend Mercy Hospital School of Nursing. The format of the program was unique for the time. Designed to prepare nurses with a diploma, we took many liberal arts courses that helped to provide a solid foundation for entry into a BSN program.

While a student nurse, I worked summers as a nursing assistant. There I met my mentor and friend, Barbara Sheehan, RN, the night shift nursing supervisor. Barbara took me under her wing and let me do things only nurses were allowed to do. Her mentorship has always been important to me and truly shaped my career. Barbara embodied what it means to be a nurse. She placed patients and families above all else, and her teachings later drove my decision to become a nurse executive.

I successfully graduated from nursing school, and as I embarked on my career as a critical care nurse, the times were tumultuous with the Vietnam War raging. Several nursing colleagues had husbands fighting in the war, and from them I learned activism. I joined the POW/MIA movement helping to batch bracelets honoring men lost at war. These nurse activists also served as mentors for the next phase of my career and life.

Being an excellent nurse was always important to me, and I loved working in critical care. And during these early clinical years, I realized that the continuous improvement of clinical practice and the environment of care needed to remain my highest priority.

It was Sr. Consuela who convinced me to go back to school and to obtain my BSN from Westbrook College (now the University of New England) and later my master's degree. She also encouraged me to take my first management position, and I became a head nurse and later nursing director, remaining at Mercy Hospital for 16 years.

I obtained my master's degree from Boston University (BU). While in graduate school, I met another strong, influential woman, Muriel Poulin, RN, one of the pioneer nurse researchers of the hallmark Magnet Hospital study. She was highly competitive and advised me that if I were going to be the nurse executive in an organization, I would need to put my ideas forward and be very clear about my objectives. She taught me that I needed to share the same business skills as the rest of the executive team. She, too, was very connected to the values of the nursing profession, always keeping her eye on the integrity of the nurse–patient relationship. She underscored the importance of the executive's role in creating an environment in which nurses' practice could flourish.

Upon graduating from BU, I took a job at Massachusetts General Hospital (MGH) as a staff specialist focused on leadership development. After nine months, I was asked to interview for a director position. As the director for Nursing Support Services, I became responsible for process improvement initia-

tives and had line management responsibility for staff support (unit secretaries and unit assistants). My major contribution was to redesign the unit-based support staff roles to ensure that the staff were more connected to care delivery. I felt it was important to move the central resources to the patient care unit, with the support staff reporting to the nurse managers instead of to me. Unity of purpose was the approach, and it was successful. The support staff loved working with the nurses, and this resulted in a common goal for care delivery. So, in just 16 months as a director, I had successfully worked myself out of a job!

But MGH was planning a new inpatient facility, and Chief Nurse Yvonne L. Munn, RN, asked me to lead the initiative for the Nursing Service. When Yvonne retired, Gail Kuhn Weissman, RN, became chief nurse. With new leadership there always comes change, and I was asked to serve as a deputy chief nurse with responsibility for multiple clinical services. In 1996, the chief nurse position became vacant, and the newly appointed CEO of the hospital, James Mongan, MD, asked me to take on this important role.

I assumed the position of senior vice president for Patient Care and chief nurse at a time when the organization was undergoing massive change. Dr. Mongan and I forged a wonderful partnership, working collaboratively to create an environment in which the workforce felt valued and recognized.

At the same time, Patient Care Services was being formed. It was important to align the coming together of nurses and numerous health professions with the hospital's new strategic direction. Throughout this transformational change, I drew upon my experience and the key leadership qualities I learned from my teachers, colleagues, and mentors, and I initiated several high-leverage strategies that I refer to as the *seeds for change*. It took years for these seeds to grow—they required ongoing care and cultivation—but today the hospital and our patients and their families are reaping the benefits. As you prepare for your own career in the finest of professions—nursing—I hope these seeds will also serve you well in the years to come.

Seeds for Change for Nurse Leaders

- *Driven by values.* I believe that all nurses are leaders and as leaders we need to be very clear about what we stand for—our actions need to be connected to our values. When I make decisions, I always focus on the impact they will have on patients and families, and of course, the nurses caring for them. Keeping my eyes on the patients and their families remains the best navigational system.
- *Communicate, communicate, and communicate.* Communication is essential to success. I seize every moment to connect with patients and families, nurses, and other colleagues to hear what's working and what's not. Being visible, accessible, and open to dialogue guides my leadership practice.
- *Exquisite listening skills.* Nurse leaders must be exquisite listeners. You have to open yourself up to hearing what patients, families, staff nurses, and colleagues are telling you. And, more important, you must hear what they aren't telling you. Becoming a good listener isn't easy—it takes practice and keen attention.

- *Importance of a strategic plan.* I have always put an emphasis on the importance of strategic planning. It is important to "know where you are headed" and to engage those with whom you work to articulate a shared strategic direction. In addition, it's just as important for a leader to be a tactical planner—to be able to identify each step the team needs to take to realize a shared vision.
- *Strike a healthy work–life balance.* As a leader in health care, it's not surprising that the more you do, the more you see there is to do. For all of us involved in health care, one of the dangers lies in not taking the time to reflect and, more important, to rejuvenate ourselves. It's key that you strike the right balance between work and your personal life. I make a conscious effort to take time off and spend time with family and friends.
- *Find a mentor and be a mentor.* I have always been surrounded by strong, determined, hardworking women. For example, my mother encouraged me to either walk past obstacles or to push through them, and to this day I call her for advice. Find a mentor who believes in you and will push you to your greatest potential. And, in the future, be certain you serve in a mentor role to pass the torch of nursing excellence to the next generation of nurses.
- *Embrace diversity.* One of the top priorities for nurse leaders is to hire and develop a workforce that mirrors its patient population and possesses the knowledge and skill to deliver culturally competent care. This requires that nurse leaders possess an enhanced understanding of diversity issues,

and that they champion healthcare and nursing diversity awareness initiatives to address them. I view a diversity program as being successful when it creates a work environment that focuses on maximizing the potential of each individual.

- *It takes a village.* I often borrow the African proverb, "It takes a village" and apply it to the work of health care. It truly takes a village to care for our patients, families, and staff. As a nurse leader, it is my responsibility to create a practice environment in which collaboration across the healthcare team is fostered and the members of that team have the skills, knowledge, and resources to do what they do best—care.

The tasks of management include championing change as set forth by the leaders, fostering teamwork in and across organizations, and focusing on customer needs and quality. Respected managers are extraordinary planners and organizers. Great managers take the time to develop themselves. There are minimally five basic steps a new manager can employ to be effective:

- As they learn the organization, they focus on priorities and identify critical issues and goals.
- They implement something every day, because this helps them stretch their comfort zone.
- They reflect on what happens and take maximum learning from all their experiences.
- They seek feedback and support from clinical staff and from leadership; they learn from others' ideas.
- They transfer learning into a plan for continued learning and assessment.

Management skill sets build on these entry-level behaviors and set the stage for development of superior managers who embrace the mission and goals of the organization and the changing environment and share the leadership vision. Managers must have administrative skills. Key skills in this area include the ability to develop long- and short-term goals, manage systems in a cost efficient manner, and recruit and hire the right individuals to build strong teams.

Because of the need for standardization and streamlining operations for work efficiency, managers develop systems and processes to get the work done, empower others, remove obstacles, and monitor progress. To facilitate work processing, managers' communication skills must be effective and strong. Components of communication are effective speaking abilities, open communication, active and focused listening, and clear, accurate, and consistent written communications.

Interpersonally, effective managers build open, friendly, and accepting relationships; display organizational shrewdness and respect; and build and use networks for advantage within and outside the organization. Managers sincerely value, foster, respect, and appreciate diversity and use differences to leverage learning. Because of these interpersonal strengths, managers are capable of handling disagreements and building consensus.

Developing organizational knowledge, such as understanding and using financial and quantitative data to enhance clinical practice outcomes, enhancing technical and functional expertise that is business oriented rather than clinically focused, and understanding the business of healthcare delivery in the organization, including broad organizational and business issues, is a new, yet critical component of the managerial role. Some of this capability is learned in graduate programs and some from immersion in a new world of the business of health care, which has clinical care as its core but focuses on the broader institutional structures and process to achieve excellence. Managers must have opportunities and support in building this new knowledge base, because it is the framework for a new and critically necessary practice within nursing.

The core abilities and skills of managers are primarily organizational. With the mission and vision as determined by leadership shaping practice and outcomes, such skills as managing profitability by making decisions with staff input become important. Managers commit to providing quality services, products, and managing standards. They focus on customer needs. Managers model quality behaviors by defining standards and develop opportunities to evaluate products, processes, and services against recognized standards.

Managers must be prepared to foster wise use of scarce resources, including nursing staff. Under the direction of the leadership, managers work to build and support additional resources and relationships. To do so effectively, managers must develop an understanding of the issues and trends in a diverse and multicultural professional and geographic community. The recognized strengths of diversity can facilitate the evolution of the organization to one that is knowledge-based and socially responsible.

Managers are role models in all their practices. Attention must be paid to how the behavior of the manager brings about trust, stability,

and change. The professional principles of the managerial role include the following:

- *Act with integrity.* Managers act with integrity when they use ethical principles in practice, build trust, demonstrate consistency in business practices, and follow through on commitments.
- *Demonstrate adaptability.* Managers demonstrate adaptability and flexibility in handling day-to-day work challenges, adjusting to multiple demands, and showing resilience in the face of constraints and frustrations.
- *Develop oneself.* Managers demonstrate learning from experience and actively pursue self-development and feedback. The feedback results in modifying behavior as necessary.

Understanding the Healthcare Delivery Organization from an Open Systems Perspective

It is clear that leaders and managers in the healthcare delivery system work from the principles of systems functioning in that the many subsystems of the whole carry out their own processes by their own standards. To be fully functional, the healthcare organization must have ways of communicating and sharing information to support its mission and goals and ensure that accurate communications penetrate all levels and silos of the agency. Whereas some subsystems may be parallel, even opposing in their goals, all work for the common expectation of success of the organization. For example, limits on staffing numbers may be a financial goal but may be a constraint for staff to advance their certifications and education.

Understanding and enhancing individual and subgroup efforts while expanding and broadening intergroup efforts becomes the mantra of the leader, with the management team reinforcing managed change to reach broad goals as fully and quickly as possible. Even the healthcare organization is part of a larger system, that is, the healthcare industry or the system of higher education. Systems and organizations within systems operate through the principles of open systems. Understanding and using the principles of open systems are keys to being a successful leader and supporting manager.

Assessments of the Organization

Knowing and utilizing the principles of open systems to enhance the functioning of the healthcare organization are tools of leadership and management alike. The ability of the leadership to assess the organization and identify areas of function and dysfunction (seen as positive and negative energy) is essential to the success of the organization to function as a cooperative and communicating whole.

Such an assessment should include the relationships of the subsystems within the organization and the organization's relationships with other systems with which it interacts. Assessing, understanding, and utilizing the energy within the system, and facilitating the generation of additional energy to achieve organization goals are overarching roles and functions of the leader, whether a leader in the nursing subsystems of the organization or in more diverse multi-department subsystems of the organization.

Where there is dysfunctional behavior within and among the subsystems, where there is extreme subspecialization, and/or where there is need for adaptation to changing or unstable environments, the leader can assess the situation and set vision and action accordingly (Levinson, 2006).

Components of an Organizational Assessment

Ascertaining as much as possible about the origins and background of the healthcare institution is key to strategic analysis and planning. The organization's roots always point to what is sacrosanct and identify the profile of services offered to the community and the employees. The major infrastructure components of the institution are the plant and equipment, the financial structure, human resources, and the product service history.

An alignment of energy exchange, communications, and balance of resources and productivity are the ideal outcomes of assessment of these components. Where there is imbalance or lack of shared information and resources, the leader and manager can develop a resolution initiative.

As the assessment proceeds, determining chief complaints and perceived problems of the organization is key. Views on key growth efforts, major changes, and organizational self-image can also help create the identity of the organization. Beyond direct and quantitative data collection, tapping into the qualitative impressions of the staff is essential.

The emotional atmosphere of the institution, for example attitudes and relationships, feelings of respect and of being valued, must be assessed. The masculine-feminine orientation, which focuses on the roles and expected behaviors of male and female members and opportunities for advancement, must be assessed. Who are the key people, and why? In addition, where and with whom do the authority, power, and responsibility lie?

An organizational assessment performed by leadership or perhaps consultants should reflect the conflicts that the institution contends with and the various strengths and weaknesses that will enhance or interfere with problem resolution. Are there latent capacities for diversification and specialization? Are there undeveloped potentials for creativity and innovation? An assessment of this nature yields enormous strength and insight for strategic planning and reinforcement of the mission and vision. It is a strong tool and reference source for leadership and management at all levels.

Once an accurate and full organizational assessment has been developed, it becomes a template for developing leadership strategies as related to areas of need and growth. All aspects and components of the organization that are affected by or under the leadership of the nurse leader are energized and supported to work as a whole and produce results greater than the sum of the individual parts. Key broad areas of the design and infrastructure of the organization include the Information Technology systems (both clinical and back office) and financial systems. The status and needs of these areas as determined from the organizational assessment, can begin to be addressed by nursing leadership to eventually enhance their performance.

To function at peak performance levels, the healthcare delivery system must have a robust, customized, fully functional and operational computerized information system. Although nurse leaders may not always be experts in the technology, they must value and use this electronic nerve center to analyze, collect, aggregate, and store data and activate data mining activities for the benefit of planning and assessing institutional functions. Information systems (IS), once planned, are developed according to

plan that both justifies cost and results in added, useful information. (Griffith & White, 2002). Some projects that can be supported by the leadership in customizing and implementing the IS can and should include creating and improving evidence-based protocols through analysis of financial and clinical information and outcomes. Such timely and cutting-edge guidelines for care are and can be hard-wired into the IS so that errors and accidents are reduced, which not only reflects higher quality care but also cost efficiency. Opportunities to automate care and the capability of comparing national data sets with current results continually enhance the value of the IS.

Wise nurse leaders stimulate and direct institutional energy toward the creation of IS standards and capabilities and provide and nurture the necessary technological expertise and information sharing abilities (i.e., reducing silos) throughout the multiprovider organization (Wolper, 2004). The expectation and necessity of developing a full-blown customized and robust IS to support the organization holds true for both clinical as well as educational organizations.

The enhancement of quality processes throughout the organization and at all levels of care is a broad-based strategy necessary for the success of the institution at all levels of operation.

Summary

Overall, the nurse leader employs strategic management principles that effectively integrate and develop all parts of the organization. Through such integration efforts, the leaders and managers are in the position to provide out-of-the-box thinking and guide shifts in courses of action so that goals are achieved. Basic to this approach is accountability and continuous learning: accountability commensurate with responsibility and continuous learning by studying prior years' outcomes and developing recognition planning are keys to the success of the leader.

The key steps in strategic management, following the establishment of organizational mission, vision, and values statements, include analysis of strengths, weaknesses, opportunities, and threats that are relevant to the organization. The roles, responsibilities, resources, and information that shape the persona of the nurse leader and the nurse manager can transport the nurse from bedside to boardroom easily, accurately, and with support and enthusiasm from the staff and leadership alike.

QUESTIONS

1. To accomplish the work that needs to be done, the nurse manager will
   a. develop systems and processes to get the work done
   b. empower others
   c. remove obstacles and monitor progress
   d. All of the above

2. To facilitate how well and quickly work is accomplished, nurse managers know that
   a. communication skills need to be clear and accurate
   b. they must do the work themselves
   c. the work must be supervised very closely at all times
   d. the environment must be quiet

3. Interpersonal strengths of an effective nurse manager include
   a. being able to oversee each step of a project
   b. open, friendly relationships with workers and peers
   c. avoiding diversity, because it detracts from learning
   d. the ability to set boundaries on a display of caring

4. It is clear that leaders and managers in the healthcare delivery system work from the principles of
   a. systems functioning, because many subsystems of the whole carry out their own processes
   b. accurate communication and leadership
   c. subsystems setting their own standards but working for common success
   d. All of the above

5. The nurse manager knows that when attempting to meet a financial goal
   a. staffing numbers must be taken into account
   b. consideration of the needs of a unit cannot come first
   c. budgets are budgets!
   d. staffing must be cut

References

Adair, J. (2006). *How to grow leaders.* London and Philadelphia: Kogan Page.

Bero, C. L., Glaser, J., & Franklin, J. (2000). Partners community healthcare extranet (PCHInet): A business plan. *Journal of Healthcare Information Management, 14*(3), 41–54.

Block, D. (2006). *Healthcare outcomes management: Strategies for planning and evaluation.* Sudbury, MA: Jones and Bartlett.

Griffith, J., & White, K. (2002). *The well-managed healthcare organization.* Chicago: Health Administration Press.

Institute of Medicine (IOM). (2004). *Crossing the quality chasm.* Washington, DC: National Academy Press.

Levinson, H. (2006). *Organizational assessment.* Washington, DC: American Psychological Association.

Studer, Q. (2008). *Results that last.* Hoboken, NJ: John Wiley.

Swayne, L. E., Duncan, W. J., & Ginter, P. M. (2006). *Strategic management of health care organizations.* Malden, MA: Blackwell.

Wolper, L. (Ed.). (2004). *Health care administration* (4th ed.). Sudbury, MA: Jones and Bartlett.

Yoder-Wise, P. (2007). *Leading and managing in nursing.* St. Louis, MO: Mosby.

Chapter 2

An Historical Overview of Nursing

Marilyn Klainberg

OUTLINE

PURPOSE

- To familiarize the reader with the impact of historical events on nursing
- To present social factors that have influenced the development of nursing
- To explore political and economic factors influencing nursing today
- To introduce nurses and other leaders in health care who have had an impact on nursing

The Impact of Nursing on the Evolution of Health Care

This chapter provides a brief historical overview of health care and identifies nurse leaders who have influenced the events that changed or improved the healthcare system within the framework of specific historical events. Additional nurse leaders who have more recently influenced the healthcare system are identified and presented throughout this book.

It is important to be familiar with the efforts of those who have gone before us, because they have a special meaning to our future. It has been said that "those who cannot remember the past are condemned to repeat it" (Santayana, 1953). Much of the early history of and information about nursing health care is based on information about ancient cultures that has been gathered by anthropologists and documented by historians (Spector, 2004).

Introduction: Ancient Cultures Before Christ

Care of the sick is not new. People have cared for their sick throughout recorded history, and we assume, before that. The term *to nurse* comes from the Middle English words *nurice* and *norice*, which are contractions of *nourice*, from Old French that was originally derived from Latin *nutricia* (Klainberg, Holzemer, Leonard, & Arnold, 1998). This term means "a person who nourishes" and often referred to a wet nurse. (A wet nurse is a woman who breastfeeds infants for those who are unable to do so.) (Klainberg, et al., 1998).

Although we often assume that life in ancient and earlier cultures may have been a basis for what we consider nursing today, care of the sick

at that time was clearly very different because of the needs of and the lifestyles in society and the impact of science and technology. Back then, palliative care was primarily provided for the sick.

Life in ancient cultures (and in some non-Western cultures today) was nomadic and was built around finding food and maintaining warmth. Health practices were varied and based upon ingenuity, prior experiences, and the environment. People used plants and herbs to heal, and they harbored the notion that evil spirits and magic affected well-being. Early people viewed illness and death as part of the natural phenomena of life, and of course there were variations of practices among cultures (Spector, 2004).

Persons designated to care for the sick—usually men—passed information verbally through the generations. Some of the information we know about these ancient cultures and their forms of health care comes from the work of anthropologists, and some comes from information that has been handed down from generation to generation.

As people's lives and environments became more developed, irrigation and waste were the first issues related to treating disease. Priests, spiritual guides, or "medicine men" were the healthcare providers for their communities. During these times, the sick became their responsibility (Kalisch & Kalisch, 1978). Sickness was often attributed to evil spirits or something that had been done to offend the priests or gods. Health care was often the result of trial and error, because science and technology as we know them today were not available. If a person ate something that made him ill, that person was told not to eat it again; if an herb made someone feel well or seemed to improve health, then that herb would be used for its assumed curative powers.

As early as 3000 B.C., the Egyptian healthcare system was the first to maintain medical records. The Egyptians were also the first to classify drugs and develop a planned system to maintain the health of their society. Rules regarding food safety and cleanliness were first attributed to the Egyptians and are still maintained today by many of the Muslim and Jewish faiths.

Babylonia was the second oldest society to maintain medical records (Donahue, 1996). During this time, the Persians, Italians, Chinese, and Indians also developed rudimentary and early attempts at the provision of health care. Greek society put an emphasis on personal health more than community health and believed that personal health was influenced by the environment. The Romans recognized the importance of the regulation of medical practice and created punishment for medical negligence.

During the Middle Ages, A.D. 500 to 1500, Christianity attempted to bring forth the notion of personal responsibility for self, as well as for others, and this was reflected in the care of the sick. Religious communities established care for the sick poor in *hospes*, places that could offer nurturance and palliative care and from which the terms *hospital* and *hospice* derive (Nutting & Dock, 1935).

From A.D. 50 to 800, these hospes, or hospitals, were usually near a church or a monastery. Men were the caregivers during this time, and women were permitted to be midwives or wet nurses and were considered witches if they attempted to usurp the role of the male healthcare provider (Ehrenreich & English, 1973).

The Crusades (A.D. 1095–1291)

War has always had an impact on the health care of society and on nursing. Woven throughout the history of humans and throughout this chapter are the impact and legacy of war upon health.

During the time of the Crusades, monks often tended to the sick. It was during this time that the Church established military nursing orders, such as the Knights Hospitalers (the Knights of Saint John of Jerusalem), made up exclusively of men who provided care for pilgrims and travelers who were in need of care (Beyond the French Riviera, 2007). Their fame was widespread, and it even influenced some crusaders to lay down their weapons and join the Knights of St. John in their work to provide for the poor, the pilgrims, and travelers (Nutting & Dock, 1935).

The Renaissance

Throughout the Renaissance period, from 1500 to 1700, growing interest in science and technology led to some advances in medicine and public health. In 1601, the Church of England mandated the Elizabethan Poor Law, which created overseers for the poor, blind, orphans, and lame (Bloy, 2002). Poverty was considered a way of life for some. The rich paid for nurses to take care of their sick at home. The Poor Law was intended to provide a place where the poor sick and orphaned would be cared for.

It was under this law that provisions for the poor to receive care in either hospitals or almshouses became available. Because many of the poor were very ill when they arrived at hospitals, and little more than palliative care could be provided for them, they often died in the hospitals. Therefore, to most people the idea of being hospitalized had negative connotations, and hospitals were considered places where people were sent to die.

Those who were sick but rich continued to be cared for at home by private duty nurses, who were privately reimbursed. Often nurses who took care of the sick in their homes were also expected to do other jobs within the household, including housekeeping, cleaning, and cooking.

The 18th Century

The industrial revolution began in the late 18th century in England (1760) and continued into the early 19th century. It was a time of technological advancement throughout the world. Early technology influenced the economy. Because of the evolution of technology, factories emerged that had the ability to manufacture and produce specific products in volume rather than goods acquired from farming, manual labor, or craftspersons. The use of machinery and the development of factories quickly spread throughout the world.

As factories evolved, people left rural and farming communities for cities to find employment. During this time, many people migrated to cities that were unprepared for a population increase; in turn, many of the new residents found themselves living in overcrowded, unsanitary housing and working in dangerous conditions for long hours. There was little protection for the worker—no sick pay or leave and poor working conditions.

Later, as science made society more aware of the relationships between hygiene and health, efforts were made to improve the poor and unsanitary conditions of overcrowding by providing places for people to take hot baths and sanitariums for the ill. Although there were persons interested in improving health care and who attempted to find ways to meet these challenges, plagues remained a major source of sickness and death.

It was not until the 18th century that any formal interventions were made by the government toward providing health care for the community. The 18th century was a turbulent time.

In 1776, the United States declared independence from Britain, and in 1789 the French Revolution began. The 18th century was also a time of scientific innovation. Benjamin Franklin invented eyeglasses that addressed both near- and farsightedness, Leeuwenhoek improved the microscope invented earlier by Galileo so that body cells and bacteria could be identified, and the functioning of the heart was described. These changes began to influence how people lived. It was during this time that the role of the nurse began to be acknowledged and schools of nursing were established.

The 19th Century

Change is often a result of challenges in the community and the world. The 19th century was also a time for innovation and reform. Throughout history those who we consider healthcare leaders have changed or influenced the well-being of a community or society. Those transformations may have been influenced by need or have resulted from changes in or outside of a system. The identification of a leader is often dependent upon how the leader creates or deals with change based upon the needs of a society. Dr. John Snow, a physician, is an example of how one person can significantly influence the well-being of an entire community by identifying and acting upon a need for change.

John Snow

In the 19th century, John Snow intervened and was able to contain a major outbreak of cholera in London. Although he was not a nurse, I mention Dr. Snow here because his role in controlling a major outbreak of cholera with little sophisticated equipment or knowledge of bacteriology was critical. Snow and his assistants calculated the actual number of deaths from cholera by going door to door and collecting information from residents about the status of health within their households. They collected information about who provided water to the homes in the various districts in London. Snow discovered that the areas supplied by the Southwark and Vauxhall Water Company had 114 deaths per 100,000, while those supplied by the Lambeth Company had few deaths from cholera.

After a tedious investigation, Snow was convinced that the source of the epidemic was contaminated water. He knew the water from the Southwark and Vauxhall Water Company was from the lower Thames, which was closer to London. London was a big city and greatly inhabited. Without sewage disposal as we know it today, waste was disposed directly into the Thames. Lambeth Company water was from an area north of London, which was less inhabited and therefore an uncontaminated area of the Thames. Because there was no indoor plumbing at that time, water was drawn for whole communities from a local pump. The pump in the Southwark and Vauxhall Water supply was from the local Thames, which was contaminated.

Upon determining this, Snow removed the handle from the pump for the water that was supplied by the Southwark and Vauxhall Company. This required the community to draw water from another source, one that was not contaminated. That simple act stopped the outbreak of cholera in London (Klainberg, et al., 1998). The pump without the handle remains in London as a tribute to John Snow's work.

Nursing Leaders of the 19th Century

The following nurses made changes in the practice of nursing in small or great ways and were among the nurse leaders of the 19th century.

FLORENCE NIGHTINGALE (1820–1910)

It was during the 19th century that Florence Nightingale forever changed the practice of nursing. Nightingale was often referred to as "the Lady with the Lamp," which was how she was described in a poem by Henry Wadsworth Longfellow in 1857. She has also been called a pioneer of modern nursing.

Florence Nightingale was a philanthropist from a wealthy English family who lived during a time when well-bred women from the upper class were not usually involved in caring for the sick. Despite convention, Nightingale wanted to study the care and treatment of diseases and afflictions, so she enrolled in a 3-month program to study nursing under the direction of Pastor Fliedner and his wife Erika at Kaiserwerth Germany (Kelly & Joel, 1996). Upon graduation from the program, Nightingale became involved in creating the organization called "Establishment for Gentle Women During Illness." Ultimately, she was appointed to the leadership position of this organization, because she was knowledgeable as a result of prior experience in the administration of hospitals and she had an expertise in nursing. As her work in nursing was acknowledged, she was consulted in the organization of training nurses; however, her efforts in the Crimean War intervened.

Florence Nightingale became involved in the Crimean War (1853–1856) after hearing about the squalid conditions of soldiers who had been injured. She organized other nurses who joined her in bringing aid, comfort, and supplies to injured soldiers. When she arrived in the Crimea what she saw was beyond her expectations. She found injured soldiers in neglected and filthy conditions with dirty rags covering their wounds. She brought clean sheets, bandages, and simply soap and water to cleanse the wounds of the soldiers, who were dying of infections caused by the squalid conditions. Because of Florence Nightingale and the women volunteers she led, the death rate from infections for wounded soldiers was almost obliterated.

When Nightingale returned home to London, she was honored as a national heroine. She remained committed to establishing a program to train nurses. In 1860, Nightingale established a training program for nurses at St. Thomas's Hospital in London, where the Florence Nightingale Museum is presently housed.

Shortly thereafter, Nightingale took to her bed until her death in 1910. It was believed that she was ill resulting from a weakened condition attributed to her work during the Crimean War. She wrote extensively from her sickbed, and many feel her writings remain significant and influential in nursing today. Her most well known book, *Notes on Nursing*, is still revered. She made nursing a profession for respectable women. Up until that time, nursing was not considered appropriate for women, and men played a major role in nursing. Nightingale died in her sleep at age 90. Every year during the week in which she was born, nurses in the United States celebrate National Nurses week in her honor.

MARY SEACOLE (1805–1861)

Mary Jane Grant Seacole was born in Kingston, Jamaica, to a Jamaican mother who was a nurse and a Scottish father who was a career soldier. Not formally trained as a nurse, she learned her nursing skills from her mother (Carnegie, 1995). As a nurse, she traveled to Cuba and Panama and worked during cholera and yellow fever epidemics. In 1836, Mary married Edwin Seacole, who subsequently died in 1844.

In 1854, after learning about the war in the Crimea, Seacole asked the war office of the British government to send her to the Crimea as an army nurse. She was refused even an interview because of her race and ethnicity (Carnegie, 1995). Seacole, determined to help the war effort, funded her own trip to the Crimea, bringing supplies with her. She soon established a hospital and respite home for wounded and fatigued soldiers in Balaclava. She worked as a volunteer and did not receive army recognition or rank in the British Army. She was known as "Mother Seacole" on the battlefield, because she nursed the wounded. Unlike Florence Nightingale, Mary Seacole received little fame or notoriety for her work or her role in the Crimean War. After the war, she returned to England destitute and in poor health. Her plight was publicized by newspapers, and eventually she was recognized in England and Jamaica for her work in the Crimea.

CLARA BARTON (1812–1912)

Clara Barton, born in Massachusetts, was a New England school teacher (Donahue, 1996). Despite not having formal training as a nurse, she volunteered as a nurse during the American Civil War. She was instrumental in organizing and acquiring needed supplies for the troops during the Civil War, often using her own financial resources. She was referred to by the soldiers she cared for as the "little lone lady in black silk" (Donahue, 1996).

Following the Civil War, she remained active in attempting to locate missing men who were in the army and helped to establish the first national cemetery for soldiers killed in war (Donahue, 1996). Exhausted following the war, she went to Europe to recover. There she learned about the International Red Cross. Clara Barton is best known for her role in establishing the American Red Cross in the United States. Barton was able to convince Congress to affiliate with the International Red Cross. This affiliation created the ability for the Red Cross to function during times of peace.

MARY MAHONEY (1845–1926)

Mary Mahoney, the first African American registered nurse educated in the United States, was born in Boston. In 1879, at age 34, Mary Mahoney graduated from the New England Hospital for Women and Children. She was the first black woman to graduate from a professional school of nursing (Carnegie, 1995). Schools in the United States at that time either limited the admission of black women to schools of nursing or did not permit admission at all. Her graduation had a tremendous impact upon the future of all black nurses.

As a nurse leader, she recognized the need for nurses to work together to improve their role in the nursing profession, and she became a member of the American Nurses Association (ANA). She was the cofounder of the National Association of Colored Graduate Nurses (NACGN) and helped make it possible for black nurses not only to be recognized but officially received by the president of the United States, Warren G. Harding. She left a legacy behind for all black nurses. She was named to the Nursing Hall of Fame posthumously, and in 1972, the United States Congress honored Mary Mahoney for her dedication to nursing.

MARY ADELAIDE NUTTING (1858–1948)

Mary Adelaide Nutting, a suffragette and nurse historian, was well known as an advocate of higher education for nurses. Born in Canada, she was a member of the first graduating class of nurses at Johns Hopkins University in 1891 and was to become the school's second superintendent of nursing. She was instrumental in creating changes to improve the education of the nursing

students at John's Hopkins Hospital by expanding the program from two to three years, allowing for greater time in the classroom, and by decreasing the number of hours the students were required to work in the hospital. (Hospitals frequently had students working long hours at the hospital in addition to their student requirements.) She realized that students needed time to study to become good nurses (Pipkin, 2001).

Subsequently, Nutting established the first higher education program for nurses as the Department of Nursing and Health, Teachers College, Columbia University, New York, and was appointed the chairperson from 1919 to 1925. She was the first woman to hold a professorship at Columbia University.

During World War I, because of the shortage of nurses, Nutting was called upon to chair the Nursing Committee for the Counsel of National Defense. It was the charge of this committee to find ways to recruit and train women as nurses for the United States Army. Nutting was also instrumental in the development and creation of the *American Journal of Nursing*.

LAVINIA DOCK (1858–1956)

Lavinia Dock was a graduate of the Bellevue Training School for nurses in 1888. She was a nurse leader who helped change and advance the profession of nursing. She used her nursing skills during the yellow fever epidemic in Jacksonville, Florida, and provided care at the Johnstown flood in 1890. Ultimately, she worked with Isabel Hampton Robb at St. Johns University. Like Nutting, Lavinia Dock was a suffragette, working for women's rights. Dock was an activist, interested in changing society. Dock worked with the New York Women's Trade Union League and walked picket lines for the Shirtwaist strike in 1913. She spoke at an

ANA convention urging nurses to support a union movement for nurses. In 1896, she joined Lillian Wald at the Henry Street Settlement, where they worked together for 20 years.

LILLIAN WALD (1867–1940)

Another nurse to bring about change during this era was Lillian Wald. Wald, a nurse and social worker born to a middle-class Jewish family in Rochester, New York, is most famous for her influence in initiating the Visiting Nurse Service of New York. She initially worked as a nurse at an orphanage. During that time, she was asked to volunteer to teach home classes for women at the Henry Street Settlement on the Lower East Side of New York, a place that educated mostly immigrant poor. At one of those classes, a young child approached Wald and asked her to come to the tenement where the child's family was living to help care for her sick mother. Wald found the place to be in a very poor state and the mother, who had recently delivered a baby, in a bed of blood-soiled clothing (Visiting Nurse Service of New York, 2007). Wald cared for the woman, cleaned her bed and room, and comforted the family.

This event changed Lillian Wald's life and health care forever. Not long thereafter, Lillian Wald began to care for sick residents of the Lower East Side and soon decided to devote her life to this cause. In 1893, along with another nurse, Mary Brewster, Lillian Wald founded the Henry Street Settlement Visiting Nurse Service, which would become the Visiting Nurse Service of New York. By 1910, the notion of the visiting nurse was supported and endorsed by health departments, the Public Health Service, and schools. The idea of keeping people healthy and not spreading disease had taken hold.

The 20th and 21st Centuries

At the end of the 19th century and the beginning of the 20th century, issues related to sanitation in relationship to the health of communities were the primary concern of healthcare planners and providers. During the 20th century, the discovery of new and more potent antibiotics and other scientific breakthroughs changed forever how the healthcare system dealt with infection.

Toward the mid-20th century, a shift in priority from the health of the community to the health and well-being of the individual occurred, and toward the end of the 20th century another shift toward care of the patient in the community occurred. Technological innovations improved and advanced how healthcare providers approached disease. The impact of health insurance also addressed and changed how healthcare providers address the well-being of the individual and the community. Furthermore, the cost of health care began to increase continually, and ethical issues arose regarding who should receive treatment based on their age or socioeconomic status; these issues continue today.

The world during these times has grown smaller with advances in transportation and the speed at which people can travel around the world. Although many of the recent technological advances have improved health and affected society positively, some, such as the rapidity in which people can travel the world, have increased the possibility of transmitting contagious diseases. The future of health care is fluid and not only depends on the advances made in technology but the economy and social issues throughout the world.

Nursing Education in the United States

Nursing education has been determined not only by the evolution of technology and advances in science, but by the needs and development of society. Initially, nursing education programs were informally part of hospitals and prepared young women to provide palliative care to patients. Courses could be completed in as few as six months. These programs trained students to provide food and a clean environment.

Hospital-based diploma schools of nursing were the first form of nursing education in the United States. These programs restricted their admission to white women. The first program to admit one black and one Jewish woman in each class was established at the New England Hospital for Women and Children in Boston, Massachusetts in 1863. It was not until 1872 that formal training schools for nurses were established and students graduating from these programs were given a diploma upon graduation (Carnegie, 1995).

The history of baccalaureate education cannot be discussed without mentioning the impact of the Flexner Report on nursing education. In 1910, Abraham Flexner, a social worker, wrote a paper identifying a profession. This report was part of work established by the Carnegie Foundation addressing medical professionalism (Klainberg, et al., 1998). Since its publication, there have been many others who have built upon the Flexner Report, adapting what stipulates a profession. The impact of this report affected many professions, particularly nursing. The amended guidelines of a profession include the following:

- Professional preparation (as opposed to an occupation)

- Preparation that takes place in an institution of higher learning, such as a college (community college or 4-year baccalaureate) or a university
- A specific and unique body of knowledge
- An affiliation with a professional organization
- Ethical codes
- Licensing
- A service orientation
- Specific educational guidelines

Diploma programs have, for the most part, been replaced by associate degree or baccalaureate programs, but there are still some diploma schools of nursing, which are nursing education programs provided by hospitals. Most nursing education programs that exist today are either in community colleges, which provide an associate's degree in science, or are baccalaureate programs from which students graduate with a bachelor of science degree. Students who graduate from any of these programs can take the National Council Licensure Examination (NCLEX) examinations to become registered nurses.

Graduate education beyond a baccalaureate education includes a variety of advanced practice roles. Master's degrees fulfill a variety of areas, such as clinical nurse specialist, nurse practitioner, certified nurse midwife, certified registered nurse anesthetist, informatics specialist, and doctorate (Doctor of Philosophy [PhD], Doctor of Education [EdD], Doctor of Nursing Science [DNS, DNSc], Doctor of Nursing [ND], and Doctor of Nursing Practice [DNP]).

The notion of clinical specialization grew as the nursing profession grew and as a result of the needs of society. It began early in the 20th century when nurses acquired specialties through hospital-based courses, and it became more complex after World War II (Mezey, McGivern, & Sullivan-Marx, 1999). In 1964, the Nurse Training Act was enacted, which provided funding to support the education of advanced practice nurses. It was not until 1965 that the first nurse practitioner program was created. There was some initial resistance to the notion of the nurse practitioner, but by the 1980s this focus became a part of master's programs. Until then, many nurse practitioners could acquire their advanced practice certification following graduation by taking an accreditation examination.

Licensure

In 1901, the first conference of the International Council of Nurses (ICN) met in New York State and passed a resolution stating that all nurses should be licensed by examination (Kalisch & Kalisch, 1978). Although licensure of nurses was met by strong opposition in most states, North Carolina was the first state nursing association to put this forward to its legislature (Kalisch & Kalisch, 1978). Subsequently, a bill was approved requiring nurses to pass an examination to practice as nurses in North Carolina, regardless of where they were trained.

New York State passed a more stringent bill shortly thereafter that required nurses to pass a nursing examination and also to graduate from a school of nursing approved by the Regents of the State University in New York State (Kalisch & Kalisch, 1978). Since then, there have been many changes in the methods of testing nurses for licensure. Today, the National Council Licensure Examinations (NCLEX) examinations are given online in the United States and in some other countries. All nurses graduating from established and credentialed nursing pro-

grams and successfully passing the NCLEX examination may practice nursing in the state in which they have applied to take the examination. Many states offer reciprocity.

The Great Depression

The Great Depression followed the stock market crash of 1929. The crash, also referred to as Black Thursday, was one of the most devastating stock market crashes in American history. The economic impact created a shift in employment and approximately 30% of the population became unemployed. This affected the economic well-being of the entire nation, creating large numbers of homeless people. Many people did not have money to purchase food or health care, and the Depression profoundly influenced how nursing was practiced.

Until that point, most nurses worked in private homes caring for patients who could afford their services. Hospitals mostly utilized students to care for the ill. Students provided cheap labor, but when they graduated they could not find jobs in hospitals, so most sought employment in patients' homes where they cared for the sick or elderly who could afford private care. Hospitals replaced graduating students with new students. After the crash and the Depression, many nurses working in homes lost their jobs, because many families could no longer afford their services. Hospitals found they could hire trained nurses for very little, because the nurses were in need of jobs, and they could be hired for either low wages or in exchange for room and board (Hott & Garey, 1988). Hospitals began to use trained nurses instead of students to provide care for their patients. Students continued to have a role in hospitals after that, but they no longer provided primary care for patients independently.

Nurses in Wars Fought by the United States

During and following the American Revolution, men served as corpsmen, providing nursing care for soldiers. Following the Civil War and before the Spanish American War in 1898, nurses in the United States Army were also men. These men were known as hospital corpsmen. They were trained at differing caregiving levels. However, there were not enough hospital corpsmen, and a need for trained nurses was evident.

In 1898, the United States Congress appropriated funds for the employment of trained nurses and for the development of the Army Nurse Corps (McGee & Hughes, n.d.). There were no restrictions on whether the nurses should be male or female. Those who applied to be trained as nurses were mostly women, and these women performed well in their role as nurses. Following this, there was little objection to women in the Army Nurse Corps. The contribution of the female nurses during the Spanish-American War and during the yellow fever outbreak positively advanced their role in the Army Nurse Corps. Female nurses along with male nurses have served in every American war since. Army Nurse Corps did not become a part of the Army Medical Department until 1901.

WORLD WAR I (1914–1918)

The United States entered World War I in 1917. Before entering World War I, the United States established the Bureau of War Risk Insurance in 1914. The Bureau of War Risk Insurance was originally intended to insure ships and cargo but was amended in 1917 to meet the needs of the returning veterans. This was to become the Veteran's Bureau.

During World War I, the number of nurses in the military grew from about 4000 to 20,000, serving both overseas and domestically. Army Nurses served in the United States, France, Hawaii, Puerto Rico, and the Philippines. Nurses also provided care on transport ships carrying wounded home across the Atlantic.

In 1917, because of its outstanding record of caring for merchant seamen and controlling disease, and despite the uncertainty of its role, the Public Health Service (PHS) was made part of the military by President Woodrow Wilson (Mullan, 1989). The Public Health Service, in addition to being concerned with issues related to the war, was dealing with other health issues, particularly venereal disease among soldiers and the Spanish flu, which killed 50,000 Americans by 1919 (Mullan, 1989). As the war generated veterans in need of health services, the PHS was furthermore asked to be responsible for returning soldiers and to oversee the Marine Hospital system, which was called upon to provide care for returning soldiers (Mullan, 1989).

WORLD WAR II

The United States entered World War II after being attacked at Pearl Harbor on December 7, 1941. At that time, the number of nurses in the Army could not meet the demand and needs of the military. Initially, this was a dilemma for civilian nurses who were torn between joining the military or continuing to work in their civilian jobs (Kalisch & Kalisch, 1978). To help encourage nurses to join the military and to prevent hospitals from being depleted of nurses, the National Council for War Service established guidelines for the recruitment of nurses (Kalisch & Kalisch, 1978). Other issues that prevented nurses from enlisting were the low salary nurses who joined the military at the beginning of the war received compared to men and that nurses received no official rank or benefits.

In May 1942, with the fall of Corregidor in the Philippines, 54 Army nurses became Japanese prisoners of war (Norman, 1999). During their captivity, they suffered greatly but continued to care for patients in internment hospitals. Under equally poor conditions, other brave nurses cared for patients under German shellfire in Europe.

In 1943, Frances Bolton introduced a bill to Congress to provide military rank for the nurses to correct the inequity between males in the military and military nurses (who were mostly female). In 1944, Congress enacted a law that provided military nurses with a temporary officer's rank for the duration of the war. Also in 1944, the military was desperately in need of nurses, and under the Bolton Act, the United States Public Health Service created the United States (U.S.) Cadet Nurse Corps to create an accelerated program to educate nurses. One hundred twenty-five nurses were admitted during the first two months and 125,000 during the next two years (Kalisch & Kalisch, 1978). The U.S. Cadet Nurse Corps program was phased out in 1948, three years after the end of the war. See Box 2–1 to read about how international events influenced one woman to join the U.S. Cadet Nurse Corps.

Box 2–1 How I Became a Nurse

Jacqueline Rose Hott

There are specific days anyone over the age of 50 always remembers: the day Kennedy was shot, November 22, 1963, and the attack on the Twin Towers, September 11, 2001. We can remember where we were and what we were doing when we heard about these national tragedies. Long before these events, though, came the day the Japanese attacked Pearl Harbor, on December 7, 1941. For me, a 16-year-old freshman at New Jersey College for Women (NJC) in New Brunswick, New Jersey, that Sunday morning in December will always stand out as a life-shaping experience. It was the day that brought me into nursing as a career.

I was not one of those women who had always wanted to be a nurse. I wanted to be a reporter, so I was an English major. I had been editor of my high school newspaper and senior yearbook; I had a column in the college newspaper. Always interested in human behavior, I also studied psychology as my minor. I knew nothing about nursing, except that my physician at home in Jersey City had married a nurse who worked at Bellevue and who occasionally helped him in his office.

Unlike me, my older sister wanted to be a nurse so that she could leave home; however, my parents would not give permission because she was not yet 17. My family tried to dissuade my sister by saying, "Nurses just carry bedpans. Is that what you want to do?" She got married instead.

I was struggling at NJC, not with studies or grades (after all, I had been my high school valedictorian), but with the cost of living on campus. I had scholarships to pay tuition, but to help my blue-collar family pay for the rest I was working jobs as a waitress in the college cafeteria, an aide in the Alumnae House, and a teacher in a religious school on Sundays. The attack on Pearl Harbor created a public relations bonanza of information about nursing and made me see that nursing could be a way to solve my economic problems in seeking an education.

I don't remember when I first saw the poster about joining the U.S. Cadet Nurse Corps: "Enlist in a Proud Profession." The atmosphere on our brother campus, Rutgers University, was heavy with the draft looming over its men. At NJC, we had special exercises to prepare ourselves physically for combat threats. I still don't know what triggered my change besides the public relations information from the U.S. Cadet Nurse Corps in pamphlets and posters that encouraged women to join the war effort. The educational bonus in becoming a nurse was continuing my baccalaureate education *for free*! As a sophomore student in the next semester, I would be able to transfer enough credits so that after graduation from a school of nursing in 33 months, I would have a bachelor's degree in nursing science (BSN), a profession, and no debt. Indeed, my next college would have *free* room, board, and tuition *and* give me a stipend of $15 a month. (Would some economist figure that out in today's prices?) *And* I would be serving my country! Now, if I would look good in that uniform . . . (I did!)

Deciding which college I would transfer to was not too difficult. I wanted a program that would accept my college credits, and NJC recommended two: Cornell University and Bellevue School of Nursing. The only thing I knew about Cornell was the song "Far Above Cayuga's Waters" and that it was a long distance from home in Jersey City. Otherwise, my doctor's wife had gone to Bellevue, it was famous for psychiatry, and it was just across the Hudson from home if I needed chicken soup. So, I became a cadet nurse at Bellevue.

Leaving NJC was hard. I was honored by the school as a Distinguished Alumnus after it became Douglass College. Surely, the roots of leadership for this woman started in a college for women and were nurtured and developed at Bellevue and later at New York University's graduate programs in nursing.

I started at Bellevue in September 1943 in one of the largest admitting nursing classes Bellevue had ever had. We had college graduates, baccalaureate students, new high school graduates, married and divorced women, blacks, Asians, Catholics, and Jews, although most students were white, Anglo-Saxon Protestants. Our faculty were all WASPs until we reached senior year in psychology.

Rigidity of rules and doing things the Bellevue way (the only way?) were the norm. Great chauvinistic pride in being a Bellevue nurse was instilled early. The goal was to be the best nurse, to give the best patient care. If we had problems, they were challenges and we were creative problem solvers. We were Bellevue nurses; we overcame. As U.S. Cadet Nurse Corps nurses, we were being prepared for combat; whether the combat was lack of equipment, personnel, or time, we persevered.

Looking back from more than 60 years later, I realize that my classmates were remarkably capable women, some just teenagers like me, others mature and seasoned. As part of our contract with the U.S. Cadet Nurse Corps, we promised to continue in nursing for three years after graduation in 1946. I am still proudly keeping that prom-ise as an independent clinical nurse practitioner in adult psychiatric nursing. The Cadet Nurse Corps poster is on the wall of my den. It still inspires me. When I left the deanship at Adelphi University School of Nursing, I left my U.S. Cadet Nurse Corps purse in the display closet as a memento. I hope that it will continue to inspire others.

By the end of World War II, 215 nurses had died in service to the United States. Their service was important to the war effort during World War II, and they were not unlike the courageous nurses who served in the Korean War, the Vietnam War, and Desert Storm and who today serve in Iraq.

Nursing Leaders of the 20th Century

MARY BRECKINRIDGE (1881–1965)

In 1925, the Frontier Nursing Service was begun in Kentucky by Mary Breckinridge, a nurse, who remained its director until her death in 1965. This service provided care for the sick poor in rural communities. Nurses traveled by foot or by horse to reach patients who would otherwise not receive the care of a healthcare provider. Nurses cared for rural and isolated families and individuals who were ill or who had been injured and also delivered babies.

During World War I, while serving as a volunteer nurse in France, Breckinridge met a British nurse who was also a midwife. When she started the Frontier Nursing Service, she realized that the frontier nurses would need this skill and sent nurses to England to study midwifery. With the outbreak of World War II in Europe, Breckinridge was no longer able to send American nurses to Britain. Realizing the importance of midwifery to Frontier Nursing Service nursing practice, Breckenridge began the Frontier Graduate School of Midwifery. The name of the school changed to the Frontier School of Midwifery and Family Nursing (FSMFN) (Kelly & Joel, 1996).

MARGARET SANGER (1878–1966)

Margaret Sanger worked as a nurse with poor women on the Lower East Side in New York City. Through this work, she became aware of the impact of unplanned and unwelcome pregnancies upon these women. She was already familiar with this on a personal level, because she was one of 11 children and saw how multiple pregnancies caused her own mother's health to suffer. She believed women should have birth control available to them.

In 1916, Margaret Sanger opened a family planning and birth control clinic in New York City. Nine days after she opened the center, it was raided by the police and Sanger served 30 days in prison. This was one of her many arrests over the years that resulted from her efforts to provide education about contraception to women. In 1930, Sanger successfully opened a family planning clinic in Harlem, New York, with support of the community, but it wasn't until 1939 that the American Medical Association officially recognized birth control as an integral part of medical practice. Shortly thereafter, the Birth Control Federation of America emerged. In 1942, the Birth Control Federation of America changed its name to Planned Parenthood Federation of America (PPFA) (Planned Parenthood, 2008). The conflict over birth control did not end there. Threats of bombing Planned Parenthood clinics continued late into the 20th century.

VIRGINIA HENDERSON (1897–1996)

Virginia Henderson attended the Army School of Nursing in Washington, DC, and graduated in 1921. She went on to Teachers College, Columbia University, graduating with a master's degree in nursing education. In 1955, with Bertha Harmer, Henderson coauthored *Textbook of the Principles and the Practice of Nursing*, a fundamental textbook. Her book and subsequent writings redefined the practice of nursing. Henderson emphasized in the book that the goal of the healthcare provider is to help people become as independent as possible (Harmer & Henderson, 1955). She described the nurse's role as threefold: "*substitutive* (doing for the person), *supplementary* (helping the person), or *complementary* (working to help the patient)" (Harmer & Henderson, 1955).

Henderson believed that "the unique function of the nurse is to assist the individual, sick or well, in the performance of those activities contributing to health or its recovery (or to peaceful death) that he would perform unaided if he had the necessary strength, will or knowledge and to do this in such a way as to help him gain independence as rapidly as possible" (Harmer & Henderson, 1955). Henderson was one of the first nurses to point out that nursing does not

consist of merely following physicians' orders. Virginia Henderson remained an active contributor to nursing and continued to lecture to groups of nurses about her philosophy until shortly before her death in 1996 at age 99.

MILDRED MONTAG (1908–2004)

Orphaned at an early age, Mildred Montag was raised by her aunt and uncle on a farm. She attended Hamline University, in St. Paul, Minnesota, and graduated in 1930 as a history major. She then decided to become a nurse and attended the University of Minnesota, in Minneapolis, and graduated in 1933 with a bachelor of science (BS) degree in nursing. She went on to attend Columbia University, Teachers College, in New York, majoring in nursing education, and graduated in 1938 with a master of art (MA) degree in nursing education.

The United States' entry into World War II resulted in an urgent need for more nurses to serve in the military. In 1942, Dr. Montag was asked by Adelphi College (presently Adelphi University), under a grant from the United States Public Health Service, to determine whether local hospitals would cooperate in establishing a school of nursing at Adelphi College. In January 1943, the School of Nursing at Adelphi College, the first program for nursing on Long Island, was established and Dr. Montag was named the director. The first 25 students were admitted under the Nurse Training Act of 1943, also known as the Bolton Act. Montag remained director of the Adelphi College School of Nursing from 1943 to 1948. As founder and director of the program, Dr. Montag is credited with developing the nursing program and making it an integral part of Adelphi College.

In 1950, Mildred Montag graduated with a doctorate from Teachers College and her doctoral dissertation changed how we educate nurses in the United States. At that time, most of the schools of nursing were 3-year diploma programs owned and operated by hospitals (Kalisch & Kalisch, 1978). In her doctoral dissertation, Montag proposed creating a 2-year program to prepare technical nurses to assist the professional nurse, whom she envisioned as having a baccalaureate degree. Dr. Montag's goal was to alleviate the critical shortage of nurses by decreasing the length of the education process from a minimum of three years to two years and to provide a sound educational base for nursing instruction by placing the program in community/junior colleges.

In 1958, as a result of her dissertation, the W. K. Kellogg Foundation funded the implementation of the project at seven pilot sites in four states (Haase, 1990). Associate degree education for nursing began as part of this experimental project at Teachers College, Columbia University, based on Montag's dissertation. In addition to creating a program that decreased the time to become a nurse, benefits of the associate's degree in nursing (ADN) program included reasonable cost and proximity of ADN programs to the community, access for diverse populations, the inclusion of adult learners, males, and married students. Seven community colleges were included in this 5-year nursing research project to evaluate the impact of an associate' degree education for nurses, and Dr. Montag was named the director of the project (Kalisch & Kalisch, 1978). Dr. Montag was the author of many publications and the recipient of many awards related to the development of the ADN program. She remained actively involved in nursing and particularly in Adelphi University School of Nursing (formerly Adelphi College) until her death at age 95.

Hildegard E. Peplau (1909–1999)

Dr. Hildegard E. Peplau, born in Pennsylvania in 1909, is known for her work and great strides in psychiatric nursing. She helped to create change in the collective way nurses and patients thought about their roles in the patient–healthcare provider relationship (Peplau, O'Toole, & Welt, 1989). Her groundbreaking work helped nurses to use their interpersonal skills therapeutically. She emphasized the nurse–patient *relationship* as the foundation of nursing practice. Peplau developed an interpersonal model emphasizing the need for a partnership between nurse and patient, and her theories were considered by many to be revolutionary. She opposed patients passively receiving treatment, as well as nurses passively acting out doctors' orders.

During World War II, Hildegard Peplau was a member of the Army Nurse Corps. Following the war, she returned to school, and in 1947, she received a degree in psychiatric nursing from Teachers College, Columbia University, New York, and went on to receive a doctor of education degree in curriculum development from Columbia University in 1953.

Ruth Lubic Watson (1931–Present)

Ruth Lubic Watson is a nurse–midwife and, in 1993, was the first nurse ever named a MacArthur Fellow by the John D. and Catherine T. MacArthur Foundation. Dr. Watson served as the director of the Maternity Center Association, which began in 1917. In 1975, she founded the first freestanding birthing center on the Upper West Side in New York City. In 1983, Watson became the president of the National Association of Childbearing Centers, which brought birthing centers to impoverished areas in the Bronx, New York, and Washington, D.C., to provide care to underserved communities.

The New York City Family Health and Birthing Center on the Upper West Side no longer exists, but Dr. Watson continues to be actively involved in the center in the Bronx and in Washington, D.C. Among many prestigious awards Dr. Watson has received, she was awarded the Institute of Medicine (IOM) Leinhard Award in 2001 for the advances she has made in personal health of others. Dr. Watson continues to speak to professional groups to promote the cause and efforts of the professional nurse–midwife.

M. ELIZABETH CARNEGIE (1916–2008)

M. Elizabeth Carnegie was a nurse historian and the author of several publications of great importance to the history of nursing, including *The Path We Tread*. Her work to advance black and minority nurses has improved the status of nursing for all nurses.

Aware of the nursing shortage in the military during World War II, Carnegie applied to the Navy and was rejected. The Army took African American nurses, but during this time said they could not recruit and take any more black nurses because they could not house them with white nurses. In an interview, she stated, "During the shortage of nurses during World War II, I applied to the Navy and just got a letter saying they were not taking colored nurses; the Army's excuse was they couldn't house black and white nurses together, could not have them in the same bunks" (Hott & Garey, 1988). Carnegie and other African American nurses protested this with a campaign in the newspapers. Eventually, the Army did take African American nurses to meet the needs of the Armed Forces (Carnegie, 1995).

Dr. Carnegie was employed by the *American Journal of Nursing* from 1953, and upon her retirement in 1978, she became the editor emeritus of *Nursing Research*. Her groundbreaking book *The Path We Tread: Blacks in Nursing Worldwide 1854–1994* is in its third edition. Dr. Carnegie initiated the nursing program at Hampton University in Virginia, was the president of the American Academy of Nursing, and was the dean of the School of Nursing at Florida A&M University. She has been a distinguished visiting professor at many universities. Up until her death in February 2008, Dr. Carnegie was an independent consultant and received countless awards and honorary degrees from universities throughout the country. Most recently, she received a lifetime achievement award from Adelphi University and the Alpha Omega Chapter, Sigma Theta Tau International.

Today

Today we think of our healthcare system as more sophisticated than that of previous generations because it is based on technology and science. However, in some ways it is not unlike the past because it is dynamic and changing. For example, today men are more prevalent in nursing than they have been in previous years, and this is because of changes in society and the evolving image of the nurse. Much of the care nurses provide for individuals and communities is based on the needs of society and is driven not only by need and tradition, but by changes in society brought on by environmental changes.

Today, as in years past, we find that many cultures and individuals maintain relationships with the persons to whom they give the power to lead them to wellness, such as nurses, physicians, or designated persons in the community. For many, these individuals serve as gatekeepers for their care. There are many communities that, either because of religious or other beliefs, require the healthcare provider to first deal with the designated gatekeeper to provide care for individuals or communities and must be considered and included when creating a plan of care.

Now, in the 21st century, there is an emphasis on the health of the individual within the community. Several factors have created this shift: the influence of insurance on the status of health and care; a decrease in resources, including fewer hospitals and fewer professional nurses; an aging population; early retirement; a shift to second careers; a struggling economy; and an emphasis on prevention, safety, and self-care.

Summary

This chapter provides a brief historical overview of health care. The nurse leaders identified influenced events that changed or improved the healthcare system. These nurse leaders played an important part in shaping nursing as we know it today. Some names, such as Florence Nightingale, are familiar and associated with nursing; the others recognized in this chapter played an important role in changing the profession. Many other nurses not mentioned in this chapter have made their mark on nursing and held a vision that affects the future of nursing. Although understanding our past and the history of nursing is important to our future, you, the reader, are the future of nursing and will also leave your footprint on the profession.

QUESTIONS

1. Mary Mahoney was the first
   a. African American registered nurse
   b. nurse to fight in the Civil War
   c. to graduate from a baccalaureate nursing program
   d. person to welcome Florence Nightingale to the Crimea

2. Mildred Montag's goal in creating the 2-year nursing program was to
   a. prepare registered nurses to replace baccalaureate nursing
   b. prepare technical nurses to assist the professional nurse
   c. lessen the burden created by the nursing shortage
   d. get evidence to complete her dissertation

3. Florence Nightingale was known as the
   a. nurse who changed nursing forever
   b. nurse responsible for the end of the Crimean War
   c. Lady with the Lamp
   d. mother of nursing

4. Dr. Hildegard E. Peplau is known for her work and great strides in
   a. medical surgical nursing
   b. nursing education
   c. psychiatric nursing
   d. caring for the sick poor
5. The first Frontier Nursing Service was begun
   a. by Florence Nightingale to help the sick poor in Wyoming
   b. by Elizabeth Carnegie in Washington, D.C.
   c. by Mary Breckinridge in Kentucky
   d. with help from Hildegard E. Peplau

References

Beyond the French Riviera. (2007). Knights Hospitalers. Retrieved October 14, 2008, from http://www.beyond.fr/history/hospitalers.html

Bloy, M. (2002). The 1601 Elizabethan Poor Law. Victorian Web. Retrieved October 14, 2008, from http://www.victorianweb.org/history/poorlaw/elizpl.html

Carnegie, M. E. (1995). *The path we tread: Blacks in nursing worldwide, 1854–1994.* New York: National League for Nursing Press.

Donahue, P. (1996). *Nursing, the finest art: An illustrated history.* St Louis: Mosby.

Ehrenreich, B., & English, D. (1973). *Witches, midwives and nurses: A history of women healers.* New York: Feminist Press.

Haase, P. T. (1990). *The origins and rise of associate degree nursing education.* Durham, North Carolina and London: Duke University Press.

Harkness, G. A. (1995). *Epidemiology in nursing practice.* St. Louis: Mosby.

Harmer, B., & Henderson, V. (1955). *Textbook of the principles and practice of nursing.* New York: Macmillan.

Hott, L., & Garey, D. (1988). *Sentimental women need not apply: A history of the American nurse* [Motion picture]. Los Angeles: Florentine Films.

Kalisch, P. A., & Kalisch, B. J. (1978). *The advance of American nursing.* Boston: Little, Brown, & Company.

Kelly, L. Y., & Joel, L. A. (1996). *The nursing experience.* New York: McGraw-Hill.

Klainberg, M., Holzemer, S., Leonard, M., & Arnold, J. (1998). *Community health nursing: An alliance for health.* New York: McGraw-Hill.

McGee, A. N., & Hughes, M. (n.d.) Women in the American Army. Retrieved October 14, 2008, from http://www.spanamwar.com/Nurses.htm

Mezey, M. D., McGivern, D. O., & Sullivan-Marx, E. M. (1999). *Nurses, nurse practitioners: Evolution to advanced practice.* New York: Springer.

Mullan, F. (1989). *Plagues and politics: The story of the United States Public Health Service.* New York: Basic Books.

Norman, E. M. (1999). *We band of angels.* New York: Random House.

Nutting, M. A., & Dock, L. L. (1935). *A history of nursing.* New York: G.P. Putnam's Sons.

Peplau, H. E., O'Toole, A. W., & Welt, S. R. (1989). *Interpersonal theory in nursing practice: Selected works of Hildegard E. Peplau.* New York: Springer.

Pipkin, K. (2001). Hopkins history: M. Adelaide Nutting shaped today's school of nursing. *Gazette*

Online, 30(16). Retrieved October 14, 2008, from http://www.jhu.edu/~gazette/2001/jan0801/08nuttin.html

Planned Parenthood. (2008). Who we are. Retrieved October 14, 2008, from http://www.planned parenthood.org/about-us/who-we-are/1930-1959-9924.htm

Santayana, G. (1953). *The life of reason.* New York: Charles Scribner.

Visiting Nurse Service of New York. (2007). Our history: Over 110 years of caring. Retrieved October 14, 2008, from http://www.vnsny.org/mainsite/about/a_history.html

Spector, R. E. (2004). *Cultural diversity in health & illness* (6th ed.). Upper Saddle River, NJ: Prentice Hall.

Chapter 3

Educational Drivers to Leadership

Kathleen M.
Dirschel

Educational Pathways to Nursing Leadership

The educational pathways to becoming a registered nurse have evolved over the last century from fully clinically oriented and ward management hospital-based training to more liberal arts and science education, which provide the underpinnings for nursing theory-based practice. Nurses receive their education in 2-year and 4-year colleges, in universities, and even now in some hospital-based schools. For the most part, colleges award degrees to graduating nurses who must then pass the NCLEX-RN examination in order to obtain their license to practice.

The 2-year graduate earns the associate degree, which is the most common preparation for nursing practice in the country. The 4-year graduate generally earns the baccalaureate degree. The members of the nursing profession have always worked actively to provide opportunities for educational advancement for nurses. Transition programs from ADN to BS (N) and from ADN and BS (N) to MS (N) are common. Programs for nonnurses to MS (N), and to one of the several doctoral program types within nursing, are also available and increasing in popularity.

The nursing theorists studied within these programs write of various views and predictions of the nurse–patient relationship. Other theories that support the development of the leadership role beyond clinical practice are described within this chapter. As aspiring leaders, it is essential that nurses actively build an integrated composite of leadership theories that focus on achieving growth and integrity in healthcare delivery systems.

Building a broad and powerful theoretical base to assess, manage, change, and evaluate both educational institutions and healthcare delivery systems, and the individuals and communities they serve, is a challenging and exciting undertaking for the nurse committed to making change at all practice levels. The nurse who can do so will be an influential and successful leader. This chapter offers some views on the various aspects of the educational pathways to nursing and the leadership roles that must be an active and growing part of our profession. Accordingly, the purposes of this chapter are threefold: to analyze educational pathways for nursing leadership from basic to advanced degrees, to analyze the theories that support effective leadership practice, and to illustrate components of a multifaceted profile of nursing leaders.

Historical Summary

Before the 1870s, nurses with any kind of education or training were virtually unknown in the United States. Indeed, the practice of nursing was seen as a menial occupation, carried out by lower-class women from impoverished or criminal backgrounds. Wealthy men and women outside the health professions who were committed to healthcare reform first advocated the need for nurses with education (Starr, 1984). Florence Nightingale described the nurse as one who would "put the patient in the best condition for nature to act upon him" (Nightingale, 1992, p. 75). Throughout the world and the ages, the idea of the nurse is based on maternal instinct, caring for the suffering, nurturing of children, and service in the community, as well as in the hospital (Donahue, 1996).

In the first 70 years of the 1800s, physicians gave lectures to nurses and midwives at state hospitals. There was, however, no formal curriculum for nurses. By the mid-1800s, there was a growing awareness of the need for schools to be formed to educate nurses to care for the sick. Early programs of study in the United States were at Bellevue Hospital, the Connecticut Training School for Nurses, and the Boston Training School for Nurses (Kalisch & Kalisch, 2004).

During the latter half of the 19th century, Florence Nightingale was the catalyst who transformed nursing into a respected and education-based field of endeavor. She wrote extensively about hospitals, sanitation, health and health statistics, and nursing and nursing education. The school she founded in 1860 offered a curriculum that included theory as well as practical experience (Ellis & Hartley, 2004). The theory portions of the schools were 1–2% of the total required hours, and the practice hours were 98–99% (Kalisch & Kalisch, 2004).

With growing pressure to meet the need for public health and school nursing in the beginning of the 20th century, and the demand for educated nurses to treat mass casualties and related disease on the battlefield in World War I, and eventually World War II, nursing education began to move to academic institutions where bachelor's degrees were given, along with diplomas.

The Goldmark Report of 1922 became a catalyst to further reshape nursing education toward theory-based practice. In-depth study of the theory of disease and the psychological and social aspects of patient responses began to shape the core of nursing education. Those graduates who were at the forefront of this nursing education revolution were identified as the leaders in the profession. The early collegiate programs generally consisted of two years of general education and three years of a conventional 3-year diploma program. Integration into a liberal arts and science-based nursing education, which led to theory-based practice, was yet to come. The nursing education programs preparing leaders of schools and colleges of nursing and nursing divisions of complex healthcare delivery systems were rudimentary at best.

The creation of a curriculum guide by the National League for Nursing Education and the demands for educated nurses for World War II escalated the training programs but not the benefits of a profession on the move. The wonder of these nurses was their ability to care for brutally injured causalities, day and night, beautiful in the midst of horror, smiling for the troops.

The Brown Report of 1948 set the stage for far-reaching changes in nursing education and nursing practice. It called for nursing as a professional education, accredited by nationally known, recognized bodies, where the outcome would be excellence in practice in a changing post-war health delivery system. This report also served as a change agent to guide the profession through the dictates of physician oversight and administrative rigidity in the practice of nursing. The Brown Report marked the beginnings of a vision of nursing leadership beyond the direct practice of patient care. The vision of managing and shaping professional nursing practice, intertwining the uniqueness of nursing with that of medicine within an administratively supportive environment, was critical to ensure the growth in depth and complexity of nursing practice and to deal with a new era in healthcare delivery.

The Brown Report came at a time when the number of nurses was declining. After the war, a nursing shortage resulted from the long and arduous working hours, low pay, and limited power and authority to shape a supportive and encouraging environment for the profession. The nursing shortage persisted through the 1950s, and efforts were under way to increase enrollment in nursing schools. Schools of nursing across the country were building stronger, more integrated baccalaureate programs, and nursing science began to emerge as the core of nursing practice, separate from the approach of a compilation of related sciences.

Modern Age of Nursing Education

Those entering practice roles in nursing are required to have specific basic educational background and usually prior professional experiences as well. All nursing leadership positions require licensure in the state of employment and a degree in nursing, traditionally the bachelor's or associate degree. More recently, nursing programs have expanded to attract those from other careers into nursing. For those who have a college degree in a nonnursing major, some programs offer basic nursing education as required for licensure in a graduate level (master's) program. However, the common core remains: the nursing license and basic clinically oriented nursing education.

Because there are several routes to achieving the common core, it is debated as to which is the most valuable and common pathway to a basic nursing education. The two most common routes are the bachelor's degree with a major in nursing (resulting in a Bachelor of Science with a major in Nursing, or BSN) and the associate degree with a major in nursing (resulting in an Associate Degree in Nursing, or ADN). Note that the degree earned may read BSN or BS, depending on what the school is authorized to award. The same interpretation is made for the MS or MSN. The growth and development of the educational and experiential credentials necessary for the practice of the nurse leader have occurred intensively over the last 50 years and reflect the evolving curricula and learning expectations at all levels of study.

In the 1950s and 1960s, basic education for nurses was offered predominately through diploma schools of nursing, which were usually housed in hospitals (Kalisch & Kalisch, 2004). However, during those years, a new version of nursing education evolved as a result of the growing interest of potential nursing students in achieving a combined general and professional education. This interest led to the creation of baccalaureate programs that were essentially competitive with the diploma school market. The growth of baccalaureate nursing programs began in earnest in the 1960s.

Around the time the surge in baccalaureate programs occurred, a new type of nursing education program emerged: the 2-year associate degree program. This new educational venture prepared bedside nurses in a 2-year period to reduce the extreme nursing shortage of the time. It also moved nursing education squarely into the American higher education system (Kalisch & Kalisch, 2004). By not requiring four years of education, as did baccalaureate programs, associate degree programs offered an approach leading to a college degree in two years that could compete with the traditional hospital-based schools.

The associate degree programs existed on college campuses, offered more theory and science as a basis for practice, and required fewer practice hours than hospital-based schools did, but geared the clinical hours toward experiences that were necessary for learning rather than apprentice-type service. Theory consisted of both nursing content and liberal arts and sciences. In those early years, two-thirds of the credits nurses earned were nursing-related, and 75% of those were for clinical practice. Although the percentages have changed over the years, the focus of modern associate degree programs remains the preparation of clinically oriented bedside nurses. A key component of the associate degree structure was that graduates were eligible to sit for registered nurse licensure. Since the 1950s, nursing school graduates from 2-year, 3-year, and 4-year educational programs can sit for the same licensure exam.

The success of the associate degree programs was evident in the fact that a large percentage of graduates passed state licensing exams on their first attempt. This program type moved nursing into the community college setting as an acceptable and common degree area. Curricula were arranged so that bridge programs to institutions of higher learning were commonplace, although sometimes complex. Because associate degree programs are offered in local community colleges, they tend to draw students from local areas and these students, once graduated, work in local healthcare delivery systems, thus continuing a cycle that alleviates a nursing shortage.

The market for associate degree programs was competitive not only because potential students were interested in a different type of nursing education, but also because hospitals that housed diploma schools were beginning to develop affiliations with local colleges and universities and to make placements for this new type of nursing student. Hospitals found ways to move nursing diploma programs to external entities. The primary driver for this exodus was the cost of supporting nursing schools, which was becoming prohibitive and causing hospitals to pass some of the costs on to patients. Affiliation agreements with local education institutes eliminated this burden (Kalisch & Kalisch, 2004).

The change in environment for nursing programs lead to a shift in the new type of nurse graduates away from the more traditional, subservient role to one of greater education and self-development. The new programs emphasized individual education and growth as well as nursing skills and abilities. Nursing education became a liberal arts–based profession. Thus began a significant change in nursing education that prevailed and continues to this day.

Nursing education came to encompass expectations for greater clinical decision making and an understanding of trends, issues, the place of research in nursing, the role of nursing in the community, and the patient teaching aspect of nursing. Both associate and baccalaureate programs, to greater and lesser degrees, provide nurse education founded on liberal arts and science education and an understanding of the independence and interdependence of the profession. In addition, both provide the educational basis necessary for graduate education.

The Issue of ADN versus BSN as Entry-Level Education to Nursing

Many members of the profession believe that the baccalaureate degree offers broader, more relevant education to practice nursing in the complexities of the current healthcare environment; it should be the only entry into practice degree. The baccalaureate degree is advocated as preparation for administrative and teaching roles, although the master's degree is often a requirement for assumption of these positions. It is also advocated for community-based roles. The baccalaureate graduate at the bedside is also an espoused goal of most clinical facilities.

There is still division in our profession about what is the appropriate entry-level degree, and why. Other members of the profession believe that the associate degree is sufficient for full entry into practice in all clinical positions, including critical care and community-based roles. In addition to the confusion within the profession, employers are also unsure as to what the differences are. The differences are not necessarily recognized in the various job descriptions and accordingly are not being formally utilized or recognized.

The question of which degree is best for different purposes and opportunities is an issue that requires research and forums for debate and discussion. Nursing is too scarce a resource and too valuable a practice to have continuous confusion and division within and outside its ranks. As a profession united in beliefs about our education and practice, nursing leaders will be better able to advance through the ranks of very complex institutions and influence achievement of fully developed theory-based practice.

Undergraduate Issues

A significant percentage of associate degree graduates do not continue their education. Approximately 60% of all registered nurses in the United States are graduates of 2-year programs, making them the backbone of the registered nurse population. In addition to the brief period for schooling and credible National Council Licensure Examination (NCLEX) results, associate degree programs offer the education at less cost than 4-year programs do. With more focus on bedside care in these intense but brief educational programs, the vision exists to prepare associate degree graduates for senior nursing leadership positions in complex, multifaceted institutions. The vision is complicated by the need for additional education and perhaps by the goal of retaining greater numbers of associate degree graduates at the bedside.

Baccalaureate education provides a strong liberal arts and science base, multiple opportunities for student leadership roles, great exposure over a longer period of time to the personal and professional benefits of higher education, and a clear vision of a future based on continuing graduate education. Associate degree education offers an intense but shortened liberal arts and science based nursing curriculum that fully prepares nursing students to sit for the same licensure as baccalaureate graduates, who are often competitive for the same positions and most likely earn the same entry salaries.

Whatever the outcome of the debate, the present status supports that associate degree program graduates enter the workforce in critical care, emergency care, and community health positions. The nursing shortage has increased the hiring of associate degree graduates into positions other than basic care, as was the original idea of such programs, and which is still stated in contemporary writings (Cherry & Jacob, 2008).

Entry-level salaries have increased over the years in nursing. What has been much slower to move upward is the ceiling for nurses' salaries. Clinical nurses who reach their ceiling salary and wish to stay in nursing and advance to teaching, administration, or advanced practice positions find, at that point, the education needed for advanced positions is time consuming, often moves in a step-wise progression, is expensive, and does not necessarily recognize prior work experience for academic credit. In 2005, of the 2.9 million nurses in the United States, less than 50,000 reported holding a master's degree. Only a very small number of nurses had earned doctoral degrees, although the number has gradually increased since the 1980s.

Master's Education Issues

Creative and credible methods of recognizing advanced learning, assessment, and evidence-based practice are developing. More opportunity than ever now exists for advanced practice education. These are strong trends to bring nursing leaders into the boardroom from the bedside workforce. These are positive trends. In an age where nursing resources are scarce, where experienced nurses sometimes leave nursing or move from organization to organization, creative, effective, and efficient solutions for advancing education are essential.

Moving nurses from clinical roles to executive level positions must be an intense priority undertaken by the profession, with a commitment to achieve clarity as to what education is necessary, and efficiency as to eliminate any redundancy in steps taken by potential leaders. The transition needs to be efficient, effective, and focused on the learning needs that executives will have as they assume the highest leadership roles in the complex, changing environments of fully integrated healthcare enterprises.

Healthcare institutions will benefit greatly by further developing roles, compensation, and scope of authority and responsibility for nurses with higher education. Institutions that develop such frameworks for success will see benefits in patient satisfaction, quality of care, and cost effectiveness.

Some are concerned that nurses are moving too far from their original calling as bedside nurses. However, leaders, managers, and teachers of nursing are essential if the profession is to lead healthcare delivery in the present and into the future. These concerns are somewhat addressed by the preparation of clinical experts such as nurse practitioners in master's level academic programs.

Academic credentials and/or professional certifications are required to ascend to leadership positions. So, while they are still evolving and becoming further refined and defined, the requirements for earned degrees and/or certifications are accepted as sine qua non within the professional role. On the one hand, the major nursing organizations, including the National League for Nursing, American Nurses Association, American Association of Colleges of Nursing, as well as the State Boards of Nursing and its overarching National Council, are key players in determining the requirements and education for clinical practice at basic and advanced practice levels.

Today there are articulation models in the form of ADN to BSN programs, and RN (usually ADN graduates) to master's degree programs in nursing. From a professional advancement standpoint, the articulation models are supportive to enhance theory-based advanced practice. The practice roles are in a variety of areas, most often for nurse practitioner roles. The focus of education roles at the graduate level is most often required for undergraduate faculty positions, and sometimes for staff development education. The management or administrative focus of graduate programs offers preparation for those in the nurse manager/director/vice president pathway.

There is still debate as to what material formal educational processes must contain to prepare the advanced practitioner to move to higher and broader leadership responsibilities. Does the formal preparation of nurses to be educators also prepare them to be deans or academic directors? What is the profession's academic mandate to shape nurses for senior academic leadership positions of vice president and president? Do the requirements for such learning belong at the master's or doctoral level of education, or both?

For nurses who wish to reach the highest levels of leadership in the clinical role, the road to practice with power has yet to be fully paved. However, there are newer efforts in this area that are worth considering. The prevailing clinical roles for the advanced practitioner have effectively become the nurse practitioner, certified registered nurse anesthetists, certified nurse–midwives, and clinical nurse specialists. The 30-year effort to move the role—especially that of the nurse practitioner—into the mainstream of the healthcare delivery system is an honorable success story for the nursing profession.

The roles of most of the advanced nursing practices are widely recognized and supported by the insurance, medical, healthcare delivery, governmental, and legal communities. The uphill battles began approximately 30 years ago to move the outlier idea for the nurse practitioner role to the mainstream where it has become a pivotal and powerful role for cost-effective, high-quality practice with a recognized outcome of patient satisfaction as well. Achievement of recognition outside the profession is evident in alterations in the practices of healthcare delivery, such as separate licensure, specialty certification, prescription privileges, and insurance reimbursement. Within the profession, recognition of achievement is by the expansion of the role from solely outpatient-based to a variety of inpatient roles, responsibilities, and titles. Nurse practitioners may practice autonomously, with or without direct physician supervision, or within institutions.

With the evolution of this nursing role, the power to control practice via independent management and decision making as a nurse practitioner is still a work in progress. The decision-making power to use institutional resources to enhance practice and/or bring together multidisciplinary healthcare teams to achieve goals for patient care such as treatment, cost efficiency, or quality improvement must expand if nursing is to lead healthcare delivery in a clinical role. To this end, what are the next formal educational pathways the profession needs to set to enhance the scope of practice and the authority of the nurse leader in a clinical role? Are there formal academic experiences that are essential to prepare the most effective nurse leader in an academic setting? How do we, as leaders of the profession, better shape the formal pathways of education for nursing leadership in the boardroom?

The Politics of the Doctorate in Nursing

The doctoral programs in nursing (Doctor of Philosophy, or PhD; Doctor of Education, or EdD; Doctor of Nursing Science, or DNS/DNSc; and Doctor of Nursing Practice, or DNP) and those that are related, in such areas in the social and behavioral sciences, provide formal education at the highest level. The primary focus at the doctoral level has long been the expansion of knowledge frontiers through the research process.

The DNP is designed to prepare nurses to provide inpatient clinical care, oversee the care of patients, and make independent decisions about care. There has been concern about whether the DNP expands knowledge through research. In partial answer to this question, it is important to note the efforts now under way by the American Nurses Association to lead support for the implementation of the role of Doctor of Nursing Practice. ANA has promulgated this role to "ensure that all patients have access to affordable healthcare benefits and services, and the ability of all health professions and organizations to innovate and improve quality of care" (American Nurses Association, 2008).

The American Medical Association has written of its opposition to this new form of nursing education at the highest level unless DNPs practice under the supervision of a physician and as part of a medical team in which the final responsibility for the patient lies with the licensed physician. Furthermore, the AMA has stated opposition to the participation of the National Board of Medical Examiners in any credentialing process for this new, highly prepared practitioner in nursing (American Medical Association Houses of Delegates, 2008a). Further potential confinement of nursing practice is stated in the following resolution: "The title of 'Doctor' in a medical setting applies only to physicians licensed to practice medicine" (American Medical Association Houses of Delegates, 2008b).

The ANA responds to these views by firmly stating that the American Medical Association does not regulate the practice of nursing, and that it is inappropriate for the organization to try to limit the scope of practice of another profession. It is essential that the two professions work collaboratively—with neither determining the scope of practice of the other—to provide an environment of quality and successful outcomes in the healthcare delivery system. The outcome of this territorial issue will eventually be resolved. With the full and consistent voices of the nursing profession, the growth of responsibility and autonomy for practice will prevail.

Education and Experience for Leadership

Entering the realm of leaders also requires that individuals bring a range of professional practice experiences to the leadership role. The responsibilities, skill sets, depth of organizational and professional knowledge, and span of control exercised by the nurse leader prior to beginning any new position are key components of the practice pathways to leadership positions in nursing. There is variability in what comprises the ideal or expected aspects of the practice component to support ascendance to the leadership role.

Nurses with a combination of graduate-level education in nursing or other fields and appropriate practice experience as advance practice nurses, nurse educators, nurse administrators, or nurse informatics specialists can become candidates for leadership positions, up to boardroom-level positions, even though their educational preparation may have been mixed with nontraditional credentials. In some sectors, there is continuing debate on how much "mixing" of nursing and nonnursing academic and practice credentials is acceptable.

There are two other components to consider in laying the groundwork for pathways to leadership roles in nursing. One is the focus and structure of the healthcare organization, which may provide patient care services, be an academic institution, and/or function as a for-profit vendor of services. Within the institution, the role of leader will reside at some level in the organization, thereby indicating the leader's span of control and where on the practice-management-leadership continuum the position resides.

The second component is the actual "meat" of the meaning of the leadership role as it relates to the institution and to the position. In all areas of nursing practice, from patient care to research, from teaching to administration, the behavior of the nurse leader reflects certain capabilities and characteristics that are identified with leadership. Examples of some common characteristics often associated with leadership are excellence in practice, strategic planning abilities, ability to make and manage change, communication skills, and ability to build an effective team.

One other consideration in creating the profile of the nurse leader, which will influence the preceding components, is the fact that the nursing leader may not move on the pathway to a nursing leadership position. Rather, such an individual may choose a leadership trajectory in a different field such as politics, law, or business. Box 3–1 introduces a nurse leader who is involved in politics, too.

Box 3–1 The Honorable Claire Shulman

Claire Shulman

Claire Shulman is a nurse and a politician. She remains actively involved in health care through her affiliation with the Queens Hospital Center. Among many awards Ms. Shulman has received, she most recently received the Lifetime Achievement Award from the Alpha Omega Chapter of Sigma Theta Tau and the Adelphi University School of Nursing.

In her own words...

"I was a nursing student at Adelphi College School of Nursing (later to become Adelphi University). As a student, I was affiliated at Queens General Hospital Center as Adelphi College had no hospital. I was a student during the war, and students ran the hospitals under the supervision of a nurse supervisor because the registered nurses were in the service. (That's why we learned so much—because we had no alternative.) Our country was engaged in World War II, and consequently we had very little in equipment. As students, we quickly learned to improvise and became nurses extraordinaire.

I graduated from Adelphi College in 1946 with a bachelor's degree, and I passed state boards shortly thereafter and became a registered nurse. My first job was in female medicine, and because of my degree I became head nurse at the ripe age of 21. I nursed until 1950 when my first child was born, and then again after the Korean War.

When my children entered school my political career began. After working in government for some time, in 1986, I became the Borough President of Queens County, New York City, and served in that capacity for 16 years. Because of my nursing experience I always paid very close attention to details, particularly in areas related to health, and was able to accomplish many things for the public including rebuilding the Queens Hospital Center, which today is the newest and best in the New York public hospital system.

My nursing experience has been invaluable in my life and has helped to govern almost everything I do. My values were created on the hospital floors as I dealt daily with life and death issues, and I have passed on these values to my family."

The pressures of the healthcare delivery system and the academic institution shape the leadership role in today's healthcare environment. These are the two major healthcare-related entities in which the nurse would typically practice. The mission and vision of the institution shape the role. The behaviors of the nursing leader are to provide vision and a strategic plan to accomplish the mission. The boardroom leader has overall responsibility to develop a resource base sufficient to support staff to meet customer needs and must commit to creating and energizing a dynamic whole within the diverse and complex staff. Overall, nursing leadership, with the help of management, has the awesome challenge of charging the energies of those around them to maintain the essence of the institution and the communities it serves.

Education and Skills for Leadership Practice

Nurse leaders must appraise the complexities and identities of the institution and the community as individual force fields. They must value and construct opportunities for energy exchanges between the institutions and the communities they serve for the betterment of both. These tasks require knowledge, wisdom, sensitivity, and a spirit of inquiry to bring ubiquitous energy together for outcomes that can be measured and valued by those involved.

The nursing leader's appraisal can focus on constructs such as diversity, community study, staff understanding, resource building, education, knowledge and skill building, communication, respect, and understanding. The focus of the nursing leader's actions is to support, assess, change, maintain, value, and select.

The tools of the leader are nursing knowledge and skills, experiences, and practices that emerge from behaviors and roles in complex institutions that serve heterogeneous populations. Analytical, judging, and investigative skills support inquiry and evaluation, questioning, and proposal development. Designing interactions to improve the providers' contributions and the customers' outcomes will occur when the integration of the preceding functions results in the ability to predict successful outcomes accurately.

The focus of graduate preparation in the academic environment is on learning requirements necessary for curriculum development, teaching and evaluation, and creatively managing student-learning needs.

Programs in administration in the healthcare delivery environment have expectations for knowledge and skill in developing and providing the resources to implement evidence-based practice protocols, managing teams, managing conflict and change, and creating an environment for care that strengthens patients and staff.

Education for advanced clinical practice prepares the nurse for a higher degree of autonomy and interdependent practice and teaches advanced clinical skills in patient assessment, treatment, and evaluation. The clinical doctorate is specifically designed for the nurse to function in clinical leadership roles in patient care situations. The newer advanced practice role in informatics focuses on Information Technology as a force within healthcare systems, designed and utilized to enhance patient care and the practice of nursing and other health-related professions. Advanced practice in informatics will enhance the creation of nursing databases and document the influence of nursing practice on patient outcomes. This information should be the basis for designing cost-effective patient outcomes while enhancing patient satisfaction and utilizing nursing abilities to the fullest.

Theories of Nursing for Clinical Practice

As nursing moved into academic settings and to professional status, one of the areas of growth was the development of theories that explained and predicted the practice. The theories of nursing, perhaps two dozen or more, focus on the nurse–patient relationship. The relationship is postulated and investigated to facilitate better understanding and to generate further postulates on achieving opportunities for healthier growth in patients and nurses. Research to test the theories to expand nursing's borders is a major focus of graduate programs in nursing.

In 1964, Martha Rogers's *Reveille in Nursing* not only marked nursing as a profession with its own scientific base, but it significantly reinforced the concept of graduate study in nursing as the sine qua non for the clinical practice of nursing and set the stage for leadership in the profession (Rogers, 1964). At last, nurses could refer to their own scientific base and build on it to explain behavior and to prepare appropriate approaches to achieve desired outcomes. In her statement, "The body of knowledge made explicit by nursing's scientists and researchers must be transmitted if the conditions of the profession are to be fulfilled," Rogers puts forth that nursing as follower or leader, in the clinical, teaching, or administrative role, has its own theoretical paradigms on which to base its assessments, plans of action, behaviors, and evaluations of nursing interventions (Rogers, 1964, p. 43). The educational pathway to leadership took a significant step forward in the 1960s and 1970s by elucidating theoretical frameworks for nursing and, equally important, clearly showing that the universe of nursing contained leadership and change agent roles in all settings and investigatory research roles.

In the 1970s, Dorothea Johnson proposed the Behavioral System Model that postulated that nursing practice should focus on the patient as an individual, rather than the disease, and should facilitate effective behaviors in the patient before, during, and after illness. Motivation, adaptation, and the change process can achieve her interpretation of the interactions in human systems and subsystems to achieve better functioning.

Sister Callista Roy put forth the Adaptation Model as a theory of nursing practice that focuses on promoting and expanding adaptive abilities. Roy's model, which evolved from behavioral and social sciences, sets a framework for clinical nursing practice to work with patients via environmental alteration to help patients develop their own adaptive behaviors leading to survival, growth, reproduction, mastery, and other aspects of transformation. The role of the nurse is proactive, to assess, evaluate, and manipulate stimuli in the patient's environment. Roy's approaches to enhance the transformation and change that occur in the person and his or her environment provide clarity to the nursing process and an important aspect of meeting patient care needs.

Martha Rogers expanded on *Reveille in Nursing* by creating a theory widely known as the Science of Unitary Human Beings. Her conceptual model emerged from the wide knowledge bases of multiple disciplines, including anthropology, biology, physics, and philosophy. She broke new ground in using these theories to explain the relationship of human beings to their environment and how the two forces interact with each other, affecting change through the experiences that occur. According to Rogers, the role of nursing is to "strengthen the integrity of the human field" and to direct and redirect "patterning of the human and environmental fields for realization of maximum health potential" (Rogers, 1964).

A more recent theory of nursing called Nursing: Human Science and Human Care, postulated by Dr. Jean Watson, identifies caring as the essence of nursing (Watson, 1985). Watson defines caring as a moral behavior and goes on to describe caring moments and the phenomena of the relationship between caregiver and patient. Her insight into the power of the relationship as the environment to enhance growth in the patient is a powerful active behavior of nursing practice. Her theory of caring highlights the creation of energy forces such as values, faith, hope, and sensitivity to self and others. These forces are drivers of health and growth in the patient and indeed in the caregiver as well. These forces generate helping and trusting relationships, and acceptance of both positive and negative feelings. The theory goes on to describe the creation of healing spaces and awareness and the development of the ability to honor what is sacred.

The theories mentioned here are but a few examples of credible and worthy theoretical constructs and paradigms written by nurse scholars. They provide a vision for knowledge-based clinical practice that, once tested and implemented, can become powerful tools for influencing and predicting positive outcomes of patient behaviors. The ability of nursing practice, based on recognized theory, to transform the patient system in positive directions strengthens our commitment to pathways to excellence in nursing care of patients and their families based on theory, the actions, and science, in turn also strengthens the profession.

Some theoretical underpinnings for the advanced practice role focus specifically on the role of the advanced practice nurse. According to Lucille A. Joel, theoretical perspectives of "structural-functionalist" and "symbolic-interactionist" will guide the advanced practice nurse (APN) to move the newer role into the mainstream (Joel, 2004). The structural-functionalist perspective guides the practitioner to the awareness that opportunities to alter roles already known (i.e., the traditional nursing role) are limited. The symbolic-interactionist theoretical perspective presents environmental forces as open to choose what they wish to react to, thereby laying the groundwork for acceptance and embracing the changing role of the nurse, from traditional to independent and proactive.

Evidence-Based Practice Approaches to Support Nursing Leadership

Advanced practice methodologies and evidence-based research, which have become hallmarks of quality nursing care, have theoretical underpinnings. They are integral to nursing practice at all levels. Practice based on researched clinical and nursing theory evidence is a powerful basis for the provision of patient care and increases the strength of predictable outcomes and observations. Furthermore, such practice enhances the power of nursing theories so that they more broadly influence practice in nursing and across disciplines. By bringing integrated theory to quantitative research testing, traditional nursing education and practice can move to the forefront in determining standards and protocols for practice that can achieve expected outcomes.

Evidence-based practice is the outcome of testing science and theory that confirms the most effective interventions and treatments for patient health issues. Evidence-based practice is based on more than the methodologically impeccable research work. It includes logic, critical thinking, and the most rational way to plan actions and make decisions (Jenicek & Hitchcock, 2005).

The major components of evidence-based practice, such as critical thinking and priority setting, are significant beyond the advanced practice role and are equally influential in graduate education and practice in education, administration, and management. The ability to think critically permeates all practice realms and can bring together the forces for change to enhance quality, access, cost efficiency, and social responsibility in the organization led by the nursing leader.

The leader is educated as a critical thinker. Disciplined, self-directed thinking considers other relevant information, uses reflective skepticism to make overall judgments about the problem or issue, and acts appropriately based on reason (Jenicek & Hitchcock, 2005). Critical thinking is a persistent effort to examine beliefs and knowledge in light of the evidence that supports it. Critical thinking has also been described by Falcione as self-regulatory judgment, leading to evaluation and inference (Jenicek & Hitchcock, 2005).

Education for leadership, via modern pathways, must actively generate decision-making behavior based on knowledge, logic, critical thinking, and communication with the communities served by the leader. From this perspective, the current efforts of evidence-based practice focus within the clinical practice realm of the leader. However, it is also important that senior academic and organizational leaders have the capabilities to make knowledge-based decisions to achieve evidence-based practice. These decisions emanate from logical, reflective analysis. Once analyzed, the decision outcomes are communicated accurately and without emotion or confusion to activate resources needed for both change and the cohesion to achieve it (Jenicek & Hitchcock, 2005).

One of the best definitions of evidence-based practice states that it is "an approach to decision-making in which the clinician uses the best evidence available, in consultation with the patient, to decide upon the option which suits the patient best" (Muir Gray, 2001).

A spin-off from the growing evidence-based practice movement is evidence-based policy making. Related to other practices besides direct patient care, evidence-based policies will use the best current knowledge as the basis for effective decision making. The creation of evidence-based policies will move further to institutionalize cutting-edge practice that is based on research. Indeed, if evidence-based practice is an important criterion for assisting decision making, then the use of this approach must extend beyond the clinical practice realm and into all areas of management and leadership where decision making is characteristic of the role (Booth & Brice, 2004).

Trusted expert knowledge systems must become the basis for solving problems and reducing the risk of poor outcomes. Healthcare outcomes such as poor-quality services, high costs, limited return improvement in overall health or functionality, and poor customer satisfaction, all can be improved with science-based actions in expert knowledge systems based on the tenets of nursing theory and evidence-based practice approaches.

For those in management or leadership roles, the use of evidence-based practice is essential to enhance effectiveness, accountability, and transparency as well as the value of costs and resources expended in achieving expected results. Indeed, evidence-based practice focuses on effectiveness. Its consequent processes are identifying evidence, critically appraising the research, incorporating the research into guidelines for practice, making decisions, and evaluating the outcomes of the decisions (Booth & Brice, 2004).

The Role of Large Theories in Leadership Development

The importance of harnessing large theories that can explain and offer predictions of outcomes of changes implemented by leadership decisions cannot be underestimated. Leadership is the ability to direct energies of the system to achieve directed change and the ability to communicate with and influence the behaviors of other interfacing and communicating systems.

Leaders have the potential to influence all aspects of the systems in which they function and over which they have control. The power of their effectiveness relates to their knowledge and understanding of unique and powerful forces within the system.

General Systems Theory

The general systems theory framework, which can be used to understand and categorize the environment of the healthcare entity and the community, is one of the broadest frameworks available to conceptualize the total organization. Nursing leaders can become skillful in interpreting and utilizing this theoretical framework to assess, compare, predict, and evaluate the world in which their influence will make a difference. Nursing leaders can develop worthwhile insight into how the organization operates and will be able to communicate those insights in a compelling fashion that will allow correction and maintenance to be ongoing with limited resistance.

Ludwig von Bertalanffy's general systems theory presents constructs of continuous energy sharing between and among sectors of open systems to attempt to achieve homeostasis, or balance, throughout the system or to achieve growth and expansion in the system, even with some disequilibrium. Energy, its transfer, and use that was not sufficient to produce growth could be dissipated and reduce the strength and effectiveness of the system, resulting in more chaos and less productivity (von Bertalanffy, 1972). In particular, general systems theory is both a model of reality and a way of viewing the living world.

The theory is overarching, and if the leader's influence is to encompass the broadest sphere of behavior, it must be overarching over all energy fields that can be included in the system of the healthcare entity and the community (von Bertalanffy, 1972).

The interactive behaviors of open systems and energy can be of considerable importance to nursing leaders in that their strategic behaviors will be directed to developing and operating successful healthcare delivery systems. To achieve that complex and continually evolving goal, the leader must be cognizant of the energy in the system—where it is coming from and how it is being utilized, transferred, and transformed. The success of healthcare organizations will depend on their ability to attract and utilize resources (energy), such as financial support of customers and the efforts (energy) of the employees.

The leadership team scans the internal and external environments and creates an environment that transforms the energies of customers and clinicians into realistic alternatives and solutions to meet the expressed needs of the customers via the skill and knowledge of the clinicians. All energy exchange must consider the characteristics of quality, value, and need for the service both from the perspective of the suppliers (the organization) and the customers (the customers and the community).

If the implemented solutions are not as good as competing alternatives, there is drain and loss of energy in the system that will weaken the healthcare delivery system. If continuous and pervasive, this could result in the organization's failure, leaving a vacuum into which competitors can expand. If implemented solutions are better than the competing alternatives, there is focused energy use and achievement of better balance with expansion capabilities; the system grows and thrives.

The key components of the system for healthcare delivery are the healthcare organization and the community. Both entities must function together as partners to achieve the development of healthcare delivery that utilizes professional energy and resources (skills, knowledge, and equipment, for example) to stimulate healthiness in the community it serves. Such healthiness can be identified as empowerment in healthcare decisions, knowledge of alternative healthcare treatments and behaviors, and opportunity to clarify and define healthcare needs that the community and individuals wish to be met through transformation of organizational energies.

Field Theory

Kurt Lewin's field theory also has relevance to leadership behaviors. It offers a perspective of a universe (the healthcare delivery system, which is the responsibility of the leader) and provides interpretation and a theoretical framework to identify and maintain or alter the "valence" of regions of concern. According to Lewin, a "positive valence" represents a region moving toward a goal, and a "negative valence" represents a region moving away from a goal (Deutsch & Krauss, 1965). Regions have tension, which is energy used for "locomotion" to achieve a change. When the goal is achieved, the regions move to a state of balance.

Using this framework, the leader has the power and could have the intent to create and clarify a "goal region" and provide the tension or expectation of goal achievement. If there is no perceived goal region, the individual's behaviors are seen as restless and movement is away from the goal, which becomes a negative valence or value as a result of the frustration and lack of direction. The creation and management of the forces to achieve change in the positive direction

of recognized need have always been a challenge for leaders. Using the tenants of field theory provides a resource to achieve vision and to support the staff at all levels in their energy use and reaching the goals they will achieve.

Chaos Theory

Chaos theory has a rightful place in the investigation of theoretical constructs that can become the tools of the successful nurse leader. Chaos theory has found its way into the nursing literature from time to time, most frequently in the psychosocial areas of nursing. Although originating from mathematics and science, chaos theory utilizes the complexities of interactions and constant change within a societal context to understand behavior. Understanding is the key to limiting the interpretation of the behavior as pathological rather than adaptive.

Chaos theory can be described as an extension of systems theory applied in it widest context. It can be the theoretical framework for assessing institutional dysfunction from all major components, such as the clinical systems, legal systems, and information systems, for example. The breakdown of these subsystems has wide and powerful effects on the individuals and community systems that depend on the support and curative services provided by the healthcare and/or educational system, which infuses energy for growth and health into the individuals and community in its network. Chaos theory can offer the skilled leader some analytical tools of insight and assessment that can validate the totality of the negative and even devastating experiences in the community of customers or the staff infrastructure of the institution.

In either case, the principles of chaos expand, and broader, more complex and powerful forces are necessary to reduce the multisystem dysfunction. Dysfunction is enlarged through diversity, and its solution is hampered by lack of knowledge and understanding.

Concepts of Social Responsibility

An evolving approach to a conceptual framework for leaders is beginning to appear in the literature under the umbrella title of Social Responsibility. From the writings beginning to emerge in this area, nursing leaders can use the viewpoints of achieving socially responsible care. Such a strategic vision will create a direction for their healthcare system that successfully and easily meets current and future needs of the organization to perform at a level of excellence. Achieving excellence in education of or directly providing care for the healthcare needs of complex and diverse communities is a significant and challenging focus for leadership in nursing.

To act in a socially responsible manner, the healthcare organization and the nurse leader inherently embody strategic approaches to management and care that is community focused. The organization develops a community relationship by assessing the following characteristics of the community it serves:

- What are the community's goals and needs, and how does the organization serve them? Determining the status of the community–healthcare organization relationship will take careful and wide scope of data collection and assessment. Interaction with community organizations and leaders on many levels will lead to some insight on this point.
- How does the healthcare organization attract the resources it needs to perform its mission? The overarching categories of resources are financial, support of its customers and expanding customer base, and quality and loyalty of its employees. What are the degrees of success and failure in each of these categories? In addition, what are the factors affecting the outcomes?
- How focused is the healthcare organization on continuous improvement? For the socially responsible institution, equilibrium is never fully achieved. Directing the process of improving quality requires skill, knowledge, commitment at a fully multidisciplinary level, and the resources to sustain continuous inquiry and problem solving.

The healthcare organization must continue to survey and interact with the environment, both internal and external, and fully develop its relationship with it. Beyond that, as a basis for a beginning, the nursing leader implements mechanisms to promote consensus among the individuals and agencies supporting the organization. A community focus creates a broad base of support to ensure that the healthcare organization will endure and be effective and responsible, even in the face of continuous change.

The Role of the Nurse Leader in Creating a Socially Responsible Organization

The nurse leader can and should be prepared to undertake and implement key actions to build and maintain the support of its influential stakeholders. Whatever the level of responsibility or power of the leader, the nurse leader can do the following:

- *Implement boundary-scanning activities.* Boundary-scanning activities include deliberate efforts on the part of leadership and management to identify providers and customers and to meet their needs by bringing them together to reach consensus.
- *Develop community partnerships.* To develop community partnerships, nursing leaders must develop relationships with community-based programs, such as mental health care centers, early development and pediatric care centers, and long-term and geriatric care centers. Developing such partnerships means citizen empowerment, which is an essential ingredient to responsive community-based social responsibility. Partnerships provide guidance to the healthcare system to ensure that it stays responsible to the citizens it is committed to serve.
- *Look inward to the purpose of outreach programs.* Are outreach programs a way for the systems to expand themselves and diminish the individualities of the communities? Are they sufficiently open to identify patient needs and fill gaps in inpatient services? Do outreach programs perpetuate paternalistic roles? Moreover, in the end, are they successful?
- *Focus on creating power among the community constituencies.* The nursing leader can challenge the nursing staff and management hierarchy to produce healthy outcomes and healthy behaviors among the

powerless and to move the constituencies from a powerless to a powerful state in deciding about their own healthcare needs and approaches. It has long been known that the health status of those with the least power is unconscionably low. The significant signs of poor health status and low power are quite universal and can be identified as follows:

Violence

Dangerous housing

Teenage pregnancies

Drug overdoses

Alcoholism

In summary, powerlessness goes along with poverty of resources and spirit. Powerlessness from any and all of the above factors leads to increasing risk factors of preventable disease. The knowledgeable and astute nursing leader, prepared by broad-based education and experience, can create a nursing and multidisciplinary infrastructure that is diverse and knowledgeable enough to interface with community leaders and community members to identify the scope of powerlessness and the capacity of the community to care for its citizens.

The Nurse Leader as Nurturer

The concept of nurturer has prevailed as a significant identifier of the nurse throughout the history of the profession. I believe it is a key one to be valued, developed, and used in our future. Using that historical view of the nurse to facil-

Box 3–2 To Better Serve: Sometimes Life Happens by Chance

Sue Buchholtz

In the 1970s, the first nurse practitioner program was developed. The effort was to provide care for an underserved pediatric population in the Midwest. There were too few doctors to serve the growing needs of communities as the population expanded. It was believed that trained, experienced nurses could act as the eyes and ears of the physician and report back abnormal findings. It was believed nurse practitioners could take medical histories and conduct physical examinations, do well-baby visits, and observe for any abnormal findings. In this way, more children could be evaluated and those that needed more treatment could be referred to the physician for further care.

Over time, the use of nurse practitioners proved so successful that it expanded to include the care of adults, maternal-child nursing, care of the mentally ill, geriatrics, and care of the frail elderly.

Multiple surveys have indicated that patients prefer the care of nurse practitioners, considering them to be more attentive, kinder, and caring. Furthermore, the use of a nurse practitioner is cost effective because it extends the care of the physician to cover a far broader range of patients than one physician can cover. Because nurse practitioners often serve in lower economic communities the service provided is invaluable to the public good and provides services that otherwise would be unattainable or unaffordable.

While working at a large state university, I became involved in writing the plan for a women's health nurse practitioner program. Although we were successful in having the program accepted, we were criticized because the three authors of the program were not themselves nurse practitioners. So, after swearing up and down that once I finished my doctorate I would never, ever go to school again, I found myself registered in a nurse practitioner program.

Returning to clinical practice from academia was the most rewarding and fun experience. I have always loved patient care. Even during my academic years, beside the didactic portion of the course, I always taught the clinical portion, wanting students to love being with the patients as much as I did. Now as a nurse practitioner I was back full time at the bedside and adoring every minute of it. I felt useful, empowered, and independent. I assessed patients, wrote orders, and followed the patients' progress. I talked to families, made discharge plans, educated those who didn't understand, and held the hand of those in need. I had extended the role of nurse to do more good, be helpful, and to serve more of those in need.

Although I never planned to become a nurse practitioner (they didn't exist when I became a nurse), sometimes life just happens that way. Sometimes you get lucky and a good thing happens so that you can do more to serve humanity and your chosen profession.

After more than 40 years of nursing, I have never had one day when I have been sorry with the decision of my chosen profession.

I have often said that for some nurses it is a job, for others it is a career, but for some of us it is a calling. It is our mission to serve the most basic needs of others to make them feel safe and comforted.

itate leadership development in today's competitive and complex healthcare environment is a challenge and an opportunity for the contemporary nurse leader. How does leadership in nursing reflect both the capacity for nurturing and the ability for visionary decision making that creates sweeping organizational and professional change in the profession, in practice, and in healthcare delivery on all levels?

The concept of the nurse as nurturer is inherent in the clinical role and the education of clinical nurses. Nurse as nurturer was the quintessential vision of the nurse. As nursing education evolved to enhance the knowledge base and decision-making abilities of nurses, there arose a turmoil that, although theory was desirable, soothing, touching, and caring were what nursing was really about. The differences of opinion on this subject in the multidisciplinary healthcare and patient community persist to this day and present an even stronger challenge and opportunity to the senior nurse leader to integrate nurturing into the executive role.

How does the nurturing nurse leader bring about changes in practice to enhance an organizational structure where nurses can develop, test, and implement approaches to evidence-based practice? What are the operational definitions of the nurturing nurse leader? What are the educational pathways that lead us to achieve that end? Or is nurturing a personality trait innate to those who become nurses, one not necessarily learned? It is largely up to the contemporary profession and its leaders and members

to reinforce the nurturing characteristic of nursing as both quintessential to its practice and integral to the science of its analysis and actions.

Summary

This chapter touches on the major components of the educational pathways to becoming a nurse leader. The development and mix of all experiences, standards of practice, and academic achievements creates a leader who is different, dynamic, powerfully rich in abilities, and changing. Early in one's career as a nurse, an individual may not envision a leadership role aligned in his or her professional direction. As the future unfolds, and this option becomes more visible, it is up to individual nurses to enhance their profiles through cultivating the strengths of knowledge, wisdom, experience, and personal growth along the lines of academic credentialing; in this way, nurses utilize theory as a basis for predicting and achieving the vision and mission of the institution that owns the leadership role.

It was through the creative and scholarly writings of nursing theorists that education for nursing leadership took on a new expanded meaning and value, yet stayed grounded in sensitive, gentle, and knowledge-based direct patient care. Through the writings and research of the 1960s through the 1990s, nursing found its center and began to use that center to create its own independent and interdependent profession. The pathway to leadership through education lies in paradigms and propositions of nursing and other theories.

The pathway of nursing education includes key stepping-stones that represent the knowledge of science and arts that support the nursing process. The value of nursing theories is that they provide tools directly related to the profession that can enhance nurses' abilities to apply the nursing process, including the ability to predict outcomes based on research findings.

QUESTIONS

1. The primary driver for beginning the exodus of diploma schools from hospitals was
   a. the cost to the hospital for supporting a nursing program
   b. an inability to attract interested students into programs
   c. a profound need for nurses
   d. women seeking new careers

2. Kurt Lewin's theory identifies tension as energy, which he relates to creating change. According to Lewin, a positive valence in change theory represents a region moving
   a. toward a goal
   b. away from a goal
   c. along a straight plane
   d. toward power

3. According to Kurt Lewin's theory, a negative valence represents a region moving
   a. toward a goal
   b. away from a goal
   c. in balance
   d. away from power

4. According to Kurt Lewin's theory, when a goal is achieved
   a. all regions disappear
   b. power will no longer be an issue
   c. the regions move to a state of balance
   d. chaos will be gone

5. Social responsibility of the healthcare organization and nurse leaders in communities is vital. Nurse leaders develop a community relationship by
   a. assessing the goals and needs of the community
   b. determining the status of health care in the community
   c. assessing how the healthcare organization attracts resources in meeting community needs
   d. All of the above

References

American Medical Association Houses of Delegates. (2008a). *Resolution 214 (A-08): Doctor of nursing practice.* Retrieved November 24, 2008, from http://www.acnpweb.org/files/public/AMA_Resolution_214_Doctor_of_Nursing_Practice.pdf

American Medical Association Houses of Delegates. (2008b). *Resolution 303 (A-08): Protection of the titles "doctor," "resident" and "residency."* Retrieved November 24, 2008, from http://www.acnpweb.org/files/public/AMA_Resolution_303_Use_of_Title_Doctor.pdf

American Nurses Association. (2008). *American Nursing Association House of Delegates Resolution 214 (A-08) "Doctor of Nursing Practice."* Retrieved November 21, 2008, from http://svnnet.org/uploads/File/ANAResponse214.pdf

Booth, A., & Brice, A. (2004). *Evidence-based practice for information professionals.* London: Facet.

Cherry, B., & Jacob, S. (2008). *Contemporary nursing: Issues, trends, & management* (3rd ed.). St. Louis: Mosby.

Deutsch, M., & Krauss, R. (1965). *Theories in social psychology.* New York: Basic Books.

Donahue, P. (1996). *Nursing, the finest art: An illustrated history.* St Louis: Mosby.

Ellis, J. R., & Hartley, C. L. (2004). *Nursing in today's world: Trends, issues & management* (8th ed.). Philadelphia: Lippincott Williams & Wilkins.

Jenicek, M., & Hitchcock, D. L. (2005). *Evidence based practice: Logic and critical thinking in medicine.* Chicago: American Medical Association Press.

Joel, L. A. (2004). *Advanced practice nursing: Essentials for role development.* Philadelphia: F. A. Davis.

Kalisch, P. A., & Kalisch, B. J. (2004). *American nursing: A history.* Philadelphia: Lippincott Williams & Wilkins.

Muir Gray, J. A. (2001). *Evidence based health care* (2nd ed.). London: Churchill Livingstone.

Nightingale, F. (1992). *Notes on nursing: What it is and what it is not.* Philadelphia: Lippincott Williams & Wilkins.

Rogers, M. E. (1964). *Reveille in nursing.* Philadelphia: F. A. Davis.

Starr, P. (1984). *The social transformation of American medicine.* New York: Basic Books.

von Bertalanffy, L. (1972). The history and status of general systems theory. *The Academy of Management Journal, 15*(4), 407–426.

Chapter 4

Leadership Theories

Mary T. Hickey

OUTLINE

Leadership Theories
    Trait Theories
    Behavioral Theories
    Current Models

Emotional Intelligence
Power
Diversity
Examples of Leadership in Action

The concept of leadership has been a subject of discussion and debate for as long as anyone can remember. There are as many definitions and classifications of leadership as there are theories and explanations. Leadership skills are important in business, politics, health care, education, community settings, and life.

Changes in today's healthcare environment are dramatic. We are faced with increased patient acuity, changes in the reimbursement system, increased outpatient services, escalating costs, and a nursing shortage. In this complex environment, health care is in need of effective leadership.

Leadership cannot be reduced to a single theory, characteristic, or behavior. It is an ongoing process that involves interactions between persons and environments. Leadership implies a relationship between at least two people: a leader and a follower. It also includes striving toward some goal. Ideally, the goal should be for the greater good; however, as history has taught us, not all leaders strive for goodness. Some use their power in leadership to guide followers down paths resulting in tragedy.

Management is a distinctly different concept from leadership. Whereas leaders can also be managers, and vice versa, the role and responsibilities of a manager are separate from the role and responsibilities of a leader. Managers often focus on the day-to-day operations for a particular department or unit within an organization. Leaders focus on a more global perspective, creating a vision and a strategic plan.

Leadership, management, and followership are all interwoven and complementary concepts: one cannot exist without the other. Each of us may be called to take on the role of leader, manager, or follower, depending on the situation.

Leadership is not something that is reserved for nurse managers or nurse executives. Anyone can be a leader. The nurse at the bedside can lead by example and work to improve patient care outcomes on a unit. The nurse manager can lead by improving staff morale and working conditions. The nurse executive can lead a department to improved patient care outcomes and patient satisfaction. Leadership is not required by a select few; each of us needs to identify and use our own leadership characteristics and strengths.

The purpose of this discussion on leadership is to reinforce principles of leadership theories and leadership styles and apply those principles to nursing and the healthcare environment. Issues regarding power in leadership are also explored in this chapter. A discussion on the need for increased diversity in health care, particularly in nursing, is included.

Leadership Theories

Many definitions and dimensions of leadership exist in the literature. Leadership is a "focus of group processes" (Bass, 1990, p. 11). Components of leadership include personality, exercising influence, power relationships, and follower compliance. Leadership can be formal or informal; a job title does not guarantee leadership. Leaders are typically viewed as agents of change within an organization, striving to reach an institutional goal. Leadership requires the combination of various skills, appropriately and expertly used in specific situations, and necessi-

tates a relationship between the leader and the followers.

Research on leadership dates back to the 1940s. The focus of the research has encompassed traits, behaviors, styles, situation, and the environment. Current views of leadership combine various elements from the research. A discussion on leadership would not be complete without considering the current thinking on emotional intelligence as a key factor.

Trait Theories

The following section describes the different leadership theories and their characteristics. Classic leadership theories and current approaches are included.

GREAT MAN THEORY

Trait theories are some of the oldest theories on leadership. The great man theory espouses that a person is essentially "born" a great leader, but this theory does not identify a specific set of characteristics. The great man theory uses historical figures as the frame of reference for this type of leader: Moses, Winston Churchill, Lenin, and Thomas Jefferson. Lee Iacocca rescued and revived a failing business; Martin Luther King, Jr., inspired the black civil rights movement; and John F. Kennedy is noted on the list of "great men."

Various business leaders of today are considered "great leaders." Surprisingly, this theory ignores the contributions of great women leaders, such as Joan of Arc, Catherine the Great, and prominent female business executives (Bass, 1990; Northouse, 2004; Yoder-Wise, 2007). Given that this is a more historical perspective, today's leaders, although often compared to great men of the past, are evaluated using more current leadership theories.

TRAIT THEORY

A leader has a certain set of qualities or characteristics that are superior and distinct from followers—this is the premise of the trait theory. This theory is similar to the great man theory in that it asserts that a person is born with the qualities that enable him or her to become a great leader. The leader must use the given talents to inspire others to work toward a common goal. This theory, like the great man theory, omits any relationship between the leader and the follower, or the leader and the situation, and has not been well supported in the research (Bass, 1990; Northouse, 2004; Yoder-Wise, 2007).

SKILLS APPROACH

The skills approach is similar to the trait approach. It focuses on three distinct skills required of leaders: technical skill, human skill, and conceptual skill (Northouse, 2004). Technical skills focus on the leader's competency in a specific type of activity, such as computer skills. Human skill is described as the ability to work with people. This requires the ability to be sensitive to the needs and motivation of others, particularly in decision making. Conceptual skills rely on the ability to have vision, develop a strategic plan, and steer the organization in a positive direction. This approach, or theory, requires the use of three domains of skills, based on the situation at hand, to be an effective leader.

Behavioral Theories

To fully understand behavioral and style theories, a discussion of motivation theories is necessary. Yoder-Wise (2007) provides a brief synopsis of each of these theories and their relationship to practice.

Maslow's hierarchy of needs was first published in the 1940s. This theory asserts that individuals are motivated by satisfaction of various needs, ranging from biological through self-actualization. Higher-order needs cannot motivate individuals until lower-order needs are satisfied. For example, in the work environment, job security must be satisfied before an individual will seek opportunities for job creativity and expanded role responsibilities.

Herzberg's theory separates motivation into two categories, or motivating factors: external and internal. External factors are described as salary, benefits, or working conditions; conditions that are not part of the individual, but part of the organization and organizational climate. Internal motivating factors are described as the desire for personal achievement or recognition for a job well done. To effectively motivate employees, there must be a balance between external and internal factors.

Vroom typically receives credit for both the development and application of the expectancy theory of motivation and its application to leadership. In this model, individual needs influence individual behavior. Positive relationships between effort and job performance reinforce particular behaviors, causing the behaviors to be repeated. These behaviors are further reinforced if rewards are associated with the behavior or outcomes. This cycle of events leads an individual to "expect" or predict that certain behaviors will result in positive outcomes, both in performance and recognition. Therefore, positive behaviors are repeated. Similarities to operant conditioning posited by Skinner are apparent.

STYLE THEORY

Style theory focuses on the behaviors of the leader rather than on personality traits. Style theory divides leader behaviors in two categories: task behaviors and relationship behaviors. Essentially, it looks at what leaders *do* in their interactions with subordinates and how they *interact* with subordinates. Northouse (2004) describes task behaviors as those that help followers achieve their goals; relationship behaviors help followers or subordinates feel comfortable with themselves, each other, and the situation.

Behavioral styles of leaders have been classified as *autocratic, democratic, laissez-faire, and bureaucratic*, each with specific behavioral characteristics. Sullivan and Decker (2005) summarize these styles. Autocratic leaders are typically described as those who make all decisions independently. An autocratic leader views follower participation as motivated by external factors or rewards; followers can be coerced to do what is required by reward or fear of punishment.

A democratic leadership style focuses more on participative decision making and follower cooperation resulting from internal motivating factors. Arriving at decisions collaboratively to achieve a common goal is characteristic of a democratic leader. Transformational leadership has some similarities to a democratic approach.

The laissez-faire leader also operates on the principle that followers have internal sources of motivation that contribute to their participation in the objective of reaching the goal. However, this leader operates by allowing the followers to self-direct and is essentially absent from the process (Humphreys, 2001).

The bureaucratic leader, like the autocratic leader, believes that individuals are motivated by external forces, such as power, punishment, or reward. However, these leaders do not trust personal decision making, by themselves or their followers. Therefore, this type of leader operates strictly "by the book," following institutional policies and rules to guide processes.

The behavioral approach to leadership style evolved to focus on two major dimensions of style: initiating structure and consideration (Sullivan & Decker, 2005). Initiating structure refers to specific managerial responsibilities. Consideration focuses on the relationship between the leader and the followers. If the leader demonstrates concern for the followers and an understanding of their needs while maintaining order and structure, in theory the followers should be more invested in the attainment of the goal (Sullivan & Decker, 2005). For example, a manager is responsible for creating the schedule for unit coverage: initiating structure. However, soliciting input from subordinates about requested days off prior to making the schedule demonstrates consideration. The interaction between these two dimensions is a component of leadership.

Often, the leader will have to employ different styles in different situations. This can be represented in the form of a grid, with behaviors occurring along a continuum (Sullivan & Decker, 2005). Integrating task and relations orientations is the most valuable way to achieve effective leadership (Bass, 1990).

SITUATIONAL-CONTINGENCY THEORIES

Situational-contingency theories are among the most heavily researched and supported theories in leadership. Much of the content of these theories is derived from the works of Hersey-Blanchard, Fiedler, and Vroom. Motivational theory has an influence on each of these proposed models.

Fiedler's contingency model is reportedly the most widely researched model of leadership (Bass, 1990). This model proposes that the leader's behaviors, the task at hand, the relationship between the leader and followers, and the personal power of the leader interact to influence the outcome. The leader's ability to reward followers, which is viewed as power, makes a significant contribution to the interactions and results.

Hersey-Blanchard began working in the late 1960s, expanding on Fiedler's work. Hersey-Blanchard proposed that leadership styles vary between leaders; leaders use either a structured, task-oriented approach, an interpersonal relationship approach, or a combination of both. The maturity of the followers significantly influences their response to the leader's approach (Sullivan & Decker, 2005; Bass, 1990). The best attitude for a leader includes attention to the task and the interpersonal relations aspect. A leader is most effective when the style of leadership matches the demands of the situation (Sullivan & Decker, 2005).

Vroom and Yetton's model of situational leadership also emphasizes the importance of adapting a leadership style to the situation or task at hand. Theirs is a prescriptive model, using a question and answer method and an algorithm approach to identify the most appropriate style for each situation (Sullivan & Decker, 2005).

The path-goal theory also includes components of personal motivation and task performance to determine leadership effectiveness (Sullivan & Decker, 2005). Leaders should be able to motivate followers and remove obstacles to success. Four specific leader behaviors are outlined in the path-goal theory: directive, supportive, participative, and achievement-oriented (Sullivan & Decker, 2005).

In summary, the situational-contingency theories demand that three factors be recognized: trust and respect between leader and followers;

degree and complexity of task structure and clarity of goal; and leader power in terms of the ability to reward followers. Also included in situational-contingency theories are a problem-solving approach, the acknowledgment of the personal characteristics and motivating factors of the followers, and the environmental demands. The leader must realize multiple components of the goal and tasks, set expectations, facilitate goal achievement, and reward followers. In doing so, followers should have increased job satisfaction and increased motivation to continue effective job performance (Yoder-Wise, 2007).

Current Models

Current theories, such as *transformational*, *transactional*, *relational*, *shared*, and *servant leadership*, have commonalities with the previously developed theories. Each of these new theories addresses the relationship between the leader and follower, the leader's ability to reward or punish followers, and the desire to achieve the common goal (Sullivan & Decker, 2005).

TRANSFORMATIONAL LEADERSHIP

Transformational theory is a newer theory that arose in the past decade, yet as noted previously, has similarities to some prior models. This theory developed as organizations were forced to reestablish and reinvent themselves in today's global market (Yoder-Wise, 2007). This model of leadership emphasizes the relationship between the leader and the followers. This leader is concerned with ensuring that both followers and leaders share the vision to change the organization, and that they will work together toward that common goal. Leaders instill a sense of moral compass in the followers, focusing on the greater good rather than individual needs. Leaders in this model also show faith in followers' ability to accomplish goals (Spinelli, 2006; Sullivan & Decker, 2005). Transformational leaders possess charisma; this characteristic draws others to the leader and allows the leader to motivate followers to reach for higher goals (Humphreys, 2001). This model incorporates elements of democratic style, motivation, and great man theories.

TRANSACTIONAL LEADERSHIP

Transactional leadership focuses on the exchange between the leader and the follower. There are two typical approaches in this model: contingent reward and management by exception. In the contingent-reward approach, each reward is contingent, or dependent upon, the follower doing what is expected. If the task, for example, is not completed, the reward is not given. In the management-by-exception approach, the leader adopts a more laissez-faire approach, only choosing to intervene, manage, or lead when followers are not performing up to expectations (Humphreys, 2001).

COMPLEXITY THEORY

Complexity theory is a current model of leadership described by Yoder-Wise (2007) and based on a systems approach and interactions between and among systems. Leaders of today are facing substantially different challenges than they did in years past. To be effective in today's world, leaders need a new set of skills, beyond intelligence, expertise, and charisma.

In nursing, the complex interactions between patients, disease processes, interdisciplinary collaboration, and communication all influence patient outcomes. This is an example of complexity science: each of the different systems both exist on their own and interact with others

to influence the outcome. In this viewpoint, there is less focus on leader control and more focus on collaboration; leaders and followers are regarded more as equals. The role of management is delegated to standardized processes; little attention is given to prescriptive direction.

Five behaviors have been identified to describe how individuals use complexity principles effectively: develop networks; encourage non-hierarchical interactions; become a leadership tag; focus on emergence; and think systematically. A tag is defined as the defining characteristics of an organization: its philosophy, values, or "personality" (Yoder-Wise, 2007, p. 14). In this model, emergence addresses interactions that foster creative problem solving. Principles of systems theory include focusing on the big picture or overarching goal, achieving a balance between short- and long-term goals, and recognizing the continual interactions in nearly all aspects of life, interdependency, and relationships. Systems theory also recognizes the value of data in making decisions and the need to evaluate all aspects of a situation.

Emotional Intelligence

Howard Gardner challenged our nation's experts to reconsider how we measure and view intelligence (Goleman, 1995). In 1983, Gardner proposed that the standard IQ test was merely a measure of one type of intelligence, one that was not necessarily predictive of success. Gardner asserts that there are multiple types of intelligence: verbal, mathematic-logic, spatial, kinesthetic, musical, interpersonal, and intrapsychic.

Daniel Goleman (1998) continued the work of Gardner and applied these principles to leadership, management, and overall success. Goleman describes emotional intelligence and examines how these principles can be effectively used in managing and leading. Using Salovey's definition, emotional intelligence can be broken down into five main domains: knowing one's emotions or self-awareness, managing emotions, motivating oneself, recognizing emotions in others, and handling relationships.

One of the fundamental tasks of leadership is for leaders to develop a positive outlook in those they lead. If followers have a positive outlook and are motivated in a positive direction, the organization as a whole will reap benefits. A successful leader has the ability to cultivate positive energy and dispel negative energy to keep the organization in a forward-moving pattern (Goleman, 2002).

True intelligence is not one single characteristic but is the combination of multiple facets and their interactions. Successful leaders have demonstrated abilities in standard IQ, expertise in a given area, and emotional intelligence. Recognizing each individual's unique gifts and strengths and maximizing that potential are important components of success.

Emotional competence is the ability to use emotional intelligence to facilitate outstanding performance: translating knowledge into action. The ability to understand, communicate, and connect with people, may, in fact, be more predictive of success than merely academic ability. In essence, the interaction between a knowledge base and the ability to connect with others significantly affects success.

Power

In terms of leadership and management, typically power is regarded as the ability to exercise influence over others to achieve goals. In its purest sense, power is used to motivate followers to achieve a common goal; power gets things done. Through the appropriate use of power, major accomplishments can be achieved.

There are two major types of power: position power and personal power. "Position power is determined by the job description, assigned responsibilities, recognition, advancement, authority, the ability to withhold money, and decision making" (Sullivan & Decker, 2005, p. 87). This type of power is legitimate, based on the manager's or leader's position within the organization. Personal power lies with the individual's personal credibility, integrity, expertise, and, sometimes, connections (Sullivan & Decker, 2005).

Interpersonal power is a more in-depth description of position and personal power. There are seven types of interpersonal power, as outlined by Sullivan and Decker (2005). Reward power is based on the leader's ability to grant rewards for follower cooperation toward achieving the set goal. Punishment or coercive power is based on cooperation from followers resulting from the fear of being penalized for noncooperation. Legitimate power is a manager's ability to exercise managerial control, based on the nature of the job title. Those leaders or managers who are experts in a field, through advanced education and experience, have expert power. Leaders who are well respected, well liked, and successful have referent power. Information power is power associated with access to important information that followers desire for personal reasons and for decision making. Connection power is based on the individual's personal connections with influential people within or outside of the organization.

Power is often viewed with gender bias. Women in positions of power are not thought of as favorably as men in positions of power. Typically, women, and particularly nurses, view power as something "ugly" (Yoder-Wise, 2007). Power, when used appropriately, helps people and organizations achieve goals.

In nursing, expert or referent power can be used to help motivate patients and families toward better healthcare practices. Expert or referent power can be used to change a practice care environment to improve patient outcomes. Nurse managers must use position power daily to distribute the workload among the staff, decide on scheduling and vacation time, and conduct personnel evaluations. Management power may be viewed in an unfavorable light by those not in positions of power. Providing that position power is used fairly, the negative feedback should be minimal.

Those not in positions of power may try to usurp the power of others. This usually involves tactics such as undermining, questioning, or challenging the message of the leader or manager. Recognizing these tactics and responding appropriately maintain a sense of order and control. Strong interpersonal skills play an important role in others' perception of those in positions of power.

Nurses are a significantly powerful population subgroup; however, this power is largely untapped. The voices of nurses are often heard quietly in hospitals and healthcare organizations, making small changes. Banded together, those voices could make significant and lasting change. Nursing organizations can use power in numbers to effect change in policy and politics as well as within their organizations. To effect change, nursing as a whole must become more informed and involved and use a collective voice.

Combining power with a mission and vision contributes to the advancement of the organization. Power is the ability to motivate others toward a common goal. To do so, the goal must be clearly identified and stated. Only then can leaders use effective leadership, management, and power to influence the outcome.

Diversity

The 2000 Census Bureau report indicates that the percentage of non-Caucasian residents in the United States is rapidly growing. Nursing must face the challenges of providing comprehensive care to patients of all races, ethnicities, cultures, religions, and languages.

The profession of nursing has always maintained a commitment to providing culturally competent care to patients and families. However, with the increasing diversity in the population, it is nearly impossible to maintain a current understanding of the various cultural responses and views about health and illness. To meet the needs of our increasingly diverse patient population more effectively, it is essential to increase the cultural and ethnic diversity of the nursing workforce.

Access to health care, financial constraints, and compliance with traditional Western medical models are significant barriers for culturally and ethnically diverse patients (Sullivan & Decker, 2005). Additionally, many U.S. residents are non-English-speaking, making it difficult for them to communicate effectively with various members of the healthcare team. In 2000, the National Advisory Council on Nurse Education and Practice noted the importance of increasing diversity in the nursing workforce to better meet the needs of our society.

Currently, the United States Health Resources and Services Administration (HRSA) reports indicate approximately 13% of nurses in the workforce identify themselves as minority.

Gender diversity is also lacking in nursing, with approximately only 5–7% of the workforce being male (Sullivan & Decker, 2005). These numbers are grossly disparate from our population demographics (Otto & Gurney, 2006).

To meet the demands of an increasingly diverse society, nursing must increase the diversity of its workforce. To do so, it is essential that leaders in nursing, particularly leaders from minority groups, seek to increase minority recruitment into the profession. It is important for current nurses from minority backgrounds to develop as leaders to facilitate recruitment efforts.

There are various strategies being implemented to increase recruitment, retention, and success of culturally and ethnically diverse students. Some programs are being developed combining recruitment of underrepresented minority students with intervention programs to facilitate success (Otto & Gurney, 2006). The financial burden associated with higher education may present a significant barrier to entry into nursing for many students. Tuition reimbursement programs through the federal government, healthcare companies, and even hospitals may help ethnic minorities to pursue nursing (Otto & Gurney, 2006).

As the nursing workforce increases in diversity, it is essential that the concern for cultural competence be extended to that workforce. Nursing leaders, managers, and co-workers must develop and implement strategies to foster cultural competence among and between employees. Maintaining open communication between all parties is essential. Leadership must be cognizant of differing cultural and/or religious beliefs and needs related to staffing patterns and general workplace assignments. Promoting a culture of collegiality and teamwork on a unit would foster collaboration among staff and encourage them to work together to best meet the needs of all patients.

It is important to recognize the unique contributions and needs of members of various cultures. Nursing leaders must encourage a culture of tolerance, openness, and respect in the workplace. Following are several methods to promote a culture of tolerance, respect, and collegiality among staff of various cultures, religions, and ethnicities:

- Respect religious observance when determining the staff schedule.
- Respect cultural holidays when determining the staff schedule.
- Make an effort to assign patients with language barriers to nurses that speak the language.
- Highlight the cultural/ethnic differences among staff at a staff meeting or party.

Examples of Leadership in Action

When I was a new staff nurse, my nurse manager demonstrated leadership skills in various ways. First, she led by example, using her clinical expertise to help out on the unit whenever necessary. She would cover patients and send the staff to any available learning opportunity in the hospital. She helped each of us develop management skills by rotating the charge nurse responsibility and demonstrating confidence in the nurse assuming that role. She was always available for support, but avoided micromanaging. She demonstrated leadership by presenting our department's accomplishments at hospital-wide activities. She fostered collaboration between all departments. The relationships and respect among and between all persons was outstanding; every member of the team was considered valuable, from housekeeping to the high-risk specialist. Open communication and respect were expected and delivered. Vision for the department was evident as she pioneered cross-training of staff to new clinical areas to allow each of us to develop more expertise, as well as changing the staffing patterns to better meet the needs of the staff, unit, department, and hospital. It was a remarkable experience working at that hospital with such a terrific leader.

Following are a few hypothetical examples of nursing leadership in action:

- A staff nurse has demonstrated tremendous growth in clinical skills. As a leader, you encourage her to consider pursuing an advanced degree. She indicates her hesitancy to do so, particularly in light of the staffing shortage on the unit. As the nurse manager, using the behavioral model of leadership, working with the staff member to accommodate her schedule demonstrates initiating structure, and encouraging her desire to advance her education demonstrates consideration.
- A clinical issue has been identified on a unit by the staff. Encouraging the staff to investigate the problem begins the process of leadership. Once the staff has had an opportunity to explore the problem and identify possible solutions, another component of leadership includes encouraging staff to disseminate findings to improve patient care on other units. As a leader, you could host a "lunch and learn" to recognize and highlight the staff's accomplishments. Continuing along that theme, the leader could facilitate the delivery of the information to other departments through an in-house conference.

Summary

Health care today demands active leadership. It is important to remember that any one of us is and can be a leader at any time. Leadership is not reserved for those in titled positions. There are various theories and models of leadership. Leadership style develops over time and is influenced by innate personality characteristics as well as a variety of skills. How a combination of skills appropriate to a given situation are executed affects leader success. The importance of interpersonal relationship skills cannot be underestimated.

Many of us face various barriers to effective leadership; time, or lack thereof, is perhaps the most significant. Most days, hospital-based nurses are struggling to get through their shift and provide adequate care to patients and families. There is little time left to focus on the larger picture or issues of leadership. It is essential that each of us take small steps each day toward growing our leadership potential and finding ways to use it in practice.

Every nurse is a leader. The nurse at the bedside is the manager and the coordinator of care for her patients. She is responsible for not only providing a service but leading by example, with caring, commitment, and concern for health and well-being. The nurse is the leader in gathering the other members of the interdisciplinary healthcare team to discuss and plan care for patients to achieve optimal outcomes. Nurses in practice can lead changes in practice by identifying an area for improvement, finding the most current evidence, and seeking to change practice.

For nursing to continue to advance in today's society and today's healthcare environment, we must develop and utilize leaders among us—leaders who can use the collective voice and collective power of nursing to advance the art, science, and caring of our profession. Nursing has a powerful impact on the health and well-being of society. We must use our leadership skills to recognize and use that power to affect the health of our nation positively.

QUESTIONS

1. Transactional leadership focuses on
   a. the exchange between the leader and the follower
   b. how well the follower copes with stress
   c. whether the follower communicates well with the leader
   d. whether the follower can be rewarded for efforts

2. There are two typical approaches in the transactional leadership model. They are
   a. both based upon Lewin's theory of environmental stress
   b. the contingent reward and management by exception
   c. determined by the environment at an agency and by leadership style
   d. the reward and punishment approach and management by reward

3. To meet the needs of our increasingly diverse patient population more effectively, it is essential to
   a. train all personnel to value every cultural group they serve within the hospital
   b. limit hospital services to those persons living within the community
   c. increase the cultural and ethnic diversity of the nursing workforce
   d. screen every patient to determine whether hospital personnel can speak their language

4. Complexity theory is a current model of leadership. A basic tenet of this theory is
   a. interdisciplinary collaboration and communication all influence patient outcomes
   b. that regardless of the patient's health issues, the nurse must focus on curing the disease
   c. that regardless of the disease process, the nurse must focus on treating the complexity of the disease
   d. that leaders, regardless of the complexity of the disease, must deal with the patient and the patient's family

5. Four specific leader behaviors are outlined in the path-goal theory. They are
   a. informative, participatory, supportive, and health care–oriented
   b. providing direction, support, development of goals, and having patient-oriented skills
   c. being goal and task oriented, helpful to novice nurses, and able to guide the way for followers
   d. directive, supportive, participative, and achievement oriented

Activities

1. In consideration of the great man theory, identify a great woman, and explain how and why she would fit the criteria for a "great woman."
2. In consideration of the skills approach to leadership, identify your strengths in a skills area that would help in your role as leader.
3. Describe which type of leadership theory or style you feel you utilize most often.
4. Is there a vision for the future in your work environment? Describe how this is communicated to and shared with employees.
5. Describe the qualities in someone you consider to have great leadership skills. Give an example of how those skills were implemented.
6. As a leader, you want to cultivate leadership skills in your staff. There is an upcoming conference in the hospital on a clinical topic of relevance to your unit. As the director of the department, you go to the nurse manager to encourage staff participation in this important learning opportunity. Although the nurse manager sees the value in this conference, she indicates that staffing the unit will present a problem. Describe how you would use leadership and management skills to address the issues of staffing and facilitate staff participation. Which style and theory of leadership did you apply?

References

Bass, B. (1990). *Bass & Stogdill's handbook of leadership: Theory, research, and managerial applications* (3rd ed.). New York: The Free Press.

Eagly, A., Johannesen-Schmidt, M., & van Engen, M. (2003). Transformational, transactional, and laissez-faire leadership styles: A meta-analysis comparing women and men. *Psychological Bulletin, 129*(4), 569–591.

Goleman, D. (1995). *Emotional intelligence: Why it can matter more than IQ.* New York: Bantam Books.

Goleman, D. (1998). *Working with emotional intelligence.* New York: Bantam Books.

Goleman, D. (2002). *Primal leadership.* Boston: Harvard Business School Press.

Health Resources and Services Administration (HRSA). (2004). The registered nurse population: Findings from the 2004 National sample survey of registered nurses. Retrieved May 28, 2008, from http://bhpr.hrsa.gov/healthworkforce/rnsurvey04/appendixa.htm

Humphreys, J. (2001). Transformational and transactional leader behavior. *Journal of Management Research, 1*(3), 149–159.

Northouse, P. (2004). *Leadership theory and practice* (3rd ed.). London: Sage.

Otto, L., & Gurney, C. (2006). Ethnic diversity in the nurse workforce: A literature review. *Journal of the New York State Nurses Association, 37*(2), 16–21.

Spinelli, R. (2006). The applicability of Bass' model of transformational, transactional and laissez-faire leadership in the hospital administrative environment. *Hospital Topics, 84*(2), 11–18.

Sullivan, E., & Decker, P. (2005). *Effective leadership and management in nursing* (6th ed.). Upper Saddle River, NJ: Prentice Hall.

U.S. Census Bureau. (2000). *Profiles of general demographic characteristics.* Retrieved May 28, 2008, from http://www.census.gov/prod/cen2000/dp1/2kh00.pdf

Yoder-Wise, P. (2007). *Leading and managing in nursing* (4th ed.). St. Louis: Mosby-Elsevier.

Chapter 5

Leadership and Management in Nursing Practice

Veronica Arikian

For the last 150 years, nursing has matured into a discipline that, incorporating concepts from the arts and sciences, has developed its own theoretical foundations for nursing practice. Of critical importance in the evolution of any discipline that serves humankind is the continued growth and perpetuation of new leaders in nursing and managers of nursing practice. What type of leader is most important to nursing in the 21st century? How is an effective manager educated? Is there a difference between a nursing leader and a nursing manager?

Leadership or Management

Nursing as part of contemporary society struggles with the distinction between leadership and management. This is a debate that has been alive and well since the industrial revolution. Contemporary and American history show evidence that scholars disagree as to the difference between leadership and/or managerial qualities when exploring qualities of many executives and political leaders such as and including presidents of the United States. Reviews of the current literature related to general leadership and management reveal that, although there are marked differences, there is a fine line between leadership and managerial behaviors.

Forty years ago, author William James (1958) made an interesting point that may help to explain one difference between leaders and managers. James contends that "once-born" personality types who have had an uneventful flow from birth through adulthood tend to be dutiful conservators and regulators of existing systems, whose rewards come from fulfilling responsibilities. On the other hand, "twice-born" personality types have lives that faced constant hardship and chaos. This latter group, James infers, have experienced a sense of loss and alienation from the larger group and have had to struggle to find a sense of identity in a disharmonious world. For the "once-born" group, extrinsic rewards in the form of acceptance by peers and comfortable conformity to the larger group or organization are preferred, whereas the "twice-born" group's reward often comes in the form of unsettling change, movement, crisis, and integration.

Perhaps then, the contribution to the development of sound leaders and managers are multifactorial: personality traits; situational and environmental influences, including the role of significant others and mentors; and life events may all play a role not just in the ability to lead and/or manage but in the desire to do so. Does this imply that leaders are born and not made? Not at all! However, distinction between "once-born" and "twice-born" personality types underscores our society's fascination with the mystique of leadership. In support of this theme, Abraham Zaleznik (1977), an eminent social psychologist and psychoanalyst, explains that most societies have two conflicting needs: one for managers to maintain the balance of operations, and one for leaders to create new approaches and imagine new areas to explore. Nursing, a profession in great need of expert managers and inspired leaders, struggles with understanding the differences between management and leadership, the development of managers and leaders, the profession's ability to appreciate the finer qualities of each role, and nurturing them.

Minimal Support: Cost to the Nursing Profession

Nursing is learning to support its own leaders and managers, but the overall situation is not tenable. At the same time that nursing is hungry for transformational leaders and highly effective managers to help nurses navigate the choppy waters of our contemporary healthcare environment, we, as a profession, are often critical of the very individuals we should be supporting, mentoring, and educating. The implications for such lack of support of nursing leadership and management among all levels of executives and healthcare workers, including nurses, are quite serious. The outcomes may include lack of motivation and productivity, poor morale and its negative impact on nursing care and patient relations, monetary loss related to absenteeism, job turnover, legal actions resulting from safety errors and lack of nursing judgment, outdated systems leading to poor outcome control, and, on an individual scale, physical, emotional, and mental stressors affecting performance and attitudes toward nursing as a long-term career. Sadly, these issues only serve to deepen the nursing shortage by discouraging potential new leaders and managers from pursuing a much-needed, viable career in nursing.

Nursing Managers:
The Beginning

The managerial role in American industrial circles developed in the 19th century as a response to massive changes in the way products and services were produced. How quickly and effectively workers could produce was studied and outlined by several experts, most notably, Frederick Taylor, the father of scientific management theory. The purpose of this scientific approach to work was to select, train, and monitor workers to maximize their efforts and make industries more profitable. However, in the process, the division between workers and their supervisors became wider and deeper, giving rise to worker dissatisfaction with relentlessly routine jobs that offered little incentive for growth or creativity.

Nurse managers are the first-line managers of nursing staff in most healthcare organizations that render patient care. Many have 24-hour responsibility for the unit, are referred to as head nurses, and charge nurses report back to them. This role grew out of the historical nursing superintendent position prevalent in physician-dominated hospitals of the late 19th and early 20th centuries. Although some superintendents (e.g., Isabel Hampton Robb) did emerge as nursing leaders, especially in the education of new nurses, most focused on day-to-day operations of patient care and supervision of both new and student nurses who actually executed the majority of patient care activities in the hospital setting. Most experienced nurses became educators or superintendents in other settings, worked in public health, or worked directly for families as fee-for-service nurses.

The strength of these early role models of nurse managers was that, in their own circles, they often demonstrated authoritarian patterns of management designed to get the job done, and they set up systems to carry out patient care efficiently. Rules and regulations were strictly enforced, and disciplinary action played a prominent role in the education of the novice nurse. The nursing superintendent was considered the final decision maker in all nursing matters, heavily relied upon by the physicians, and certainly, in addition to her expert (knowledge-based) and reward power (ability to reward good nurses), she also had coercive power (ability to punish poor nurses) and the legitimate power bestowed on her by the physicians in charge (Reverby, 1989).

Because it was no longer possible for one person to oversee the minutiae of all care issues, hierarchies of supervision developed over time with superintendents becoming directors and appointing selected staff to head nurse positions in the expanding healthcare organizations of the 20th century. The weakness of the head nurse role model was that new management was trained in the role to mirror the qualities of the traditional superintendent, with new nursing staff and students often on the receiving end of difficult assignments and long hours with little relief, little support, and even ridicule and punishment. "The rigid hierarchy of the military and familial model reinforced both distance and harsh discipline. . . . As in the military, special uniforms, badges, pins, and caps, as well as elaborate ceremonies to acknowledge or deny advancements, served to reinforce the disciplinary aspect of the hierarchy" (Reverby, 1989, p. 53). It was the exception for head nurses of the early and mid-20th century to receive special education in managerial theory or techniques; therefore, on-the-job training, role modeling, and selection for the role through favoritism, influenced nursing's long tradition of "eating one's young." Unfortunately, some of these characteristics still linger, even in the best nursing environments.

The Nurse Manager Today— What Is Needed Now

It is an old saying that one can't move forward if one doesn't know where one has been. With our short visit to nursing history, we now understand the context within which the nurse manager grew over the last half of the 20th century. During the 1960s, in response to the need for formal instruction in management theory and managerial practices, many baccalaureate programs incorporated management classes and practicum experiences into their curricula. This has been very advantageous during periods of nursing employee shortage, when many baccalaureate graduates are called on to fill managerial roles within a short time after graduation.

Exposure to management principles, however, is not a prerequisite for a nursing management position. In fact, depending on geographical location, local need, and attrition, many nurses are promoted to managerial positions with no more than on-the-job training and sporadic role modeling and mentoring. Today, the educated nurse manager can benefit from several management theories that have been promoted in business circles since the 1940s. Since the 1950s, nursing scholars have used many of these theories to explain, analyze, and observe managerial and leadership behaviors that are most effective in producing positive outcomes.

Management is a unique subset of behaviors that require leadership characteristics. Zaleznik (1977) wrote, "Managers tend to view work as an enabling process involving some combina-

tion of people and ideas interacting to establish strategies and make decisions. Managers help the process along by a range of skills, which include calculating the interests in opposition, staging and timing of controversial issues, and reducing tensions. In this enabling process, managers appear flexible in the use of tactics: they negotiate and bargain, on the one hand, and use rewards and punishments, and other forms of coercion, on the other" (p. 71). Managers, then, are people who are problem-focused, requiring an ongoing balance of power that often results in compromise within a known set of predictable circumstances.

Zerwekh and Claborn (2006) describe management as a problem-oriented process that is linked to the nursing process and that has four functions that can be executed continuously and often simultaneously:

1. Planning what is to be done
2. Organizing how it is to be done
3. Directing who is to do it
4. Controlling when and how it is done

The management style used to perform these functions is also described by Zerwekh and Claborn (2006) as existing on a continuum that ranges from the strictest autocratic method to the most flexible laissez-faire approach. As introduced in the previous chapter, the autocrat leader/manager has an authoritarian manner, makes decisions unilaterally, puts tasks before people, but operates well in crisis situations such as cardiac arrest codes.

The moderate manager offers staff more choices in management decisions so that some are made with staff input. The more democratic the manager, the more input the staff can offer. This manager is people-oriented more than task-oriented and appreciates the power of group dynamics. Good management supports communication rather than being a top-down-driven event. Communication moves both ways, giving staff opportunities to make some decisions, with the most democratic managers offering staff the most encouragement to make informed decisions.

The laissez-faire manager, as described in the previous chapter, creates the most permissive climate and provides little direction, giving staff liberal opportunities to implement major decisions. However, for this to be effective, the manager who uses this style must create an environment and select a staff that are highly independent and motivated.

One current approach to managerial theory and practice incorporates the theories of several management scientists (Clark, 2009). A behavioral science approach to management uses Maslow's hierarchy of needs, Argyris's theory of humanistic and democratic values, McGregor's theory X and theory Y, and Herzberg's motivational theory. Using these combined behavioral methods addresses human needs, group dynamics, communication, and motivation and offers these essential guidelines for effective management. The following approaches apply these combined theories in the workplace:

1. Staff must have basic needs (e.g., physical and safety needs) met before higher-level needs can be satisfied (e.g., creativity, self-development).
2. A sense of belonging to a staff and organization is critical to finding meaning in the job.
3. Staff potential should be developed in an exciting work environment that offers a psychologically safe, logical, and predictable atmosphere.
4. Staff satisfaction with work will foster commitment to the organization, which will produce higher productivity.
5. Staff should be encouraged to accept responsibility and use untapped intellectual potential.
6. An interesting and meaningful job, recognition, and promotions are more important to staff than are monetary rewards.

Today's nurse manager who follows these guidelines must apply them to a myriad of situations and skill sets. Because nurse managers encounter fluctuations in job requirements on a daily basis, multiskilling and constant readjustment to a changing environment are often necessary. These fluctuations and changes may take the form of staff absences, understaffing, high patient acuity, changes in upper management or policy, and alterations in upper management's expectations of middle managers. The well-prepared manager should expect to adapt to these environmental and staff changes, and it is this characteristic, adaptation, that makes the manager effective. Nurse managers must establish work systems on their units, collaborate with other healthcare professionals and workers, coordinate unit activities with the needs of the patients, address communication issues, help to resolve conflicts between staff members and between staff and patients/families, delegate tasks and roles appropriately, counsel employees discreetly and with confidence, invoke policies and standards when necessary, handle mistakes and errors, and strategize short-term solutions to short- and medium-range issues.

Nursing Management: The Attraction

Management is doing things right; leadership is doing the right things.

—Peter Drucker (Cooper, 2008)

The motivation to fulfill the role of a nurse manager may be based on several factors including desire to improve working conditions, commitment to the larger organization, belief that one can do a better job than one's predecessor, drive to enhance one's career path and eventually earn more money, and the challenge of a new role. Bondas (2006) identified four paths to management/leadership roles:

- The path of ideals (where the manager creates the ideal work unit)
- The path of chance (whereby one stumbles upon the manager role by accident)
- The career path (the ladder that leads to more authority and power)
- The temporary path (which occurs when the nurse takes a managerial position but has the option to give it up)

Bondas's research reveals unsettling findings among a group of nurse managers: many nurse managers considered themselves educationally ill prepared to implement organizational, leadership, or economic skills. These findings support the continuing lack of formal nursing management/leadership education, leaving nurses who aspire to managerial positions to acquire these skills in a haphazard manner that is subject to gaps in knowledge and poor role modeling.

Nevertheless, in the face of the dismal paucity of formal managerial education and the lack of psychological preparation for the staff nurse who is promoted to nurse manager (often on the same unit), nurse manager candidates are identified and placed on a course that will likely prove to be exhausting and emotionally challenging. Their longevity in such positions is a testament to the willingness of nurses to adapt to the transition from staff to manager and their resilience in the face of upper management obstacles to unit success in the form of assisting and protecting staff members to whom they often feel a caring obligation.

The Nurse as Leader

> To be able to lead others, a man must be willing to go forward alone.
>
> —Harry Truman (Cooper, 2008)

We have established that there is a fine line between leadership and management, and that line blurs from time to time. There are leaders who are effective managers and managers who emerge as inspirational leaders, and there are many leadership theories to explain leadership behavior and related phenomena. Why is it important to learn about leadership theory? Just as it is so important for nursing to educate and prepare new generations of effective managers, it is critical for nursing to take charge of the development of its future leaders. Bliech (1999) points out that all professional nurses must use leadership-type behaviors when caring for patients. Not every nurse will have the title "nurse manager," but every nurse can fulfill some type of leadership role.

Nurse managers have learned, over time, to acquire impressive organizational and time management skills, many learned on the job. In addition, they have taken on multiple roles in the healthcare system: case manager, coordinator of care, conflict manager, mediator, collaborator, counselor, evaluator, teacher, motivator, team builder, supervisor, and both staff and patient advocate. Managers need a template for practicing management skills, and leaders need a philosophical map to guide their choices of leadership styles.

We can use an aircraft analogy to see an important difference between managers and leaders. The pilot who guides the aircraft is the leader. The pilot does not know the details of what is routinely happening in the cabin of the aircraft but does know the direction in which to guide the aircraft, atmospheric changes that may help or impede progress, and predicted takeoff and landing conditions. The attendants in charge of the cabin are kept informed by the pilot of general progress and any problems that might emerge during the flight that could affect the passengers. The flight attendants also know who needs food, who can't get to the bathroom without help, and who is a minor traveling alone. The attendants work as a team but look to the attendant in charge (the manager) for guidance and help in unforeseen situations.

There are several major theories that are clustered under theory types: traits, style, situational, and transactional/transformational theories. In the following paragraphs, we examine a few of these theories. Many studies on leadership have been conducted in the last 30 years. Barker (1992) points out common themes that have emerged:

- Past leadership theories are not enough to help organizations move through uncertain, rapidly changing times.
- Working people want to have jobs that give them a sense of self-worth and meaning.
- New leadership styles are very much needed for nursing and for other critical areas as well. The most successful organizations are those that have innovators at the top. These leaders are effective because they are aware of how their own behaviors and beliefs about human nature, "about the relationship between leaders and followers, becomes a self-fulfilling prophecy" (Barker, 1992, p. 41).

The great man theory, discussed in Chapter 4, supports the myth that leaders are "born, not made and is probably the basis of Trait Theory." Clark (2009) explains another older theory—trait theory—researched more recently by McCall and Lombardo (1984), which—identifies four critical traits that contribute to leader success:

- *Calmness under pressure.* In a crisis this leader remains calm and in control
- *Admitting mistakes.* All people make mistakes from time to time, this leader does not attempt to hide these mistakes, but rather admits the error and goes forward
- *Ability to persuade others without negative pressure.* This leader attempts to educate others in a positive manner to influence them and acquire their support
- *Having a broad-based expertise rather than a narrow one.* This leader in not insular in their approach to leading others

Other traits of the effective leader include energy, enthusiasm, initiative, keen intelligence, creativity, good health, decisiveness, self-confidence, dependability, and friendliness (Tomey, 2000). Yoder-Wise (1999) also adds these traits: coach, communicator, counselor, boundary setter, flexibility, trustworthiness, motivator, competent, and capable of rapid learning in changing situations. These theories do not specifically address environmental influences, but James's (1958) "twice-born" personality type does takes a step further, acknowledging that situational factors, such as adversity and alienation, play a role in leadership development. Since then, other theories were developed to explain leader behavior.

Likert's (1967) leadership theory identified four decision-making styles. These follow a continuum from high to low control:

HIGH CONTROL

LOW CONTROL

1. authoritarian	2. benevolent
3. consultative	4. participative

1. The exploitative authoritative style is the most aggressive and uses fear and coercion to keep followers under control. Direction is top-down driven, with little consideration given to the individual.
2. The benevolent authoritative style uses a "benevolent dictatorship," where rewards and praise are given, but the approach is paternal, and most decisions are made by the leader.
3. The third leadership style is the consultative leader who also makes most of the decisions, but communication flows from the staff up, and the leader listens to followers' opinions.
4. The participative leader encourages followers' decision-making processes and facilitates effective working relationships. The nature of decisions to be made affects the amount of participation by staff (Clark, 2009).

Another significant theory is situational leadership theory (Hersey & Blanchard, 1999), which addresses relationship, task issues, and maturity level (Tomey, 2000). This theory considers the interactional influences of both leaders and followers. These may take the form of stressors on the group, collective and individual moods of group members, the motivation and knowledge level of the staff, and the organizational environment. The leader who places high emphasis on relationships and task completion may be working with a staff that responds well to a democratic leadership style, whereas the leader who is very task-oriented and puts little emphasis on relationships would utilize an autocratic approach to staff. A laissez-faire leadership style puts less value on both tasks and relationship and takes a "hands-off" approach to staff, allowing employees to construct their own working style and environment.

In general, according to Hersey and Blanchard (1999), staff that are most mature require less structure and more emotional support, and staff that are less mature require more structure and less emotional support. Overall, this theory focuses less on the attributes and more on the skills the leader needs to employ and the situations to which the leader must adapt to deal with the needs of the group. In fact, Johnson determined that leaders should adapt their style to where the followers are in terms of competence and motivation (Clark, 2009).

Other theories emphasize motivations and rewards, such as the path-goal theory (House & Mitchell, 1974) and the leader-member exchange theory (Graen & Uhl-Bien, 1995). The theories that capture the imagination for nursing are the transformational and authentic leadership theories. But do these theories capture the difference between authentic and transformational leadership theories? And how can these theories help the future of nursing?

Transactional and Transformational Leadership

The theory of transactional leadership implies an agreement between the leader and the followers, whereby the leader knows the followers' needs and provides rewards based on adequate performance to meet those needs. This style often fuels competition among followers, focuses on performance tasks, and leans heavily on mutual benefits, contingent rewards, and shorter term operations (Tomey, 2000). Using a transactional leadership style is one way in which the leader can motivate employees to get the job done for the organization.

Transformational and authentic leadership take a different path. Clark (2009) offers three assumptions about transformational leadership:

- People will follow a leader who inspires them.
- A visionary leader must maintain personal integrity, use rituals and ceremonies to mark special occasions, and motivate through organizational culture symbols.
- Infusion of enthusiasm into the staff is critical to getting things done. Nurse leaders offered a list of traits they believed contributed to successful leadership: thoughtfulness, responsiveness, commitment, creativity, resilience, vision, scholarliness, courage, and innovation (Houser & Player, 2004).

Several writers have pointed out that managers follow the rules and leaders often break the rules. Managers as adapters are stable and reliable, whereas innovative leaders stimulate radical change and intellectual inquiry, look for new solutions, and eagerly meet crises with energy and stamina. At the same time, innovative leaders are sensitive to what inspires others, use optimism as a powerful motivator, encourage the creativity and learning of followers, and make their vision real and meaningful for their constituents (Clark, 2009; Tomey, 2000). The environment these leaders create is stimulating, change-oriented, supportive of ideas, and highly communicative.

Authentic Leadership

Authentic leadership is closely related to transformational leadership, and these leaders are characterized as having definite purpose, known values, "heart," positive relationships, self-discipline, and credibility (Clark, 2009; Kouzes & Posner, 2003; Shirey, 2006). Authentic leaders foster close relationships with their followers; it is a bond based on trust, not rules. These leaders role-model "heart" to their followers: fearlessness, a sense of hope, and belief in self. They know that followers who believe in themselves will be more confident and productive and that if they are encouraged often, they will grow. Authentic leaders are psychologically engaged with their followers; they coach and educate their followers, encouraging continual self-improvement. These leaders made it a point to publicly reward and compliment their followers, essentially giving meaning to work.

Kouzes and Posner (2003) give specific examples of how effective authentic leadership is executed:

- Authentic leaders set clear standards; they know that if goals are real, make sense, and are attainable with hard work, followers will commit to them, putting their values into action.
- Authentic leaders expect the best, but not in a vacuum. They are artists in that they create a vision for every follower so that each one has a goal to work toward and can exert his or her best efforts.
- Physical presence is critical; authentic leaders pay close attention to their followers, providing them with ongoing feedback, keeping them on goal. However, this attention is not negatively focused but looks for what is positive in performance.
- Personal recognition is effectively used by authentic leaders, modeling a thoughtful environment that sets the tone for the workplace.

- Authentic leaders are master communicators. One of the most effective methods of communication is storytelling. The leader tells a compelling story of what has happened, what is happening, and what will happen, further motivating and moving followers.
- Celebrating together is another way the authentic leader builds the work community. Celebration fosters commitment and happiness; followers like being in that workplace and are more likely to remain and work more energetically.
- The authentic leader sets an example and is credible—they do what they want and expect their followers to do. There is no room for empty platitudes and promises; the authentic leader delivers and expects others to do the same.

Role modeling is critical to successful authentic leadership; such leaders use self-discipline to care for themselves, and they model these behaviors to their followers. These leaders are aware that burned-out, mentally and physically exhausted people will become pessimistic, cynical, depressed, and ultimately, ineffective. Self-care is not selfish, it is vital; self-care takes the form of individual pursuits, such as meditation, vacations, hobbies, and group events such as dinners, parties, and reward celebrations.

Finally, transformational, authentic leaders are agents of change. Zaleznik (1990) characterizes effective leaders as "being able to overcome the conflict between order and chaos with an authority legitimized by personal magnetism and a commitment to their own undertakings and destinies" (p. 16). Change agents who are effective leaders do not leave their followers scratching their heads, worrying about what's coming next. Instead, these leaders inspire oth-

ers to manage the uncertain with a level of trust, to seek creative solutions in an intellectually empowering environment, and to "keep their eyes on the prize (the goal)," while managing the day-to-day tasks of the work during unstable times. The leader who communicates confidence and caring during difficult times generates a high level of trust and loyalty among people who will work even harder toward the vision.

Clark (2009) reports that, in 2005, the American Association of Critical Care Nurses (AACN) stated that healthy work environments should be safe, healing, humane, and respectful for nurses, patients, and their families. In addition, both the American Organization of Nurse Executives (AONE) and the American Nurses Association recognize the importance of leader-supported healthy work environments. The AONE 2002 study of 21 hospitals produced exemplars for best practices; leadership development and effectiveness were found to be critical success factors.

The American Nurses Credentialing Center's Magnet Hospital Program, started in 1983, also recognized the need to reward positive work environments. This highly competitive program recognizes those organizations employing nurses that meet criteria for nursing excellence. These are desirable working environments that attract and retain expert and highly professional, caring nurses. "The full expression of the Forces (of magnetism) embodies a professional environment guided by a strong visionary nursing leader who advocates and supports development and excellence in nursing practice. As a natural outcome of this, the program elevates the reputation and standards of the nursing profession" (American Nurses Credentialing Center, 2008). These magnet hospitals offer beacons of light; their leaders have inspired their staff to the highest levels of nursing excellence. In our current, uncertain, rapidly changing healthcare environment, it is important for all nursing leaders and managers to continue learning leadership skills from the exemplars in our nursing community, and for the best leaders to teach and mentor all of us so that we may, in turn, teach the best leadership behaviors to the next generation of nursing leaders.

Summary

This chapter reviews how we develop roles of leadership and identifies qualities of good leadership. The content in the chapter discusses the differences and similarities of nurse managers and leaders. The chapter furthermore explores transactional and transformational leadership theories and role and style of authentic leaders.

QUESTIONS

1. Nurse managers each day encounter many changes in their job requirements. One skill that helps the nurse manager success is
   a. the ability to master many skill sets
   b. an autocratic management style
   c. frequent change of staffing
   d. a changing environment

2. The well-prepared manager should expect to adapt to
   a. support from the organization
   b. environmental and staff changes
   c. the monotony of the job
   d. successful interactions with staff

3. Authentic leadership is characterized as
   a. being educationally prepared at the master's level
   b. remaining aloof and distant from followers
   c. fostering close relationships with followers based on trust, not rules
   d. demanding high standards from followers

4. The nurse who is an authentic leader knows that
   a. followers who believe in themselves are more productive
   b. followers who believe in themselves are more confident
   c. it is important to coach and educate followers
   d. All of the above

5. The great man theory supports the following:
   a. All leaders are educated to lead.
   b. Leaders are "born, not made."
   c. Leaders must have a master's degree.
   d. All men are leaders.

References

American Nurses Credentialing Center. (2008). Program overview. Retrieved October 17, 2008, from http://www.nursecredentialing.org/Magnet/ProgramOverview.aspx

Barker, A. M. (1992). *Transformational nursing leadership.* New York: NLN Press.

Bliech, M. R. (1999). Managing and leading. In P. S. Yoder-Wise (Ed.), *Leading and managing in nursing* (pp. 2–20). St. Louis: Mosby.

Bondas, T. (2006). Paths to nursing leadership. *Journal of Nursing Management, 14*(5), 332–339.

Bullough, B., & Bullough, V. (1972). *The emergence of modern nursing.* New York: Macmillan.

Cesarina, T., & Wagner, L. (2007). Change agent. In K. A. Polifko (Ed.), *Concepts of the nursing profession* (pp. 266–278). Clifton Park, NY: Thomson Delmar.

Clark, C. C. (2009). *Creative nursing leadership and management.* Sudbury, MA: Jones and Bartlett.

Cooper, S. (2008). Our top 25 leadership quotations. *Slideshare.* Retrieved November 21, 2008, from http://www.slideshare.net/simoncooper/leadership-quotations-presentation/

Diamonte, T., & Giglio, L. A. (1992). The durability factor: A systems approach to managerial endurance. *Leadership and Organization Development Journal, 13*(4), 14–19.

Ellis, J. R., & Hartley, C. L. (2005). *Managing and coordinating nursing care* (5th ed.). Philadelphia: Lippincott Williams & Wilkins.

Gordon, S. (1991). *Prisoners of men's dreams.* Boston: Little, Brown.

Graen, G. B., & Uhl-Bien, M. (1995). Relationship-based approach to leadership: Development of leader-member exchange (LMX) theory of leadership over 25 years: Applying a multilevel multi-domain perspective. *Leadership Quarterly, 6*(2), 219–247.

Hersey, P., & Blanchard, K. H. (1999). *Leadership and the one minute manager.* New York: William Morrow.

Hersey, P., Blanchard, K. H., & Johnson, D. E. (2008). *Management of organizational behavior: Leading human resources* (9th ed.). Upper Saddle River, NJ: Prentice Hall.

House, R. J., & Mitchell, T. R. (1974, Fall). Path-goal theory of leadership. *Contemporary Business, 3,* 81–98.

Houser, B. P., & Player, K. N. (2004). *Pivotal moments in nursing: Leaders who changed the path of a profession.* Indianapolis, IN: Sigma Theta Tau International.

James, W. (1958). *Varieties of religious experience.* New York: Mentor Books.

Kirkpatrick, S. A., & Locke, E. A. (1991). Leadership: Do traits matter? *Academy of Management Executive, 5*(2), 48–60.

Kouzes, J. M., & Posner, B. Z. (2003). *Encouraging the heart: A leader's guide to rewarding and recognizing others.* San Francisco: Jossey-Bass.

Likert, R. (1967). *The human organization: Its management and value.* New York: McGraw-Hill.

McCall, M. W., & Lombardo, M. M. (1984). *Off the track: Why and how successful executives get derailed.* Greensboro, NC: Center for Creative Leadership.

Muff, J. (Ed.). (1982). *Women's issues in nursing: Socialization, sexism, and stereotyping.* Prospect Heights, IL: Waveland Press.

Nelson, S., & Gordon, S. (2006). *The complexities of care.* Ithaca, NY: ILR Press.

Polifko, K. A. (2007). *Concepts of the nursing profession.* Clifton Park, NY: Thomson Delmar.

Reverby, S. M. (1989). *Ordered to care.* New York: Cambridge University Press.

Shirey, M. R., (2006). Authentic leaders creating healthy work environments for nursing practice. *American Journal of Critical Care, 15*(3), 256–267.

Steers, R. M., & Porter, L. W. (1991). *Motivation and work behavior.* New York: McGraw-Hill.

Tomey, A. M. (2000). *Guide to nursing management and leadership.* St. Louis: Mosby.

Yoder-Wise, P. S. (1999). *Leading and managing in nursing.* St. Louis: Mosby.

Yukl, G. (1989). *Leadership in organizations.* Englewood Cliffs, NJ: Prentice Hall.

Zaleznik, A. (1977). Managers and leaders: Are they different? *Harvard Business Review, 55*(5), 67–78.

Zaleznik, A. (1990). The leadership gap. *Academy of Management Executives, 4*(1), 8–22.

Zerwekh, J., & Claborn, J. C. (2006). *Nursing today* (5th ed.). St. Louis: Saunders Elsevier.

Chapter 6

Professional Organizations, Quality Care Standards, and Ethics

Marilyn Klainberg

OUTLINE

Professional Organizations

Any organization is a group of people who join together and have shared interests, a mission, or similar goals. A professional organization is an association whose members also have common goals or interests; however, there are additional benefits to membership in a professional organization. A professional organization provides professional standards of practice, guidelines for ethical or legal behaviors, and a professional code of conduct. Some professional organizations also act as a credentialing agency.

Professional organizations serve their membership on many levels. Their goal is to ensure that the profession provides society a high quality of service. Professional organizations exist in most professions to judge their members as professionally competent. Therefore, professional organizations serve an important purpose not only for the profession itself, but also for the general community. They set standards and provide mentorship and networking for their members. They also provide services such as continuing educational opportunities and leadership to members. Other services, such as newsletters with updates on both professional and political issues, insurance programs, advocacy programs, and resources for information are offered to their members.

Professional organizations furthermore serve society by advocating and lobbying for the highest quality of professional and ethical standards to benefit the public. A recent issue for which professional organizations have lobbied is against mandated overtime. Many professional organizations have political action committees (PACs) dedicated to dealing with issues such as mandated overtime. PACs represent professional organizations at each level of government.

Each organization has its own structure and culture, which are the framework for its work and mission. Organizational culture is an example of the norms and values of the membership. Members vote to elect leadership and policies that are reflected in the mission and goals of the organization. Each organization has a philosophy, mission statement, and goals and objectives. Of course, the culture of an organization is not stagnant but vibrant and alive. Therefore, mission, structure, and culture, which are based upon the needs of the greater society and the impact on the membership, may be affected as norms and values within a society change. So, organizations, then, are fluid and change with the needs of their members. Active membership in the organizations that represent our profession is extremely important.

Nursing has many active nursing organizations that represent different specialties of the profession, such as the Association of Women's Health, Obstetric and Neonatal Nurses (AWHONN), and some that represent specific ethnic groups, such as the Black Nurses Association, the Philippine Nurses Association, and the National Hispanic Nurses Association. Some of the specialty organizations such as the Oncology Nurses Society offer certification examinations for their membership.

Some organizations, such as the American Nurses Association (ANA) and the International Council of Nurses (ICN), are generalist organizations representing registered professional nurses. Many include subgroups that represent specialty groups and state and district organizations. These often set standards for professional behaviors and provide and support research. Professional organizations serve and protect the community in maintaining standards of care, providing information that protects patient safety, and representing and protecting the membership.

Many state organizations have subgroups that assist their membership by providing continuing education, professional development, and support services. An example is the New York State Nurses Association (NYSNA) Statewide Peer Assistance for Nurses program (SPAN). SPAN is a resource for nurses in New York State who are coping with chemical dependency (alcoholism and/or drug addiction). SPAN works with nurses, provides them with support and rehabilitation services, and represents impaired nurses with the State Education Department through the Office of Professional Assistance Program and the Office of Professional Discipline. Many other states offer similar services for nurses.

Nursing Organizations

Membership in a professional nursing organization is essential to the strength of the nursing profession. Membership not only supports the profession of nursing, but it creates a stronger profession by banding nurses together, giving them a more powerful voice in guiding the direction of the profession.

American Nurses Association

The ANA is a national organization whose main purpose is to address issues related to licensure, collective bargaining, and political concerns. An important role of the ANA is to provide standards for the nursing profession. The ANA also publishes the *Nursing Code of Ethics with Interpretive Statements*, which is based upon the International Council of Nurses' Code for Nurses (Hook & White, 2003). Founded in 1899, the International Council of Nurses (ICN) is an international organization made up of 120 international nursing organizations and is dedicated to uniting all nursing organizations (International Council of Nurses [ICN], 2000).

The ANA is represented in each state by the state and district organizations, such as the New York State Nurses Association (NYSNA) and the ANA-California Nurses Association (ANA-CNA). There was a fracture in the support of the California Nurse Association (CNA), and they voted to secede from the ANA. However, sufficient members wanted to be represented by ANA and formed the ANA-CNA.

National League of Nursing

Headquartered in New York City, the National League for Nursing (NLN) was founded in 1893 with a goal of promoting excellence in nursing education (National League for Nursing [NLN], 2007). The NLN was the first nursing organization and was originally called the American Society of Superintendents of Training Schools for Nurses (NLN, 2007). Its membership includes nurse educators, schools of nursing, and healthcare agencies. You can be a member through your agency or as an individual. It is presently an accrediting agency primarily for 2-year nursing education programs. The NLN is committed to providing educational services that provide quality education programs for all nurses. The NLN and the ANA work collaboratively with each other. ANA is the official voice of nursing, and the NLN functions to support and unite interests of nursing. It provides professional development through educational programs, continuing education, meetings, and workshops.

American Association of Colleges of Nursing

The American Association of Colleges of Nursing (AACN) is a national organization that accredits baccalaureate and higher education nursing programs through the American Nurses Credentialing Center (ANCC). It also provides credentialing for specialization in areas or expertise (American Association of Colleges of

Nursing [AACN], 2004). Nurses wishing to become certified in an area and who provide evidence of meeting requirements of education may sit for a national examination.

AACN also provides it members with educational programs that support research and data collection. It provides support to deans, directors, and associate deans through meetings and publications and ultimately students (AACN, 2004).

Sigma Theta Tau International

Sigma Theta Tau, the national honor society for nursing, is an international nursing organization. Unlike other nursing organizations, members of Sigma Theta Tau must be nominated and then may be accepted for membership by demonstrating that they meet the membership criteria developed by the organization. Sigma Theta Tau is a nonpolitical organization that promotes scholarship and research.

The National Organization of Nurse Practitioner Faculties

Since 1974, the National Organization of Nurse Practitioner Faculties (NONPF) has been an organization specifically for nurse practitioners (NPs) at the national and international levels. Its mission is to develop NP curriculum guidelines, and it is the leading organization for NP faculty (National Organization of Nurse Practitioner Faculties [NONPF], 2008).

International Council of Nurses

The International Council of Nurses (ICN) is an international organization that provides a code of ethics and standards for nursing practice throughout the world. Additionally, the ICN supports international research standards and policies for nursing practice (ICN, 2000).

Association of Women's Health, Obstetric and Neonatal Nurses

The Association of Women's Health, Obstetric and Neonatal Nurses (AWHONN) is a nursing organization that addresses issues related to the health care of women and newborns through advocacy, research, publications, and the creation of high-quality, evidence-based standards of care (AWOHNN, 2008).

Hospice and Palliative Nurses Association

Established in 1987, the Hospice and Palliative Nurses Association (HPNA) is an organization for nurses who provide care for patients in a hospice setting and provide palliative care. HPNA is a nationally recognized organization for nurses working at various levels of nursing care (HPNA, n.d.).

National Student Nurses Association

The National Student Nurses Association (NSNA) is a professional organization for students. NSNA membership begins at the student level. Although a fully independent organization, it works closely with the American Nurses Association. Each state has its own state professional organization that is related to the NSNA (NSNA, n.d.b). NSNA offers workshops, national meetings, networking, educational services such as NCLEX–RN review sessions, and has its own student Bill of Rights (NSNA, n.d.a).

The National Student Nurses Association (NSNA) is an organization geared for undergraduate nursing students. The NSNA mentors future nurses and provides leadership opportunities and career guidance. Many schools of nursing have their own student nursing organizations that address day-to-day activities for the individual student nurses in their program, but membership in the National Student Nurses Association (NSNA) provides a unique focus for student nurses.

The Work of Professional Nursing Associations and Organizations

Organizations such as the American Association of Colleges of Nursing (AACN), the ANA, the NLN, and the NONPF are simply a few of the professional organizations available to nurses. There are specialty groups such as the American Association of Critical Care Nurses. The mission of many of these organizations includes the following:

- Maintaining professional standards and ethical issues
- Providing testing for credentialing
- Dealing with current issues while maintaining tradition
- Lobbying to improve the health of society
- Political involvement, such as through political action committees (PACs)
- Collective bargaining
- Networking
- Promoting a safe and healthy workplace

To fulfill the mission of a political action committee (PAC) or a lobbying group, the professional organization must be strong and represent large numbers of members. Therefore, supporting your professional organization as a member is important. Support will bring you the power of numbers, because an organization with a large membership represents many and has a greater voice. This is particularly true when attempting to make legal or political

impact. Legislators intend to represent their constituents, and the larger the number of constituents, the greater the impact they can have on their legislators.

Professional organizations that represent specific clinical interest groups are important for the following reasons:

- They maintain professional standards.
- They deal with current issues while maintaining tradition.
- They improve the health of society.
- They provide networking opportunities.

The dilemma of having so many organizations is that membership has become fragmented and the ability to be a strong lobbying organization often becomes diluted.

Unions and Nursing

Collective bargaining is an important method of negotiation and is part of the mission of many nursing organizations, particularly the ANA. It is a process of negotiation that is regulated by state and federal labor laws under the National Labor Relations Act (NLRA). The NLRA was first established in the 1930s to protect the rights of workers to organize and engage in collective bargaining. The notion of unionization became strong in the United States in the late 1930s, following the Depression and as part of the National Industrial Recovery Act. Nationally, this meant that child labor laws, minimum wages, and a 40-hour workweek were established for all American workers.

However, although the idea of unionizing professional nursing is not new, it remains controversial for some. Because nursing is a profession, some nurses are not comfortable with unionization and collective bargaining. However, medicine has become more of a business as a result of the impact of health insurance, and in turn the role of nurses has grown and needs to be represented in collective bargaining.

The ANA was a leader in helping its state affiliates to organize collective bargaining units. Although not all states participate in this, and neither do all hospitals, it has changed how nurses' roles are represented. Today, other unions have begun to represent nurses as well. If you work in a hospital that is represented by any collective bargaining unit, it is important for you to become familiar with what is in your contract, issues such as who is represented by the union, how the union represents you, and who to contact with concerns.

Quality of Care and Standards of Care

Issues related to the provision and quality of patient care are most important to healthcare providers and have driven the methods upon which patient care is assessed. The need to give safe, appropriate care in facilities in which nurses work is a commitment and a goal toward providing excellent patient care. The following section explores how the quality of care is assessed, as well as the measurement of the standards of care.

Providing Safe Patient Care: Standards of Care

Quality of care refers to the suitability and safety of the care provided to patients. How we evaluate or view quality of care is influenced by issues related to whether care is offered in a timely, efficient, and effective manner. In addition, the perception of patient satisfaction with the care they receive must be factored into how we measure quality of care.

Issues of safety are particularly of concern, and many feel that safety issues are related to the nursing shortage. Nurses' work must be dedicated to patient safety, and whether this occurs is indicated by how the institution responds to quality issues, which include adequate staffing, equipment, and training, as well as appropriate hospital policies. Issues of concern are related to and aimed at the prevention of errors in care, such as medication errors; prevention of patient falls; fragmented care; care coordination and teamwork; infection control and prevention; care of the frail (particularly the elderly); and specialty areas such as operating rooms and emergency departments (Finkelman & Kenner, 2007). Another issue of concern relates to the impact of technology on health care, particularly medical informatics. Until recently, the concept of providing quality care revolved around identification of errors in care but has shifted and moved from quality assurance to the improvement of the provision of health care.

Why Move from Quality Assurance?

The concept of managing and maintaining quality and excellence in health care so as to provide safe and efficient patient care is not new. Healthcare providers have for a long time attempted to impart excellence in the delivery of health care. Until recently, the system of doing this was quality assurance (QA). QA is a method of evaluating healthcare agencies and systems using identified and recognized standards of care. This process was established to detect errors and inefficient behaviors in the provision of health care. The methodology of QA includes the evaluation of chart audits, the review of incident reports, and observations made within healthcare facilities. The goal is to identify areas in need of change.

However, the notion that we could ensure quality health care by using these methods was difficult to accomplish. QA agencies could not fulfill the promise of ensuring quality, because QA provides only a method of inspection and identification of problems, but not improvement. QA focuses on identifying problems in performance and outcomes. It assesses whether a care standard has been adhered to or not. QA offers no direction for what to do about an existing problem. Because it is an externally initiated and driven process, QA tends to provide reactive rather than proactive changes to a system. QA often marginalizes accountability for quality because it is more of a "watchdog" rather than a tool to use to collaborate to find solutions and provide quality care. Because QA reviews are periodic inspections scheduled for a specific time, staff and agencies could work toward preparing for a QA visit, and then afterward slip back to old routines of care.

In 1996, the Institute of Medicine (IOM) of the National Academies began to focus on assessing and improving the nation's quality of care. In 1998, the first phase of its quality initiative began with a report that dealt with quality cancer care (IOM, 2008). In subsequent studies, the IOM intended to improve all areas of health care and during 1999–2001 produced two papers addressing the issue of quality of health care titled, "To Err Is Human: Building a Safer Health System" and "Crossing the Quality Chasm: A New Health System for the 21st Century" (Finkelman & Kenner, 2007). These reports became the impetus for the healthcare system to turn to Continuous Quality Improvement (CQI) as a method of assessment of healthcare agencies.

CQI, also referred to as Total Quality Management (TQM), provides a greater span than QA does because it evaluates performance and outcomes continuously, which is a more encompassing and realistic approach to providing and implementing quality care. CQI incorporates QA but brings it to a higher level. CQI is more proactive in the identification of actual or potential problems as well as promoting a plan for solutions that are the bases for improvement of care. It operates within a framework of system thinking, is internally driven, and takes into account interactions and interrelationships among all components of a system. Therefore, CQI is not the responsibility of one discipline or department but accepts input from all and shares accountability. It is proactive, part of daily operations, and focuses on improvement.

CQI or TQM includes activities and the process of quality assurance, and then goes beyond QA to include programs geared at improving the quality of care and prevention.

Does It Work?

Whether CQI improves an organization's productivity and viability is not yet clear, because many assessments of CQI are mostly anecdotal evidence. However, it is believed that the movement toward CQI is an improvement from the QA system of evaluation.

Organizations That Monitor and Improve the Quality of Health Care

The Joint Commission

Since 1951, the Joint Commission (TJC)—formerly known as the Joint Commission on Accreditation of Healthcare Organizations (JCAHO)—has been the most important evaluating agency that accredits most healthcare organizations and programs in the United States.

It monitors standards for healthcare organizations and accredits healthcare agencies. The Joint Commission is a not-for-profit voluntary organization established to monitor and evaluate healthcare agencies. It requires agencies to conduct a root cause analysis of events defined as errors that result in physical injury, a psychological event, or death. Root cause analysis is designed to search for the basic or unique cause of an event to prevent future occurrences. TJC also evaluates organizations' compliance with standards and other accreditation or certification requirements that focus on improving the quality and safety of care. The Joint Commission examines policies and procedures as well as outcomes of care.

The Agency for Healthcare Research and Quality

The Agency for Healthcare Research and Quality (AHRQ) funds research for issues related to quality care, medication error prevention and reduction, and policies that promote safe patient care.

The Community Health Accreditation Program

The Community Health Accreditation Program (CHAP), a not-for-profit agency, was established to provide accreditation for community health and home care agencies.

National Committee for Quality Assurance

The National Committee for Quality Assurance (NCQA) is a not-for-profit agency that evaluates health maintenance organizations (HMOs). It established the Health Plan Employer Data Information Set (HEDIS). The data obtained from HEDIS allow employers and consumers to compare HMOs. The goal of NCQA is to establish information related to outcomes and prevention.

Ethics and Professional Behavior

Ethics is a branch of philosophy. Ethics includes moral reasoning or moral principles of conduct. Defining ethics is complex because ethics are intensely personal and often a reflection of people's culture or the rules or guidelines of a society. Moral principles are the basic standards for what we consider right or wrong.

In their goal to provide safe care, restore health, ease pain and discomfort, promote well-being, and prevent illness, nurses must be aware of ethical issues that affect the care they provide their patients.

The following list defines some basic terminology used in the discussion of ethics:

- *Autonomy.* Independence or self-determination
- *Beneficence.* The obligation to do good
- *Nonmaleficence.* To avoid harm
- *Confidentiality.* An obligation to uphold a patient's privacy and maintain information in confidence
- *Justice.* Treating people equally and fairly
- *Distributive.* Fairest distribution according to need
- *Egalitarian.* Equality in access
- *Utilitarian.* Giving first to who needs it most

The Nursing Code of Ethics

A code of ethics is a text that provides the guiding principles for a profession. A code of ethics is how a profession regulates itself. It is a written document intended to be used by the pro-

---

Box 6-1 Personal Message from a Contemporary Nurse Leader

Marilyn H. Oermann

Dear Students:

You could not have made a better career choice. You have heard in many of your courses how nurses make a difference in health care, and that message is true. Did you know that the public considers nursing to be the profession with the highest ethical standards and the most honest of all the professions (Gallup, Inc., 2008)? In study after study, patients indicate consistently that nurses are key to quality patient care. You will find nursing to be a rewarding profession and one with much flexibility in terms of career path and work schedule. With a nursing degree, you can provide direct patient care; gain specialized preparation for roles as a nurse anesthetist, midwife, nurse practitioner, and clinical specialist; be a manager or an administrator at various levels of an organization; teach patients, staff, and students; and move into many other healthcare roles. What other career path lets you work on a weekend as a full-time job or schedule your work around school and family?

I did not always want to be a nurse, but my strengths in science led me to a nursing career. I received my BSN from Pennsylvania State University and was in one of that university's first nursing classes. It is hard to believe, but in 1967 when I went to the main campus of Penn State, there were few women on campus. After graduating, I practiced and taught in the nursing program at Reading Hospital (Reading, Pennsylvania). It was then that I realized my interest in establishing a career path in nursing education. One of the keys to developing a career is thinking ahead of what you want to be doing in five and ten years from the present and preparing yourself strategically for that role. A career in nursing education requires advanced education, and for this reason my next step was to obtain a master's degree in nursing education from the University of Pittsburgh (Pittsburgh, Pennsylvania). You need to carefully select your educational programs, because in many areas of nursing the program you attend will determine the positions to which you can apply. Choose carefully with your 5- and 10-year goals in mind. After completing my master's degree, I immediately began a PhD program, which I finished five years later, after attending both my master's and doctoral programs as a full-time student.

I then needed experience as a nurse educator. During my graduate program, I taught part time at St. Margaret Memorial Hospital School of Nursing (Pittsburgh, Pennsylvania) and at the University of Pittsburgh, gaining skills in clinical teaching. I realized the importance of finding a mentor with whom I could work to develop my career as a faculty member. I decided to take an assistant professor position at Wayne State University (Detroit, Michigan) because of the opportunity to work with Dorothy E. Reilly, who was one of the leading nurse educators at the time. I learned early on the importance of looking ahead and knowing what defines success in the role of nurse educator. In an academic setting, success is measured by teaching effectiveness, research and scholarly productivity, and contributions to the school, university, and nursing profession. By identifying my 5- and 10-year career goals and knowing what qualities defined success, I focused on those, was promoted from an assistant to an associate to a full professor, and served in many different faculty and administrative positions.

I spent the majority of my career at Wayne State and began writing about clinical teaching, evaluating student learning and performance, and other nursing education topics. From that early time to the present, I have authored or co-authored 11 books and more than 180 articles and chapters about nursing education and other topics in nursing. A few years ago, I began a new position as professor and chair of Adult and Geriatric Health in the School of Nursing at the University of North Carolina at Chapel Hill. In this new position, I work closely with faculty on their career development, rather than on my own.

As you develop your career in nursing, be clear about where you want to be in five and ten years, learn what defines success in that type of nursing role, and do what it takes to be successful. *You* are in charge of your career, and *you* need to plan for it.

Sincerely,

Marilyn H. Oermann, PhD, RN, FAAN, ANEF
Professor and Chair, Adult and Geriatric Health Division
School of Nursing
University of North Carolina at Chapel Hill, Chapel Hill, NC
Editor, *Journal of Nursing Care Quality*, www.jncqjournal.com

fessional and the public as a guide to how the profession functions and as a regulatory plan for the profession's membership.

In the provision or delivery of health care, nurses, not unlike other healthcare providers, are often involved in ethical issues. Many of these ethical dilemmas may deal with unclear areas of logic or gray areas related to your own or your patient's beliefs. The nurse and other healthcare providers can be very clear about their own ethical and moral beliefs related to a situation, but these may be in conflict with the situation or the personal beliefs of the patient.

To deal with ethical or moral dilemmas, it is important to become aware of your own values. This is known as values clarification. Knowing your values is an essential part of making an ethical decision. What we value is dependent on many external influences: our environment, family influences, culture, education, time, and place of residence. Our values can change over time, and as healthcare professionals we can learn to accept other people's right to be guided by their own values in ethical and moral decisions.

Moral principles guide your action in a moral dilemma. They are influenced by many factors, such as society, family, and environmental needs. They deal with principles like autonomy and justice. Moral decision making is a social process that involves reflection upon your moral perspective. It requires the ability to practice moral reasoning. Moral reasoning initially includes the ability to be aware that an ethical situation exists. It requires an ability to reflect on ethical decisions and organize the details of a situation based upon an ethical perspective to develop a moral point of view and the ability to articulate and explain this point of view. Some, such as Dr. Carol Gilligan, believe that moral reasoning is influenced by gender and should be taken into account (Huff, 1998). Gilligan's work has found that men and women use different approaches to moral reasoning. According to Gilligan, the male approach is justice related and leans toward individual rights and the respect of those rights. Women's approach is that people are responsible for others and is responsibility oriented (Cypher, n.d.).

Professional vs. Personal Ethical Behaviors

Professional ethical reasoning and decision making are dependent on many things. Our personal moral values, culture, traditions, and religion affect our decision making and are the root of moral values. Many of our ethical behaviors and decisions are based on our personal value systems and religious influences, but these are additionally affected by our professional moral guidelines. Some feel gender may also affect moral reasoning and values.

Moral choices are also influenced by society and environment. Therefore, the professional environment plays an important part in how we implement our professional ethical decisions. The *Code of Ethics* of the American Nurses Association sets the standard for the nursing profession.

Whistle-Blowing: Is It Ethical, or Not? That Is the Question

Whistle-blowing is a term that refers to a situation in which a member of an organization discloses information that exposes an organization's or a person's inappropriate behaviors that are a danger to society and that have been hidden by the organization or by fellow workers. Whistle-blowing, according to Tim Porter-O'Grady, is "about righting a wrong—a wrong that is believed to be deceitful or that results in the mistreatment of others" (Porter-O'Grady & Malloch, 2007, p. 175).

Whistleblowers are often long-time employees who have great loyalty to an organization and who may be conflicted in exposing deficiencies in the organization or about a peer. Usually, the whistleblower attempts to go through the organization to report or disclose a situation. Whistleblowers are often conflicted in their decision to "tell," because they are afraid of losing their job or are concerned about their own or their family's well-being. In the past, whistleblowers were unprotected, but the whistleblower now has legal protection and the federal government encourages reporting of fraud related to Medicare and Medicaid. However, whistle-blowing remains a risk-taking behavior.

Nurses in particular are ethically bound to report issues that put either the patient or other nurses at risk. In an organization that is ethically responsible, whistle-blowing should not have to occur, because there should be mechanizations in place to remediate or fix a situation. The nurse is responsible for seeing that no harm comes to a patient or a peer.

ANA Code of Ethics

In nursing, the ANA *Code of Ethics* is the benchmark by which nurses and legal associations view ethical decisions made in professional settings. In 2001, the ANA House of Delegates voted to accept the nine major provisions of the *Code of Ethics*, which were then approved by the Congress of Nursing Practice and Economics (ANA, 2008).

The ANA *Code of Ethics with Interpretive Statements* is the latest update approved by the ANA.

It contains nine ethical provisions and interpretive statements. The interpretive statements are intended to clarify the provisions. These are published and available from the American Nurses Association, or you can view the *Code of Ethics with Interpretive Statements* online at http://nursing world.org/ethics/code/protected_nwcoe813.htm.

Bioethics

Bioethics is the study of ethical issues that have arisen with the advancements made in health care. Although it is a fairly new term, decisions concerning the provision of health care are not new. This area of study related to critical choices made in health care and medicine is also referred to as biomedical ethics.

Only fairly recently have nurses been included and represented on bioethics committees in healthcare agencies. A bioethics committee is an interdisciplinary team in a healthcare agency that deals with ethical decisions affecting the provision of care. Today it is not uncommon for nurses to serve on bioethics committees in healthcare agencies. But until the last decade, nurses were not included on most ethics committees. Bioethics committees serve to assist hospital staff and professionals with ethical dilemmas. An ethical dilemma is when an individual must choose between two unfavorable alternatives.

The International Council of Nurses Code of Ethics

Since 1953, the International Council of Nurses (ICN) *Code of Ethics* has served as a worldwide standard and guide for nurses (ICN, 2006). In 2006, it was revised. The standards are reviewed to accommodate the changing needs of society and to meet the impact of changes in health care. The *Code* is available online in a variety of languages in PDF format at the ICN Web site. It addresses the need for nurses to respect human rights and for patients to be treated respectfully.

Summary

The work and mission of a professional organization is to serve as the framework for the profession's structure and culture. Organizational culture is the norms and values of the organization's membership and profession. Professional organizations set standards for professional membership behaviors, quality improvement, and ethics for the entire profession. Many professional organizations maintain PACs to lobby for political issues and for legislative change. Membership in and support of professional organizations are important; however, with so many organizations, support may become fragmented.

QUESTIONS

1. Nurse M. belongs to the American Nurses Association. She knows that her membership is important because membership in a professional organization will
   a. act as a union to protect the nurse in professional matters
   b. provide the nurse with representation in legal matters
   c. enable the nurse to become a travel nurse
   d. serves the profession as well as the general community

2. Carol Gilligan believes that
   a. the ethical standards of men and women are the same
   b. men have greater ethical standards than women do
   c. women have greater ethical standards than men do
   d. the ethical standards of men and women are different

3. You are the triage nurse in an emergency department. Several patients arrive at once, and you must decide who will be cared for first. The hospital where you work has a policy that mandates that persons with chest pain or head injury receive care first. This policy is an example of which ethical principle?
   a. justice
   b. distributive
   c. egalitarianism
   d. utility

4. You have decided to join a political action committee (PAC) as part of your state nursing organization. On a PAC, you might be asked to do which of the following:
   a. write to your state senator in support of particular legislation related to health care
   b. represent your organization at a meeting with legislators
   c. attend a rally in your state capital to support legislation related to health care
   d. All of the above

5. A nurse is part of a Continuous Quality Improvement team. The team works throughout the year, because
   a. its goal is to ensure quality care for patients
   b. it evaluates performance and outcomes continuously
   c. it is ethically required to do outcome evaluation
   d. All of the above

Activity

This activity is intended to help you clarify and get in touch with your values. There are no right or wrong answers to this exercise. Imagine that you have just won or inherited a million dollars. Using a paper and pencil, list (prioritize) in order of importance 10 areas where you would spend your money and how much you would give to each item on the list. It must total a million dollars in the end. After you do this exercise, try to analyze how you made your decisions and how you prioritized the list.

References

American Association of Colleges of Nursing (AACN). (2004). *About AACN*. Retrieved July 22, 2008, from http://www.aacn.nche.edu/ContactUs/index.htm

American Nurses Association (ANA). (2008). *About the code*. Retrieved July 15, 2008, from http://www.nursingworld.org/MainMenuCategories/ThePracticeofProfessionalNursing/EthicsStandards/CodeofEthics/AboutTheCode.aspx

Association of Women's Health, Obstetric and Neonatal Nurses (AWHONN). (2008). *Promoting the health of women and newborns*. Retrieved November 24, 2008, from http://www.awhonn.org

Becker, L. C., & Becker, C. B. (1992). *Encyclopedia of ethics*. New York: Garland.

Cypher, A. (n.d.). Notes on "In a Different Voice" by Carol Gilligan. Retrieved September 17, 2007, from http://acypher.com/BookNotes/Gilligan.html

Finkelman, A., & Kenner, C. (2007). *Teaching IOM: Implications of the Institute of Medicine reports for nursing education*. Silver Spring, MD: American Nurses Association.

Gallup, Inc. (2003). Public rates nursing as most honest and ethical profession. Retrieved August 15, 2008, from http://www.gallup.com/poll/9823/Public-rates-nursing-most-honest-ethical-profession.aspx

Hook, K. G., & White, G. B. (2003). *The preface to the code*. Retrieved July 22, 2008, from http://www.nursingworld.org/mods/mod580/cecde03.htm

Hospice and Palliative Nurses Association (HPNA). (n.d.). *Welcome*. Retrieved July 8, 2008, from http://www.hpna.org

Huff, C. (1998). *Gilligan's "In a different voice."* Retrieved August 15, 2008, from http://www.stolaf.edu/people/huff/classes/handbook/Gilligan.html

Institute of Medicine (IOM). (2008). *Crossing the quality chasm: The IOM health care quality initiative*. Retrieved July 31, 2008, from http://www.iom.edu/CMS/8089.aspx

International Council of Nurses (ICN). (2000). *Code for nurses*. Retrieved November 8, 2008, from http://www.gale.cengage.com/pdf/Appendices/BioethicsAppend.pdf

International Council of Nurses (ICN). (2006). *The ICN code of ethics for nurses*. Retrieved August 16, 2008, from http://www.icn.ch/ethics.htm

National League for Nursing (NLN). (2007). *About the NLN*. Retrieved July 20, 2008, from http://www.nln.org/aboutnln/index.htm

National Organization of Nurse Practitioner Faculties. (2008). *Welcome to NONPF*. Retrieved November 8, 2008, from http://www.nonpf.com/

National Student Nurses Association (NSNA). (n.d.a). *Bill of Rights and Responsibilities for Students of Nursing*. Retrieved August, 16, 2008, from http://www.nsna.org/pubs/billofrights.asp

National Student Nurses Association (NSNA). (n.d.b). *Welcome to the NSNA*. Retrieved August 16, 2008, from http://www.nsna.org/index.asp

Porter-O'Grady, T., & Malloch, K. (2007). *Quantum leadership: A resource for health care innovation* (2nd ed.). Sudbury, MA: Jones and Bartlett.

Unit Two

Career Development

Chapter 7

The Nurse Leader and Teams

Deborah Ambrosio
Mawhirter

OUTLINE

Understanding Teams

A *team* is a group of people who assemble with a common goal. In a recent article titled "What CNO's Really Want," Chiverton and Witzel (2008) write, "Building a high-functioning collaborative team of nurses is one of the most important tasks for any nurse leader" (p. 33). This is an important concept to keep mind when reading this chapter.

This chapter offers insight into types of teams, team function, team building, team outcomes, and the role of a nurse leader in the team environment. Most healthcare organizations have high expectations for nurses' involvement with teams. Teams' focus can include quality improvement, staff action, shared governance models for unit function, and patient focus. This chapter can help you obtain a clear understanding of healthcare team structure and how to discover an individual's potential as a team player or leader.

Manion, Lorimer, and Leander (1996) describe the culture of healthcare organizations as team-based. Teams in health care provide opportunities for organizational improvements, increased employee and customer satisfaction, as well as improved patient outcomes. The implementation of an effective team helps to forge relationships among multiple disciplines to improve health care.

The word *team* is used commonly, but Katzenbach and Smith (1993), state that "not all groups are teams" (p. 113). Teams are distinguished by shared leadership, collective work, commitment, purpose, and mutual accountability. According to research done by Katzenbach and Smith (1993), a *workgroup* is a collection of individuals who gather for a joint effort, but they rely basically on the individual contributions of each member with individual effort. In a team, the effort is a collective work that is greater than any one individual's efforts. It is the effect of the collaboration and synergy that defines a team—the team's communal labors are greater than the sum of its individuals' efforts.

Katzenbach and Smith (2002) define a team as "a small number of people with complementary skills who are committed to a common purpose, performance goals, and approach for which they hold themselves mutually accountable" (p. 45). This definition focuses on the elements needed to produce a highly effective team (com-

plementary skills, the commitment to the organization, responsibility, accountability, and a common purpose or goal).

A favorite definition is Maxwell's (2002), "A team is many voices with a single heart" (p. 28). This is a profound definition that explains why teams can achieve amazing results when they work together for a common purpose or goal. It is this "single heart" that makes the difference between a workgroup and a team.

An example is a sports team: the team members work together, but how do they act collectively? Teams may have the right players, but without a strategy, without a plan, without practice they will not win the game. With effective teamwork and collaboration, a group of individuals becomes a team that can win a championship. "Groups of health care personnel thrown together" in an office, a clinic, or a hospital unit are generally called teams, but "they need to earn true team status by demonstrating teamwork" (Grumbach & Bodenheimer, 2004, p. 1246).

Types of Teams in Health Care

In the 21st century, healthcare professionals deliver patient-centered care by each individual working as a part of an interdisciplinary team. An *interdisciplinary* team is one in which all members participate in the team's activities and rely on one another to accomplish the goal of improving the patient's health.

Interdisciplinary Teams

The interdisciplinary model of care provides a collaborative approach for all members of the healthcare team to share information and knowledge to affect the treatment and plan of care for the patient (Manion et al., 1996). The interdisciplinary team responsible for the patient's plan of care in a hospital may consist of many professionals: the nurse, the social worker, the case manger, the physical therapist, the pharmacist, and the physician. These groups tend to function as working groups rather than teams, the difference being the sense of accountability, the "single heart." Frequently, they do not become true teams because they do not have a sense of collective accountability and instead function with a sense of individual accountability.

A true team needs to have synergy to produce an effective outcome. Ideally, the patient and family should be included in the team process to jointly develop actions for the plan of care. At a team conference, all members present their assessment findings and collaborate to develop or update the patient's plan of care. There is communication, coordination, and cooperation among the professionals performing for the one purpose (the goal) of improving the patient's health (Manion et al., 1996).

Multidisciplinary Teams

Members of multidisciplinary teams provide care to the patient independently and share information with other members of the team; the patient is merely the recipient of care. Each of the professional disciplines has specific goals for the patient's care needs (Manion et al., 1996).

Performance Improvement or Quality Teams

Another team structure is quality improvement teams. These teams have been a part of health care since the 1980s. These teams are usually designated by an organization's administration and hospital steering committees to improve or evaluate a process or issue. The purpose is to analyze problems, generate solutions, and make

changes in an institution for positive outcome. The origin of this structure is in the Total Quality Management (TQM) or Continuous Quality Improvement (CQI) philosophies of Edward Deming. In health care, the terms *performance improvement* or *continuous quality improvement* are used because health care must always strive to continuously improve performance. This means doing a good job and always trying to do it better (McLaughlin & Kaluzny, 2006).

Organizations often assemble personnel from multiple departments to assess an issue or examine a complex problem. Most quality improvement teams are developed to promote change to improve a system. One of the popular analysis processes used today was developed by W. Shewhart. The Plan-Do-Check-Act (PDCA) methodology or some variation is employed in most healthcare systems (McLaughlin & Kaluzny, 2006). Analysis is always data driven. CQI has a direct impact on the quality of patient care. Systems are often designed or redesigned to provide cost-effective improvements in care.

In 2000, the Institute of Medicine published a report titled *To Err Is Human* that discusses patient safety issues and the need for improvements in the system to provide better care. This made quality teams essential to meet the Joint Commission's (JCAHO) standards. Hospitals choose indicators to analyze and make improvements. The Joint Commission review process includes accreditation standards in the areas of patient safety, medical errors, and adverse events. Analysis of data and performance improvements that brings about change within a hospital system is essential to meet current standards.

Quality measurements are imperative in health care to identify areas to improve patient care. Specifically, in 1999 the American Nurses Association developed nursing-sensitive indicators to understand the extent to which nurses affect the improvement of patient safety and healthcare outcomes (Montalvo, 2007).

Nursing-sensitive care indicators are based on the "principles of measure, evaluate and improve practice" (Montalvo, 2007, p. 2). Institutions collect data on patient-centered outcome measurements such as pressure ulcer prevalence, falls prevalence, falls with injury, and restraint prevalence (Montalvo, 2007).

McLaughlin and Kaluzny (2006) discuss five benefits of CQI applications: "intrinsic motivation, capturing the intellectual capital of the workforce, reducing managerial overhead, increasing capacity and creating lateral linkage" (p. 55).

- *Intrinsic motivation.* Employees have input into the improvement to provide better care and work on processes to "do the right thing."
- *Capturing the intellectual capital of the workforce.* Managers are aware that the front-line employee knows the process better than management does and allow all levels to have input in improvements.
- *Reducing managerial overhead necessary to bring about managerial change.* As CQI teams are empowered to review processes, less is spent on consultants to identify issues.
- *Increasing capacity.* Professionals are involved to support the quality effort to do process analysis.
- *Creating lateral linkages.* Lateral linkages refer to having information move across the organization as well as up and down the chain of command (anyone can identify a problem or process in need of an improvement). (McLaughlin & Kaluzny, 2006).

Quality improvement teams are empowering to employees and are exciting to be part of because they facilitate change to improve care within an organization. Continuous quality improvement efforts are critical to decrease errors in health care and to provide a safer environment for patients.

Team Nursing

Traditionally, nurses have functioned as team members. The term *team nursing* is defined by Odegaard Turner (1999) as a "staffing method that provides a staffing mix of personnel with different skills, competencies, and licensure who work together to provide care for a specified number of patients" (p. 291). This differs from functional nursing, which is based on a task-oriented philosophy, where each employee has a specific task that he or she must perform. For example, the medication nurse focuses only on administration of medication to the patient. Team nursing is a more unified model; the members of the team focus on the goals of the patient with the coordination of a team leader. The team leader must have effective communication and delegation skills to facilitate optimal care. A team conference among team members is crucial to having a high-performing team (Catalano, 2006).

Communication

Everyone has a right to, and an obligation for, simplicity and clarity in communication.

—Max DePree, *Leadership Is an Art*

Nurses and leaders need effective communication skills and the ability to understand teammates. According to Max DePree (2004), individuals must be respected for their diverse gifts. Leaders must communicate their own personal philosophies of respect for others. This is not a policy or acquired skill but is inherent in the way good leaders treat members of their teams (DePree, 2004).

Covey (1989) states, "Communication is the most important skill in life. We spend most of our waking hours communicating. But consider this: You've spent years learning how to read and write, years learning how to speak. But what about listening?" (pp. 237–238). In his book *The 7 Habits of Highly Effective People*, Covey devotes a chapter to empathic listening. Nurses are taught therapeutic communication and the skills of empathic listening to communicate effectively with patients, and these skills can also be used to understand colleagues. Covey's leadership model suggests that every good leader should use this skill to "seek to understand" people; he believes that we usually first seek to "misunderstand" (p. 239). He suggests that we are so busy focusing on ourselves that we rarely try to understand what another human being is communicating.

As leaders, we must take time to actively listen. Covey suggests that we listen at one of four levels: ignore the other person (not really listening), pretend to listen, practice selective listening, and attentive listening (concentrating on the words being said). What leaders and team members must practice is empathic listening, "with the intent to understand" (p. 240). "Seeking to first understand another person's frame of reference. You see the world the way they see the world and you understand how they feel" (p. 240).

Empathic Listening

"Empathic listening is so powerful because it gives you accurate data to work with, instead of projecting your own autobiography and assuming thoughts, feelings motives and interpretation" (Covey, 1989, p. 241). This concept is important when working with teams and as a nurse leader, by listening to the person's thoughts and dealing with the reality of the other person's heart and head. Listening to seek understanding of the person's perspective is imperative to being effective and successful.

Effective communication is essential in the workplace, and it requires skill and practice. Nurses in leadership roles must refine their own interpersonal skills to communicate clearly, openly, and honestly with respect for others' ideas, thoughts, and opinions. During team interactions, members must be clear and establish rules of behavior to communicate effectively. The mission and goals of the team should be defined, and all individuals must understand that their contribution is valued.

Conflict Resolution

Conflicts help growth and the formation of ideas for creative solutions to team interpersonal issues. McLaughlin and Kaluzny (2006) note that friction among members may develop as a result of interprofessional rivalries or two individuals dealing with solving a difficult problem. An effective tool for conflict resolution is Riley-Balzer's (2008) CARE confrontation model. CARE, which stands for Clarify, Articulate, Request, Encourage, includes the steps necessary to develop a win-win approach to conflict because negative words are not used and blame is not placed.

Riley-Balzer (2008) in *Communication in Nursing* describes the CARE model as follows:

> Clarify *the behavior that is problematic. Be specific about the aspect of behavior that is self-destructive or destructive to others. The behavior*

to be changed should be the focus so that it is clear you are not attaching hurt. Articulate why the behavior is a problem. Articulate how their behavior is likely to hinder them or irritate others or how it makes you feel. Request a change in client's or colleague's behavior. Your suggestion should be offered tentatively and respectfully. Encourage a change by emphasizing the positive consequences of changing or the negative implication of failing to change. (p. 274)

Team members should be taught conflict resolution techniques, to empower them and build collaboration in the team. Drinka (2000) suggests that recognizing and addressing team conflict are important to foster creativity and "innovation in group decision making. . . . Establishing safe venues for expressing conflict is one of the most useful things that a team can do" (p. 158).

The leader must support the team in learning how to handle conflict constructively. Be aware that causes of conflict include "poor communication, differences in values, beliefs, or goal, personality clashes and stress" (Arnold & Boggs, 2007, p. 319). The nature of conflict in a team could be caused by unclear goals, content issues, relationship issues, and power struggles. Power struggles are caused by individuals acting for their own self-interest, not the team's. Individual differences in behavior may lead to conflict. Members who do not understand the group norms or specific processes at the organizational level may also be the source of conflict.

How people communicate the message can cause conflict. Conflicts can flare up based on individuals' perception of others or the discussion topic or may even be sparked by the tone of voice used by a member. Relationships within the group can sprout a conflict. Communication is influenced by the way people feel about themselves and the subject matter being communicated.

Developing Teams

Leaders must decide on the group membership, how large a group, and which people are to be invited to the group. Katzenbach and Smith (1993) observe that "large numbers of people have trouble interacting constructively," and they recommend teams of 12 or fewer members are effective. In their study, larger teams developed subgroups and did not work together as one unit. In larger groups, it becomes more challenging to share viewpoints and confront issues, and members often become frustrated. These large groups cannot develop a sense of synergy (Katzenbach & Smith, 1993).

Team leaders must consider the environment for the team. Having an appropriate place for meeting facilitates group interaction, and people must feel comfortable. The room must have enough space and limited interruptions. Seating should be comfortable and arranged for members to have face-to-face discussions to allow for open communication. To encourage communication, team members should sit in a circle or around a table to help to equalize the members' positions and power (Arnold & Boggs, 2007).

The membership characteristics depend on the mission of the team. Bennis (1997) states, "Greatness starts with superb people" (p. 197). This means choosing the right people with the correct skills (technical and creative skills) who are committed to the project. Team members must buy into the cause and believe in the project goal. Members of great groups are dedicated "to the love of the work" (p. 200). "Great groups are made up of people with rare gifts working together as equals" (p. 199). Gratton and Erickson (2007) discuss the need for diversity among team members. They found that "the greater the proportion of experts a team had, the more likely it was to disintegrate into nonproductive conflict or stalemate" (p. 102). Commitment, collaboration, and dedication are qualities needed to help form effective teams that achieve their goal.

"The richer the mix of people, the more likely that new connections will be made, new ideas will emerge" (Bennis, 1997, p. 197). Diversity in the group helps to form collaboration in the group; notably, all members must understand that the team rules include respect, tolerance of each other, sharing information, and a unified purpose of achieving the agreed-upon team goal.

Collins (2001) stresses great leaders recognize that the "right people" are assets if they are in the position to do what they do best. He uses an analogy of a bus. He found that great leaders "first got the right people on the bus, the wrong people off the bus, and the right people in the right seats—and then they figured out where to drive it" (p. 13).

The right combination of persons is an important concept when considering choosing team members. What is the "right" job/seat for a person based on his or her expertise, talents, and skills? What mix is needed to accomplish the goal? Katzenbach and Smith (1993) suggest that the most important factors that influence a team's success is including the right mix of skills. The skills the team members need are "technical or functional expertise, problem-solving and decision-making skills" and demonstrating good "interpersonal skills" (p. 115).

Stages of Team Development

Tuckman (1965), based on empirical research, introduced his theory on the developmental sequence of groups and coined the popular terms "forming, storming, norming, and performing" (p. 396). Tuckman looked at relationships within the group and with the leader. In 1977, Tuckman and his coauthor Jensen published an article titled "Stages of Small-Group Development Revisited" and introduced the termination phase of the group as *adjourning*. Tuckman and Jensen observed group behavior in different settings and identified how people came together and began to function. Tuckman's model explains team development (Smith, 2005).

Forming

The initial phase is *forming*; the members need guidance and direction. The leader/facilitator must be aware that members of the team may be anxious. Tuckman (1965) identifies this as the "orientation" stage (p. 396). Members have questions regarding roles, responsibilities, and function of the team. It is important for them to understand the external relationship of the team with the organization.

The forming phase is considered the testing and dependence phase (Tuckman, 1965). The group members try to get to know each other and find commonalities. Individuals gather information and impressions of colleagues/team members. Communication is often superficial chitchat. The leader needs to take an active role, helping members feel accepted, answering questions, defining the goal, giving clear direction, and facilitating interaction in the team. Team members should feel valued. Ice-breaking exercises can help members get to know each other and have an enjoyable experience.

ICE-BREAKING EXERCISES

Ice-breaking exercises are a fun way to help people introduce themselves to each other. (See Box 7-1.) Games can also help to identify members of the team that enjoy competition. The Internet is a great source for finding simple examples of ice breakers. PopEd.org is a Web site that has many ice-breaking exercises.

The role of the leader/facilitator when using an ice breaker is to clarify the team's goal and purpose, delineate responsibilities, and set up the ground rules (Yoder-Wise & Kowalski, 2006). The behavioral expectations of the members should be discussed such as mutual respect, attendance, and the ability to listen openly to what others have to say. This stage is like the first day of school. Everyone is polite, a little anxious or cautious because they're not sure what to expect, and most of the time it is pleasant. Everyone is waiting for the teacher to explain what is expected, such as the class rules, and of course to find out more about the people in the class (NYS Governor's Office of Employee Relations, n.d.). "You may ask yourself do I feel comfortable participating, can I be myself in the group?" (Arnold & Boggs, 2007, p. 275).

Storming

The next phase is *storming*, or the conflict around interpersonal issues (Tuckman, 1965). Members of the team are coping with position and control issues. Disagreement is normal. It is common to observe challenges among members, defensiveness, and competition. Some members are not willing to talk openly and others are not willing to listen actively. Decisions in the group are not

---

Box 7-1 Ice Breaker Exercises

One excellent and unique way to have members introduce themselves is by having them proclaim to be their favorite food. This exercise keeps the group laughing. An interesting Web site is About.com on the topic of adult education ice breakers. Peterson (2008a) writes step-by-step directions on how to use ice breakers effectively. An additional favorite is "If you had a magic wand," for which individuals state their name and department, and then tell the group what they would change in the organization as it relates to the focus of the team's purpose if they had a magic wand. It is a fun and insightful exercise that develops some of the team goal from the group's input on what processes need to be changed.

Peterson (2008a) also describes the popular ice breaker "Who would you take with you if you were marooned on a deserted island?" A variation is "what five things would you take if stranded on a deserted island?" The individuals can take people or things. The group always finds it amusing and interesting to learn what their colleagues value and to identify similarities and differences among group members. These 20-minute exercises help to develop a sense of who people are working with and encourages team spirit.

made easily during this time. Team members have a need to establish themselves in relations to the others in the group. Cliques or alliances may form with power struggles. To avoid these emotional issues, leaders must keep the group focused on the goals and the value of each member.

It is the team leader's responsibility to discuss with the team the need to have a win-win approach to conflict. Conflict can be beneficial because it can help encourage creative and innovative solutions to problems. Drinka (2000) suggests that recognizing and addressing team conflict are important to help foster creativity and "innovation in group decision making. . . . Establishing safe venues for expressing conflict is one of the most useful things that a team can do" (pp. 157–158). All members of a team should be taught conflict skills to promote constructive confrontations to advance the team's goals. When resistance is overcome, the group will learn to compromise and move into the third phase of norming.

Norming

Norming is the term used for the development of cohesiveness in the group. Manion, Lorimer, and Leader (1996) refer to this stage as the "pleasant and teamwork phase" (p. 82). Evolution has taken place and new roles are emerging. People feel comfortable expressing opinions. People work cooperatively and accept each other. The group accepts responsibility and agreement on how to achieve goals. Team learning takes place. Decisions are made; commitment and unity are strong. "Common agreement develops about the behavior standards expected if the group is to achieve its goal" (Arnold & Boggs, 2007, p. 277). There is general respect among members. The function of the group as a whole is important.

Performing

Norming leads to the *performing* or the achievement stage where the focus is on the performance and results (Manion et al., 1996). The team is cohesive, functioning according to its own rules and goals. Members are accountable; there is a collective caring and a positive feeling among members. The group often exceeds their own expectations. All members have a mutual respect with a high degree of support and value for each other. The energy of the group is to accomplish the goal. It's the same sense of cohesiveness seen in winning sports teams. A true team leader or player when given accolades for a job well done will share that recognition by saying, "I could not have accomplished this without each and every member of the team." In health care, as in sports, it is not the designated leaders or individual acting alone; it is the team that accomplishes the goal. This was best said by Harry Truman: "It is amazing what you can accomplish if you do not care who gets the credit."

It should be noted that during the group development process groups may be productively norming and performing; if a new member is added to the group, it may cause the group to move back into storming. The process is dynamic, and leaders need to be able to help understand members and help the group stay focused and move forward to performing. New members should clarify their roles and assess the culture and the group dynamics (NYS Governor's Office of Employee Relations, n.d.).

Adjourning

The final phase of the process is *adjourning*; this is about completion and disbanding. It has also been referred to as the "de-forming and mourning stage of the process." The group, although proud of its accomplishments, feels a sense of loss. Leaders must be sensitive to the loss and look to reward or recognize the team for a job well done (Grzeskowiak, 2008).

Not all teams progress through all phases. In most cases, if the team does not advance, they may not achieve their goal. Many factors can cause the team not to progress or even to regress, such as unclear goals, change in objectives by leadership, lack of management support or ineffective leadership, and lack of trust and accountability of team members.

Teamwork

> Teamwork is the ability to work together toward a common vision. The ability to direct individual accomplishments toward organizational objectives. It is the fuel that allows common people to attain uncommon results.
>
> —Andrew Carnegie

Teamwork is an active process involving health professions working together for a common goal. As Katzenbach and Smith describe in their landmark 1993 article, "The Discipline of Teams," for teamwork to be effective it must include four elements: a common commitment and purpose, performance goals, complementary skills, and mutual accountability.

Xyrichis and Ream (2007) state, "Teamwork is accomplished through interdependent collaboration, open communication and shared decision-making, and generates value-added patient, organizational, and staff outcomes. . . . Attributes of teamwork are concerted effort, interdependent collaboration and shared decision making" (p. 239).

Wiecha and Pollard (2004) further describe characteristics of teamwork as the 12 Cs of teamwork:

1. Communication
2. Cooperation (empowerment of team members)
3. Cohesiveness (team sticks together)
4. Commitment (investing in team process)
5. Collaboration (equality in the team)
6. Confronts problems directly
7. Coordination of efforts (ensuring actions support a common plan)
8. Conflict management
9. Consensus decision making
10. Caring (patient-centered outcomes)
11. Consistency (with one another and the environment)
12. Contribution

The authors suggest that application of the 12 ingredients most likely produces a synergetic effect as well as fosters creativity, learning, and innovations.

Even the best teams experience conflict. Conflict can be a constructive process for teams. Brandt (2001) states, "When differences arise among individuals who know how to collaborate, conflict can prove constructive rather than destructive. Teamwork facilitates understanding and leads to a true appreciation of differences, creating a system that values shared decision making and communication. To ensure that collaboration prevails, nurse leaders can create cultures of caring in which staff feel compelled to make cooperation part of their routine" (p. 32).

Briles (2005, p. 32) states, "Eliminating conflict enhances teamwork, and teamwork can help wipe out conflicts." It is a reciprocal process:

for the team to function effectively communication must be clear, and members must act collaboratively, understanding group norms of respect for all individual team members. The team leader must be prepared to help handle conflict and practice effective communication.

Hader (2005) describes an essential element in the successful team: trust between team members. Effective teams have members that "maximize his or her colleague's strengths" (p. 4). This means having the ability to keep the focus on achieving the goal and recognizing the specific talents of members. Teams that trust each other do not let competition among members become an obstacle. The ground rules are clearly defined with expectations for all members. "High standards of behavior and personal commitment must be inherent in all teams" (Hader, 2005, p. 4). In the process of teamwork, egos and personal agendas are put aside and the team goal is the priority.

Kaissi, Johnson, and Kirschbaum (2003) found that nurses "perceived teamwork as important for reducing errors and for better decision making" (p. 216). Nurses value teamwork to help make better decisions and viewed teamwork as important as technical competency for patient care.

DiMichele and Gaffney (2005) used nine management principles to create a proactive nursing team:

1. Identify the team's strengths and weaknesses.
2. Build trust.
3. Focus on the positive.
4. Create a common vision.
5. Market the vision.
6. Make the vision a reality.
7. Foster open, honest communication.
8. Encourage creativity.
9. Foster an environment of constant renewal. (p. 61)

They used these principles to develop a proactive and positive team. It is important to embrace the vision to create an effective team. The vision of the team must be in direct congruence with the organization mission and values to be successful. Culture of the organization should be considered when developing the team vision.

Team members need to be adaptable, meaning that they must be flexible, teachable, creative, emotionally secure, and service minded (Maxwell, 2002). Maxell states that "working together precedes winning together" (p. 10). Collaboration is the essence of teamwork. Maxwell suggests that it is more important to achieve the goal than compete with each other. He states that "commitment comes as the result of choice, not conditions" (p. 24).

In health care, nurses are committed to improving the patient's health; this is something we value as a profession. Team members must be committed to the goal and believe in its value to be successful. This is the source of the team's energy and creates excitement, which is the team's driving force. Denis Waitley (in Maxwell, 2002, p. 77) asserts that "enthusiasm is contagious. It's difficult to remain neutral or indifferent in the presence of a positive thinker."

In today's changing healthcare environment, nurses need to be positive thinkers to improve and build our teams. "The people's capacity to achieve is determined by their leader's ability to empower" (Maxwell, 1998, p. 126). Teams that are empowered are effective high-performing teams able to accomplish goals. Leaders empower the team by encouraging and allowing creativity and developing trust. Teams need to be cheerleaders for the goal, willing to stand up and be heard. It takes hard work, dedication, and leadership for teams to be productive.

Recognition of Team Accomplishments

The nurse, as part of a team, performs meaningful work that improves patient care outcomes. The use of teams further helps improve organizations in cost-effective ways, by providing safety and customer satisfaction and meeting external standards for excellence. So, we need to celebrate! Who doesn't like a party, a reward, a pat on the back for a job well done? These celebrations do not have to be elaborate. Recognition can be as simple as administrational leadership thanking the team for accomplishing the goal or making the change. It could be a thank-you letter from the institution's board of directors or a team recognition lunch or an after-work party.

Recognition can be as simple as printing a picture of the team in the institution's or hospital's newsletter praising their work, holding a pizza party for fun, or giving a coupon for lunch in the cafeteria. It is an acknowledgment recognizing the team's hard work. Bethune, Sherrod, and Youngblood (2005) suggest that recognizing staff helps to keep them happy and should be used as a retention practice. They give examples of creative messages acknowledging staff for jobs well done. Some examples include "hand out peppermint patties and tell staff, 'You're worth a mint!' Give out Almond Joy candies with a note that states, 'You're a joy to work with!'" (p. 26).

Leaders need to recognize the value of teams. Having a meal together can especially foster celebration. Administrative leadership should share in the celebration. This serves two purposes: team members feel valued and rewarded, and hospital leadership acknowledges how much hard work is going into the project. Leadership cares about the team and shares its interest.

Because hospitals are intent on cutting costs, there may not be money in budgets to reward the team. Cohen (2006, p. 14) believes, "Respect, recognition and appreciation are all perceived as a reward" and states, "Nonmonetary rewards show your employees that you recognize their accomplishments and appreciate their hard work and time" (p. 10).

One institution developed a points incentive program based on rewards, similar to bonus points earned on a credit card (points were redeemed for various rewards). This helped motivate staff to fill open shifts and increased job satisfaction. "Rewards are more tangible and encourage employees to work toward a specific goal" (McKnight, McDaniel, & Ehmann, 2006, p. 42). Jones (2008) writes that teams celebrate victories, and the top performers know "that partying must be deserved," and "without victory, celebrations are meaningless" (p. 127).

Jones (2008) notes differences among team members: some are high achievers and some strive to be superior, the "elite performer" (p. 127). The driving force for best performers includes honest, constructive feedback and a celebration for a job well done. He suggests this is the difference among athletes, for example, that some are merely good and some go on to be Olympic athletes.

Nelson (2005) cites studies that directly tie recognition activities to employee motivation and satisfaction. He suggests that best personal praise is timely, sincere, and specific. He describes eight ways to praise teams. A favorite is, "Have members create awards for each other. Invest in team mementos and symbols of a team's work together, such as t-shirts, or coffee cups with a team motto or company logo" (p. 155). Nelson quotes many CEOs in his book, *1001 Ways to Reward Employees*. Robert Crandall, former CEO of American Airlines, said, "There's nothing more important than making certain that each employee feels respected and valued" (p. 166).

As nurse leaders, the best way to say thank you is one that fits personal leadership styles and the team. A small token, such as a decorative pen, is simple but effective.

Leadership: What It Takes to Work with Teams

Maxwell (1998) writes, "Only secure leaders give power to others" (p. 121). Leadership must take on responsibility to facilitate the development of clear goals and build a sense of mutual accountability among team members. Mutual accountability is present in a team when the team refers to the "we" of the group and not the "I" (Katzenbach & Smith, 2001, p. 155). The focus of the team is collaboration, working together. Leadership's role should be supportive, empowering, and respectful of the group's collective talents and commitment to the team goal.

Respect

In this changing, hectic, healthcare arena and today's economic market, most people just want to get the job done. Everyone wants to be the star, save money, and accomplish the task. Success should not be achieved at the expense of others but done with respect and value for the teammates. Each person has individual talents and should be appreciated and mentored. It is as easy to be nice to others as it is to be mean-spirited. A positive attitude can make everyone feel as good, including the people that work with you. (Complaining about each other is a waste of time.) Bennis (1997) refers to great groups to examine how "collective magic is made" (p. 3). He speaks of creative and respectful collaboration in great groups. That creative collaboration is developed when "work is pleasure" and the group finds "joy" in problem solving (p. 8). He suggests that leaders and organizations should respect groups for their talents and achievements. People work hard in great groups when they are empowered and supported by the organization and allowed to achieve (p. 9–12).

Empowerment

"The people's capacity to achieve is determined by their leader's ability to empower" (Maxwell, 1998, p. 126). Nurse leaders want to create a positive culture and working environment. Empower the team and watch them accomplish more than their goal. Fostering trust and good communication skills with a focus on the goal is part of the nurse leader's role. Leaders can accomplish more with colleagues and staff by being genuine, meaning being humble and treating people with value and respect. Outhwaite (2003) concludes that leaders explore their "own values and beliefs and strive to develop their self awareness" (p. 375).

Gracious Communication

Collins (2001) in *Good to Great* studied Fortune 500 leaders and found that the great leaders, the successful ones, have qualities of "personal humility and professional will" (p. 20). That means that if you are on a team or you are the team leader, you did not accomplish the goal alone. Acknowledgment and credit should be given to the team. Yes, some individuals will shine, but they are shining for the purpose and the team. Acknowledge the team's effort, the role of each member on the team, and their contribution to accomplishing the task or goal. This is done with a simple thank you.

Genuine communication skills are nurse leaders' tools for being successful. Communicate in a way that is clear, honest, and gracious. For example, say, "Thank you, (*person's name*), for keeping us on task at the last meeting. We were able to (*state the accomplishment*)." Your support, direction, and influence are valuable resources. Lead by example and be a positive role model—it is contagious. Keep in mind these few words when working with teams: "None of us is as smart as all of us" (Bennis, 1997, p. 1).

The Future of Teams: Virtual Teams

Advances in information technology and communication are changing healthcare teams. The use of technology, such as the Internet, e-mail, digital imaging, video, teleconferencing, mobile phones, Web cams, and software is creating new abilities for teams to be composed of people outside the walls of a specific institution. "Virtual teams are groups of people who work interdependently with shared purpose across space, time, and organization boundaries using technology to communicate and collaborate. Virtual team members may be located across a country or across the world, rarely meet face to face, and include members from different cultures. Virtual work allows organizations to combine the best expertise regardless of geographic location"

(Kirkman, Rosen, Gibson, Tesluck, & McPerson, 2002, p. 67).

Virtual teams can be formed and can meet online. They can use "synchronous collaborative technologies, such as online chat systems, video- and/or audio conferencing, interactive whiteboards, or a combination of them" to brainstorm or have group discussions (Wallace, 2004, p. 163). The team members and the organization must be prepared to work collaboratively through the use of technology and adapt to new ways of working (Conner & Finnemore, 2003).

For example, a nurse working in the emergency department in the middle of the night can easily contact the radiologist, who is at home, to read a patient's MRI. Technology brings the experts closer without requiring them to be in the same room physically. The meaning of the word *team* is expanding to include a virtual team that is composed of people who may not even be in the same time zone.

The development of e-health teams is empowering the healthcare industry to provide more effective systems to care for patients. Research is now providing data that interdisciplinary virtual teams who do "virtual integrated practice" (Rush University Medical Center, 2008, p. 222) are providing care to chronically ill patients, reducing the patients' need for emergency room visits. Virtual integrated practice links patients to physicians, pharmacists, nurses, social workers, and dieticians via phone, fax, and e-mail to coordinate the patients' care. This study reported cost-effective positive outcomes for patients.

Interdisciplinary e-health clinical teams come together for the benefit of the patient to provide expert care via technology, not hands-on care. "The Internet is a logical platform for supporting interdisciplinary teamwork" (Wiecha & Pollard, 2004). Web-based learning will also advance health education of the public. Children and adults have access to educational material specific to their illness and support groups.

Virtual teams are being used to promote better health, and the possibilities are endless if we use our imaginations and are creative. Hurling and associates (2007) used the Internet as a medium to stimulate healthy behavior and concluded that providing access to the fully automated Internet and a mobile phone–based physical activity program had a positive impact on patients' activity levels. Patients exercised more and became active participants in their health program.

The use of virtual teams around the globe will allow institutions to recruit the best people in the organization or the world to be on the team. Technology has made communication quicker and easier for virtual teams to work; they are the future (Katzenback & Smith, 2001).

Challenges of Virtual Teams

Virtual team members encounter challenges based on the way they communicate. Because the team members rarely have face-to-face meetings, it may be difficult to develop trust and cohesiveness among members. Kirkman and colleagues (2002) report that "trusting someone in a virtual team is linked directly to their work ethic. The trust has been built through the task-based relationship" (p. 69). Another obstacle virtual teams deal with is that members may feel a sense of isolation. There is a lack of social interaction; members do not receive verbal and nonverbal cues when communicating. There is a lack of team-building activities to engage the group in team spirit or synergy.

Leadership must be creative to overcome the obstacles of the virtual team. Kimball and Eunice (1999) suggest having a team photograph so that all members can "see" each other; creating a "virtual water cooler" (p. 59), an electronic space in which to share stories and feelings; and developing team norms by sending "hot news" bulletins for which the norm is to respond to provide support (p. 60). These are just a few creative ways to overcome the challenges of virtual teams. The aim is to keep the team connected to each other and the purpose of accomplishing the goal.

Nurses, as futurists, must contemplate additional applications of virtual teams and how they can improve health care.

Summary

Healthcare organizations and leaders today recognize the benefit of high-performing collaborative teams. Teams today are organized to make decisions, solve problems, and improve and manage patient care.

Dye and Garman (2006) summarize teams by stating:

> *Developing teams means you select executives who will be strong team players, actively support the concept of teaming, develop open discourse and encourage healthy debate on important issues, create compelling reasons and incentives for team members to work together, effectively set limits on the political activity that takes place outside the team framework, celebrate successes together as a unit, and commiserate as a group over disappointments. (p. 108)*

A nurse's career encompasses many teams, and roles include leader (coach) and team player (cheerleader) to help accomplish the team's goal. Each role is not about individual accomplishment or performance, but about collaboration, working together as a whole. The goal in many cases is to make an improvement in the system and/or a change in practice to provide optimal care for patients.

This chapter provides foundational wisdom about how to develop and work with teams, taking into account Katzenbach and Smith's (2002) six principles: the number of members should be fewer than 12, team members should have complementary skills, the team must understand their purpose, the team must have specific performance goals, the team must have commonly agreed upon team rules for working, and all members must be mutually accountable (p. xvii). Using these guidelines helps teams perform and have positive outcomes, which should always be celebrated.

Organization commitment is necessary for the team to be successful. Teams should have a purpose and goal with clearly defined roles and tasks for team members to work together. All members must be devoted to respecting one another. The team communication is open and conflict resolution skills are developed. The team as a whole is "one heart" and accountable as a unit for accomplishing the goal. Organizations and teams must celebrate success.

To be a true team, teams must work through developmental phases to develop cohesive relationships that collaboratively reflect the sense of team spirit and synergy. Working together with colleagues is a rewarding experience; embrace it, be enthusiastic, and team goals will be achieved! Become the kind of team member or leader everyone wants to work with.

QUESTIONS

1. Teamwork is very important, especially in a healthcare environment. The nurse knows that
   a. caring and commitment of team members to work together are important in the cohesiveness of the team
   b. collaboration and coordination of work are important factors in how a team functions successfully
   c. how members communicate, including confronting each problem directly and to manage conflict, is important
   d. All of the above

2. In today's world, use of technology is important in the care of patients. Some healthcare facilities
   a. are using virtual teams to promote better health
   b. are avoiding the use of technology in some areas
   c. know that technology should be limited because it deters nurses from their work
   d. All of the above

3. When attempting to deal with problematic situations, an important goal of the nurse who is a team leader should be to
   a. use and project her own experiences with similar situations to attempt to help the team because her experiences are the most accurate
   b. be a good listener and not project her thoughts or experiences onto understanding the needs of team members because their input is most accurate
   c. not listen to the person's perspective because it is not necessary to be effective
   d. present solutions to the team because this saves time and can be effective

4. Using the CARE confrontation model for conflict resolution, the nurse would do the following when two workers are in a situation that is resulting in conflict:
   a. insist that the persons who are having difficulty dealing with each other sit down and speak to each other
   b. request that the persons having difficulty working together leave the unit until they resolve their problems
   c. speak with the persons in conflict to first clarify behaviors and articulate how the behavior is irritating, request change, and encourage them to work out their issues
   d. identify who the person is who is causing the conflict and request that person be moved to another unit

5. A nursing team method approach to patient care is different from a functional task-oriented approach in that it
   a. is a staffing scheme in which employees perform tasks that are complementary to each other to provide patient care
   b. provides a staffing mix of personnel with different skills and competencies who work together to provide patient care
   c. focuses on administrative input as a guide to patient care
   d. requires the team to take over all functional tasks

References

Arnold, E., & Boggs, K. U. (2007). *Interpersonal relationships: Professional communication skills for nurses* (5th ed.). St. Louis: Saunders Elsevier.

Bennis, W. (1997). *Organizing genius: The secrets of creative collaboration*. New York: Basic Books.

Bethune, G., Sherrod, D., & Youngblood, L. (2005). 101 tips to retain a happy, healthy staff. *Nursing Management, 36*(4), 25–29.

Brandt, M. (2001). How to make conflict work for you. *Nursing Management, 32*(11), 32–35.

Briles, J. (2005). Zapping conflict builds better teams. *Nursing, 35*(11), 32.

Catalano, J. (2006). *Nursing Now! Today's issues, tomorrow's trends*. Philadelphia: F. A. Davis.

Chiverton, P., & Witzel, P. (2008). What CNO's really want. *Nursing Management, 39*(1), 33–47.

Cohen, S. (2006). Compliment your staff with nonmonetary rewards. *Nursing Management, 37*(12), 10, 14.

Collins, J. (2001). *Good to great.* New York: HarperCollins.

Conner, M., & Finnemore, P. (2003). Living in the new age: Using collaborative digital technology to deliver health care improvement. *International Journal of Health Care Quality Assurance, 16*(2), 77–86.

Covey, S. (1989). *The 7 habits of highly effective people.* New York: Simon & Schuster.

DePree, M. (2004). *Leadership is an art.* New York: Currency Books.

DiMichele, C. M., & Gaffney, L. (2005). Proactive teams yield exceptional care. *Nursing Management, 36*(5), 61–64.

Drinka, T. (2000). *Health care teamwork: Interdisciplinary practice and teaching.* Westport, CT: Auburn House.

Dye, C., & Garman, A. (2006). *Exceptional leadership: 16 competencies for healthcare executives.* Chicago: Health Administration Press.

Gratton, L., & Erickson, T. J. (2007). Eight ways to build collaborative teams. *Harvard Business Review, 85*(11), 100–109.

Grumbach, K., & Bodenheimer, T. (2004). Can health care teams improve primary care practice? *JAMA, 291*(10), 1246–1251.

Grzeskowiak, M. (2008). Group Dynamics. Retrieved July 20, 2008 from www.medhunters.com/articles/groupDynamics.html

Hader, R. (2005). Put the 't' back in team [Editorial]. *Nursing Management, 36*(2), 4.

Hurling, R., Catt, M., De Boni, M., William, B., Hurst, T., Murray, P., et al. (2007). Using Internet and mobile phone technology to deliver an automated physical activity program: Randomized controlled trial. *Journal of Medical Internet Research, 9*(2).

Institute of Medicine. (2000). *To err is human: Building a safer health system.* Washington, DC: National Academy Press.

Joint Commission. Provision of care, treatment, and services: Overview. Retrieved July 30, 2008, from http://www.jointcommission.org/NR/rdonlyres/D315C586-0D2B-4DB4-A9E4-FFC7681A55CC/0/LTC2008PCChapter.pdf

Jones, G. (2008). How the best of the best get better and better. *Harvard Business Review, 86*(6), 123–127.

Kaissi, A., Johnson, T., & Kirschbaum, M. (2003). Measuring teamwork and patient safety attitudes of high-risk areas. *Nursing Economics, 21*(5), 211–218.

Katzenbach, J. R., & Smith, D. K. (1993). The discipline of teams. *Harvard Business Review, 71*(2), 111–120.

Katzenbach, J. R., & Smith, D. K. (2001). The discipline of teams: A mindbook-workbook for delivering small group performance. New York: John Wiley.

Katzenbach, J. R., & Smith, D. K. (2002). *The wisdom of teams: Creating the high performance organization.* Boston: Harvard Business School Press.

Khurana, S. (2008). Andrew Carnegie quotations. Retrieved May 17, 2008, from http://quotations.about.com/od/stillmorefamouspeople/a/AndrewCarnegie1.htm

Kimball, L., & Eunice, A. (1999). The virtual team: Strategies to optimize performance. *Health Forum Journal, 42*(3), 58–62.

Kirkman, B., Rosen, B., Gibson, C., Tesluck, P., & McPerson, S. (2002). Five challenges to virtual team success: Lessons from Sabre, Inc. *Academy of Management Executives, 16*(3), 67–79.

Manion, J., Lorimer, W., & Leander, W. J. (1996). *Team-based health care organizations: Blueprint for success.* Sudbury, MA: Jones and Bartlett.

Maxwell, J. C. (1998). *The 21 irrefutable laws of leadership: Follow them and people will follow you.* Nashville, TN: Thomas Nelson.

Maxwell, J. C. (2002). *The 17 essential qualities of a team player: Becoming the kind of person every team wants.* Nashville, TN: Thomas Nelson.

McKnight, B., McDaniel, S., & Ehmann, V. (2006). Try point incentives for employee reward and recognition. *Nursing Management, 37*(12), 42–45.

McLaughlin, C., & Kaluzny, A. (2006). *Continuous quality improvement in health care.* Sudbury, MA: Jones and Bartlett.

Montalvo, I. (2007). The national database of nursing quality indicators (NDNQI). *Online Journal of Issues in Nursing, 12*(3), 1–13.

Nelson, B. (2005). *1001 ways to reward employees* (2nd ed.). New York: Workman Publishing Company, Inc.

Nelson, B., & Economy, P. (2003). *Managing for dummies* (2nd ed.). New York: John Wiley.

NYS Governor's Office of Employee Relations. (n.d.). Fundamental team and meetings skills. Stages of team development. Retrieved July 20, 2008, from http://www.goer.state.ny.us/Train/online learning/FTMS/200s1.html

Odegaard Turner, S. (1999). *The nurse's guide to managed care.* Gaithersburg, MD: Aspen.

Outhwaite, R. (2003). The importance of leadership in the development of an integrated team. *Journal of Nursing Management, 11*(8), 371–376.

Peterson, D. (2008a). Ice breaker: If you had a magic wand. Retrieved August 10, 2008, from http://adulted.about.com/od/icebreakers/qt/magicwand.htm

Peterson, D. (2008b). Marooned. Retrieved August 10, 2008, from http://adulted.about.com/od/ice breakers/qt/marooned.htm

Polzer, J. T. (2008). Making diverse teams click. *Harvard Business Review, 86*(7/8), 20–21.

PopEd Toolkit. (2005). Opening exercise and ice breakers. Retrieved August 10, 2008, from http://poped.org/icebreakers.html

Riley-Balzer, J. (2008). *Communication in nursing* (6th ed.). St. Louis: Mosby Elsevier.

Rush University Medical Center: Reduced emergency room visits for elderly patients attributed to virtual health care team approach. (2008, May 26). *Diabetes Week,* 222.

Smith, M. K. (2005). Bruce W. Tuckman: Forming, storming, norming, and performing in groups. *Encyclopedia of Informal Education.* Retrieved May 4, 2008, from http://www.infed.org/thinkers/tuckman.htm

Tuckman, B. (1965). Developmental sequence in small groups. *Psychological Bulletin, 63,* 384–399.

Wallace, P. (2004). *The Internet in the workplace.* New York: Cambridge University Press.

Wiecha, J., & Pollard, T. (2004). The interdisciplinary ehealth team: Chronic care for the future. *Journal of Medical Internet Research, 6*(3).

Xyrichis, A., & Ream, E. (2007). Teamwork: A concept analysis. *Journal of Advanced Nursing, 61*(2), 232–241.

Yoder-Wise, P., & Kowalski, K. (2006). *Beyond leading and managing nursing administration for the future.* St. Louis: Mosby Elsevier.

Chapter 8

Nursing Leadership and Assumptions

Barbara Stevens
Barnum

OUTLINE

Leadership issues or confusion often arise from one's assumptions. That is because assumptions are those stealth things that sneak in, unasked and often unexamined. They are seldom questioned or even identified, and nobody pays much attention to them—at least not until things go wrong.

Historically, one way to be considered a leader in nursing is to be a nurse manager. Because of this, nursing has always had some confusion over who its leaders are and who its managers are. Sometimes both roles coincide in the same nurse leader. Vice presidents of nursing in practice organizations and deans of colleges or schools of nursing are examples of how these roles may be combined because the nurse leaders in these positions are often required to be both nurse managers and leaders. Positional leadership extends downward to head nurses and

department chairs. These nurses also have a great opportunity to exercise leadership, if they have vision and the ability to convert vision into action. Conversely, there are managers who provide little leadership, who have formal titles but who might simply be called functionaries. They fill job descriptions without really leading anyone anywhere.

For the purposes of the rest of this chapter, I seldom differentiate between leaders and managers. My case studies involve nurse leaders in executive positions. Similarly, I refer to all models as leadership models, whether they specifically concern leadership or other aspects of management, for example, administration or organization.

Nursing has a long history of seeing around the next corner through the eyes of leadership models created in the business literature. Insofar as nursing delivery of care and education are business, this has served nursing well. Often, not-so-original leaders are perceived to be out in front as they reiterate the latest theories to come down from various business schools and apply them to nursing.

It is clear, however, that some business models are a better fit for nursing than are others. Some of those models include the following:

- An individual delivery point
- A personal one-to-one interface with patients
- A complex delivery environment
- A continually changing technology
- A continuous threat from diverse alternate professions and occupational groups
- A need to serve patients in distress

Nursing also takes place in an environment that requires much negotiation (and therefore good interpersonal skill are vital) with other delivery groups and patients.

In the history of nursing leadership, the adaptations from the business literature have been relatively predictable. As a new and popular model arises in business, we adopt and adapt it. We have applied and evaluated everything from management by objectives to transformational leadership to research-oriented practice. In essence, when a model acquires a certain level of acceptance in business, nursing is likely to adapt it. Some adaptations from business clearly are management models, while others are leadership models (in a more limited sense). The application of a model in nursing is often burdened with assumptions that the model is clear or adaptable.

Assumptions and Leadership Case Study 1

The subject matter, the effect of assumptions on leadership, is presented in case studies. My first case study has to do with a natural nurse leader who suffered from a lack of knowledge of all management models.

I was asked to consult with a nurse leader who found herself in a crisis situation. This was a leader who, almost single-handedly, brought into existence an organization devoted to public and professional education concerning serious health conditions. She worked tirelessly to find donors for start-up monies; she wooed major public figures on to the board of directors; she planned fund-raising events; and she got commitments from exciting speakers who could stimulate membership growth.

This leader had a sparkling personality, drive and motivation, and an enormous capacity for problem solving in bringing the organization into existence. In essence, she created a big, successful organization primarily by her own effort. As she reported to me, aside from her family, this organization was the most important thing in her life. This nurse leader had what I call a creative personality. Her approach to building anything, in this case, an organization, was to get involved in all aspects of growth, balancing all the activities required, never dropping the ball. She brought the organization from an idea to a major corporation with a president and a management staff, an operational staff equal to the objectives of the organization, and a prestigious board of directors, of which she was a member.

Then, suddenly her world fell apart. Twice in rapid succession, the organization's president spoke to her about her being a poor representative for the organization. He reprimanded her for causing trouble and upsetting important staff members. On a third meeting, he informed her that he had enough board support to remove her from the executive board when her term was up at the end of the year.

This is when she called me in for consultation. She was virtually unable to understand how such a thing could have happened. After all, it was the organization that she began. She had spent the best part of five years of her life bringing it into existence. She assumed her place on the board of directors would go on in perpetuity. She was stunned by such ingratitude and determined to fight to keep her place in the organization.

On hearing this, I recognized a familiar scenario, one that has played out in many organizations. She could not believe that the president (whom she had helped to select) would do this to her. The president, as she described him, was a radically different type of leader than she was. Indeed, he had what I often call the "seamstress personality." My vision of this type of leadership likens it to that of sewing a patchwork quilt. Each element, or square, has its own purpose, its own function in the overall pattern; someone heads each element with accountability for that function. The organization was large by this time, and the president had designed a well-functioning pattern of interfaces. He was a good seamstress; the pieces fit together seamlessly.

I helped the founder examine the instances where he called her a poor representative of the organization. In one incident, she had an opportunity for an important interview in a major newspaper. The reporter was an old friend she had cultivated early in the creation of the organization. In the second incident, she had convinced a major celebrity to speak at the next upcoming fund-raiser. These activities, in her eyes, were major victories for the organization. In her mind, she was doing what she had always done for the organization: building, building, building. However, the president insisted that she had stepped on the toes of the Vice President for Public Relations and that she had done the same to the Vice President for Events Planning. Hardly understanding why, she apologized to these individuals. She did so but could not comprehend how she was wrong. In her thinking, she had access to major players that these vice presidents could not approach.

One could, of course, propose that the president had narrow vision and was failing to appreciate what benefits the founder was able to contribute. However, his thinking was exactly what one would expect from a seamstress personality. The problem involved several steps from a consultant's point of view. First, I had to bring the founder to see that the broad ranging creative functions, so essential in a young and growing organization, assumed a different flavor in a large, mature organization. She had given no thought to the notion that the organization might have changed over time, and she resisted this reality. It was difficult for her to accept that her organization had, as organizations do, metamorphosed and grown into a different entity.

When we looked at her assets (as she wanted to do) in preparing a challenge to the threat to remove her from the board of directors (BOD), we discovered several hard facts. First, given the way she originally set up the donation system, she maintained no control of the resources that came into the organization. Similarly, in structuring the BOD and its policies, she had made no rules that would ensure her ongoing reappointment. In fact, in her creative efforts, she gave no thought to even the possibility that she might need to protect any aspects of her ownership.

We looked at the policy by which the BOD voted members in and out and realized that she was vulnerable to a simple majority vote. When I asked, she had no idea who might vote for or against her reappointment. The president said he had the necessary votes against her. She had not even questioned whether this might be a reality. I introduced her to the concept of assessing votes before the election. She said she would canvass members as best she could before the vote. I explained that she needed to assess this immediately to work toward gaining support of BOD voters. I also explained to her the need to avoid creating further organization turf battles.

She was confused about the outcome regarding the newspaper interview. Her reasoning for accepting the interview had to do with the ultimate good of the organization. How could, for example, a good interview in a major newspaper be bad for the organization? Her thought process, like those of any creative-type person, was focused on the good of the organization as a whole, not on its internal parts. I had to help her see that the organization had changed and its needs were no longer those reflected in start-up functioning. It was difficult for her to understand that, although she might be correct concerning the final outcome of the interview, she couldn't overlook internal effects on the organization itself. For her, this sort of thinking was like learning a foreign language.

Eventually, we talked about her place on the BOD and how she would have to change her leadership type; she could no longer be an autocratic leader and ride "roughshod" over assigned managers. We talked about the difficulty of playing from one's weaknesses rather than one's strengths and that she would have to do two things: she would have to exert political pressure to keep her post and she would have to change her leadership style. I encouraged her to think about the possibility of adopting a new cause, of using her creative strength for another start-up venture, especially when I felt the depth of her resistance to changing her leadership style.

The lack of basic knowledge of organizational and leadership theory had made her vulnerable to major mistakes. Yet this kind of behavior is typical of many creative types caught up with the acts of initiating a "great cause." Understanding theory of organizations and leadership behaviors would have prepared her for what happened. At least she could have learned cautionary steps, perhaps clearing her activities with appropriate department heads.

She could still act in a way that would help her cause, but she would have to back up and learn a new style of leadership, or she could capitalize on her natural style of leadership—however, it would probably have to be in a different organization, at a different stage of growth.

What is the message of this case study? Here was a charismatic and effective creative leader who was instinctively successful at what she did. Her style was perfect for *creating* an organization. Yet her performance was uninformed by a knowledge of either organization structuring or leadership styles. She might talk about the ingratitude of the organization; she might talk about the unfairness of casting aside the organization founder, and all of this is true. However, knowing this changes nothing. Neither is that pattern unique to this one situation. Ironically, she was a victim of her own success; the larger she enabled the organization to grow, the more she was bound to clash with a team of managers who had a different definition of success. It never occurred to her that different assumptions underlie different definitions of success.

Instinctive leadership is good; informed leadership is enduring. This case demonstrates the delicate intermix of leadership theory and organization theory. They can be studied separately, but, as this case demonstrates, problems arise in the way they intermix in real cases. This nurse leader, despite building a growing organization, assumed that nothing would change: her skills would be valued forever. This clearly did not occur.

Assumptions and Leadership Case Study 2

In this case study, we see a different type of leadership failure. In this scenario, the nurse leader failed to examine her assumptions and was ineffective in assessing the organization. In this case, in contrast to the first case, the nurse was inundated with theory, but that fact itself became an obstacle.

In this situation, a nurse vice president (NVP) in a community hospital in a suburb of a large northern city had come to her current position from a successful career managing a nurse-run wellness clinic in the West. She was appointed to a new position as NVP with a much larger local organization. This was essentially her first role in a relatively big hospital.

The nurse leader assessed that the staff in her new position had great stability, probably because they preferred local employment to going into the city. The average age of her head nurses was 45 years old. A large proportion of

the head nurses and staff had graduated from a local diploma school that had been out of existence for 20 years. However, half of the head nurses had completed their Bachelor of Science degree. The other half had been grandfathered into their position.

The previous Director of Nursing (DON) was never given the NVP title and had completed a bachelor's degree in health administration. She retired after having been in her role for 30 years. Hospital administration and the physicians admired her and hoped the new NVP would be as effective as her predecessor. The staff had been very loyal to the DON, so the new NVP was particularly glad that the DON had retired and had not merely stepped down. Patient care was excellent and new staff projects included cross training of nursing aides so that they could work effectively on two different units and a project to start a nursing advisory committee to review the Departmental Procedures and Practices manual.

Prior to this appointment, in her previous role, the new NVP was most proud of building a staff of nurse practitioners who functioned independently with their patients and in close collegial relationships. Much of their practice dealt with holistic care measures such as therapeutic touch, visualization, sound therapy, Rolfing and craniosacral therapy, aromatherapy, psychotherapy, and nutrition counseling, among others. The practice was popular, productive, and financially profitable.

This nurse leader had a very special interest in spirituality and had used the Beck and Cowan (Spiral Dynamics) model (Beck & Cowan, 1996). Following early work by Graves, Beck and Cowan described a spiral dynamic of ascending management/environment styles that spoke to ever-increasing levels of humanism and ultimately spirituality. They labeled these styles as memes, constellations that speak to interaction between philosophy and environment, in other words, the psych-cultural DNA of the managerial systems. Each of these eight meme systems represents a philosophic way of seeing the world, a collection of compatible elements, a valuing system, a description of psychological reality, and the way in which a leader thinks and operates with that system. Beck and Cowan arranged these meme systems in hierarchy, where each higher meme shows a more developed sense of ethics and, in the higher ones, spirituality. For simplicity, a color scheme was added to differentiate levels of development.

The new NVP operated within the green and yellow memes in her old group. The green meme values included the well-being of the group and building of consensus. Members of this meme strive to feel accepted by their peers, to share and participate rather than compete. They seek peace for the inner self, with caring and reconciliation dominant. The yellow meme provides for flexible and knowledge-based operations. Function and competency are more important than rank; people do the things that fit with their natural talents. These meme values had been particularly important to the nurse leader in her original practice, a system primarily staffed by holistic nurse practitioners.

When asked about her management style during her job interview for the position of NVP, this nurse leader said that she ran the practice on business models that included sensitivity to human needs and spiritual elements, more specifically the green and yellow memes of the Beck and Cowan model. This got nods from the team that interviewed her, probably because they knew little or nothing about the Beck and

Cowan model. The NVP assumed that she was signaling to the interviewers her commitment to high levels of organizational design, focusing on spiritual values.

When she began the new job, the first thing that she noted was a tendency of staff, even of her supervisors and head nurses, to check everything with her before doing it. If she had measured it on the Beck and Cowan scale, she would say that there were too many behaviors down in the red meme, where the leader keeps all the power and has control over the rewards and punishments of others (Beck & Cowan, 1996). Or perhaps the blue meme, where the focus is on service, duty, and punishment for failing to follow the rules, that is, the one right way, the meme where loyalty and tradition are most important. She vowed to change this behavior for staff to act independently.

In her previous practice out West, nurses thrived on this level of freedom. Carefully, she designed her management behaviors to direct this new group toward the same level of independence. For example, when they asked for direction, she would tell them to make their own decisions. She was aiming for yellow meme behaviors. Staff needed to position more of their practice on a knowledge basis, and she needed to make them realize that function and competency were more important than rank was. Based on Beck and Cowan's work, she believed people were happier when they did the things that fit with their natural talents.

As she got to know the staff, she appointed several staff nurses to head important committees (most of which were newly created by her). The managers needed to learn that a head nurse or a supervisor might be a better committee member than a leader. Some of their young staff nurses began to thrive with the changes, but the head nurses and supervisors were slow to make the changes. There came a day when this NVP was shocked to find herself out of a job without notice. This occurred just when she was starting to build a spirit of group membership among some of the younger nurses. She was amazed when the organization president said she was showing no leadership, leaving her mangers immobilized, unable to move, with no direction.

This woman was out of her position with no time for a consultant, no way to fight back. What she shares with the leader in the first case study in this chapter is a sense of righteous indignation, a sense that what she was doing for the organization was the "right thing." Yet, where the leader in Case Study 1 failed to understand organization theory, this leader overestimated what a theory could do in the abstract. She failed in assessing her environment. Because her preferred philosophy had worked beautifully in the previous environment, she assumed it would be good in the new setting. Not a good assumption in this case!

She failed to assess that her new staff, particularly her managers, were used to highly hierarchal structure where all orders came down from the top. The environment, the philosophy, all came from the blue meme level at best—the level that rewards loyalty, tradition, and following the rules, especially the rules of the leader. Where she thought she was setting them free to do creative management by functioning at a higher meme, she was actually casting them free, but without an anchor. Her managers also had their assumptions about what made up good management. Their assumptions and her assumptions weren't even close.

In any system, one can probably find a mixture of memes, with change taking place toward a higher level of development. Although the meme system is not illustrated here in all its complexity, it is an important system in that it changes the assumptions underlying each level and type of management. It shows that philosophy and environment are inextricably mixed. Its advantage is that many things that are normally invisible (assumed and not questioned) are specified in this example and shown to have great influence on the outcomes. If, for example, the leader recognizes what behaviors a system rewards, the leader can adapt or even challenge the system more effectively. This is particularly important if the leader wants to foster change. You can't change something that you don't understand.

In the situation in Case Study 2, the NVP's zeal for a set of values is an example of false assumptions that led her to believe that the values she espoused would be equally important to her new staff. This mistake ignored the normative standards in this organization. She failed to consider staff expectations. She should have considered the degree to which this staff operated because of the top-down highly directive style of the previous director. The situation is a clear example of the old adage that leadership has to involve the second half of the dyad, the followership. There is no leader without a following. There are some basic things one can say about any leader in relationship to their followers. First, someone too far ahead of the would-be followers may be called a visionary, but usually much later on, perhaps when that person is deceased! Someone with such advanced insight seldom becomes a leader because the followers cannot keep up with him or her.

The motto for 21st-century leadership is to have vision for the near future first, with the far future to follow. What this realistically means is that the leader has to be ahead of the followers, but not too far ahead.

This NVP was attempting to move her staff from a very low level meme to a very high level meme without any consideration of whether they were capable of or prepared for such a radical shift. The NVP tried to move them from crawling to dancing without any of the steps in between. Her vision was too advanced for where this group was in the here-and-now.

This case shows what happens when one is committed to certain goals without a clear recognition of the present state of those who will be affected. The NVP simply assumed this new staff could follow where she led.

Summary

These cases are examples of how assumptions may defeat leadership. In most cases, the following are important factors for the leader to consider:

- *The environment.* The organizational environment is particularly important. How is the organization structured? What are the hidden messages (assumptions) beneath this structuring?
- *The followers.* In the case of organizations, the followers will be barriers—staff members, individuals, and groups. What are their respective values? What do they see as their best interest?
- *The power brokers.* Who in the organization or environment controls important resources? Who has the power to make decisions? How do they feel about these

powers? For example, do they see themselves as stewards of the organization or as important people with control over others? What are the motivations and values on which they act?
- *Oneself.* What is driving me? What makes me vulnerable to ignoring messages from other domains? What values and beliefs do I hold? Do I assume that others are like me or different?

Because it is impossible to check every pertinent assumption, we've created phrases to stand for a good assessor: common sense, good instincts, horse sense—that one calls up crazy images—and a good business head. Some people simply are better than others are at knowing which assumption to examine. However, here are some clues. The next time you have to analyze a situation, take the preceding categories and systemically scan them. Use the negative approach to capture the elusive assumptions. Ask, for example, what is the very worst the organization could do to me if it turned nasty? Ask the same question about every power broker. What would he do to thwart my goals? Then, ask what if I did the dumbest thing possible? What would it be? What would happen if I tread on toes? The negative sometimes gives more insightful answers than the positive. Negatives are trick questions that provide warnings that you might miss otherwise.

Beware of the things you love in your work; they give a dangerous pull and a skewed perspective. Look at the two case studies as an example: the first nurse leader loved her organization, and she could not let go. The second nurse leader loved a theory so much that she could not see the nature of the followers.

QUESTIONS

1. Nurse Jones refuses to take on a nurse manager role in her hospital because Nurse Jones knows that
   a. management and leadership can never be considered as one entity
   b. she has good leadership skills and will not be able to advance in the organization
   c. she may have good management skills, but she does not have leadership skills
   d. she has no management skills, although she is a good leader

2. Important factors that a leader must consider when in a leadership position are
   a. the environment and the followers
   b. the followers and the power brokers
   c. the power brokers and oneself
   d. All of the above

3. Much of how nursing leadership operates is
   a. dependent on an industrial model
   b. built upon a business model
   c. original and unique to nursing
   d. not organized

4. It is important for the nurse leader in an organization to be aware of
   a. how the structure of the organization changes to function within its boundaries
   b. changes that occur in the organization that do not precipitate changes in the nurse's role
   c. the environment in which the nurse works
   d. the role of the nurse leader in specific situations

5. The application of a new model in nursing is often burdened with the
   a. reality of the model
   b. appropriateness of the application
   c. newness of the model
   d. clarity of the new model

References

Barnum, B. (1999). *Teaching nursing in the era of managed care*. New York: Springer.

Beck, D. E., & Cowan, C. C. (1996). *Spiral dynamics: Mastering values, leadership and change*. Oxford, UK: Blackwell Publishing.

Dossey, B. M. (1997). *Core curriculum for holistic nursing*. Gaithersburg, MD: Aspen.

Dossey, B. M., Keegan, L., & Guzzettta, C. E. (2000). *Holistic nursing: A handbook for practice* (3rd ed.). Gaithersburg, MD: Aspen.

Tonges, M. (Ed.). (1998). *Clinical integration: Strategies and practices for organized delivery systems*. San Francisco: Jossey-Bass.

Chapter 9

Time Management and Critical Thinking

Marilyn Klainberg

OUTLINE

Time Management
    Strategies for Effective Time Management

Critical Thinking Skills

Time Management

The term *time management* refers to how we manage time in our personal and work lives. Good time management is how effectively and efficiently we use our time. Procrastination, spending excessive time on a project, or wasting time are examples of poor time management. However, that being said, there are times when what might be interpreted as misspending time actually may be appropriate to a situation, even if it is viewed as not being productive. There are occasions when it may appear that we are wasting our time, but in those moments we may need to be less productive to accomplish a greater goal. An example of this is sitting and talking with a patient, and although this may seem less productive at the moment (only if this

is not neglecting another patient or causing another patient harm), this time spent may be more productive in the overall care of the patient with whom you're spending the extra time. The constant act of doing "something" noticeable may not be as productive as taking a quiet moment with a patient. Taking a few moments for oneself may not seem productive, but if you need to refresh your body and spirit, it may be time well spent. Taking time for yourself helps to discourage burnout.

Burnout is the term that refers to an emotional or psychological condition that occurs when stress causes you to feel or become emotionally exhausted. Burnout is usually considered to be related to work. It can come from doing the same job for long periods of time or stress related to chronic disorganization.

Organizing your time helps to combat burnout. Symptoms of burnout range from physical exhaustion to mild fatigue to sometimes flu-like symptoms and emotional turmoil.

Managing and balancing your workload can also be helpful in deterring burnout. Burnout can cause your problems to seem overwhelming and you may become unable to function and to do the job that needs to be done. This is true in relationship to work, as well as in your personal life (Smith, Jaffe-Gill, Segal, & Segal, 2007).

As a student, you already have some skills concerning time management. You have been successful in managing your time being a student. You have had to learn to manage time for study and class preparation, time for your family, socialization, and to make decisions on prioritizing the importance of the demands on you and how much time to devote to them. Some of you have juggled school, work, and family obligations while being a student. This is good practice for your first job, which will require you to manage not only your personal time, but also work and how you care for patients. These decisions will affect the care you provide your patients, and if you are stressed from one part of your life, it will influence the other parts. If you are exhausted because you have not planned your time well, you may not be able to provide safe care to your patients.

To get hold of how you handle your time, you must first begin to understand your own work habits. You also must know something about your physical needs. This includes eating, fluid intake, and sleep cycles (your circadian rhythms). You must honestly look at how your time is currently being spent. Learn to prioritize, and develop goals. When caring for patients, prioritizing may be easier because

often patient needs are clear. In developing goals, it is important to explore long- and short-term goals in relationship to prioritization needs. Factors that interfere with time management despite good planning and prioritization in the workplace can include unexpected interruptions, excessive paperwork, red tape, and meetings. Sometimes poor communication and disharmony with co-workers can interfere with getting the job done.

Time orientation may affect your management of time. Much of time orientation is related to culture, society, and environment (Schein, 1996). Time orientation refers to the way we view time, and it varies in different cultures (Spector, 2004). Some cultures are future-oriented, and others tend to more present-oriented. Members of future-oriented cultures are more concerned with long-range planning and issues of prevention than present-oriented believers. Someone who is future-oriented will set up appointments in advance and plan activities, such as the trip to the physician's office. A present-oriented person is more spur-of-the-moment and may not be on time for an appointment or even plan ahead to make an appointment. The care we give our patients is extremely tied to time management and orientation, and so we must be aware of the different ways in which our patients manage their time. Therefore, particularly in the workplace and in your professional life, time management must supersede an individual's time orientation.

Time management strategies include prioritization of events. Nurses must be high achievers to give the best patient care possible. In managing your time, you must consider appropriate delegation of work and working with teams. Chapter 7 discusses teamwork in greater depth.

Strategies for Effective Time Management

Following are several strategies you can use to help manage your time effectively:

- Planning is of the utmost importance to managing your time efficiently.
- Establish what needs to be done and when it needs to be done.
- Set long- and short-term goals.
- When appropriate, learn to delegate.
- Learn to ask for help from your peers, nurse manager, or nursing assistants.
- Set priorities for urgent and nonurgent care.
- Become aware of how long things take to do because this is helpful for you as well as if you delegate work to someone else.
- Remember that time communication is important to those with whom you work and to the patient. Let everyone know your time frame. Miscommunication in time communication can slow up how you get your work done.
- In planning for the care you will provide, gather materials and arrange them so that you can proceed without stopping and starting to collect items. Starting and stopping during care can be a major time-waster.
- Learn to set boundaries. Setting boundaries mean to learn to say *no* when you are overburdened with work.
- Be prepared for change. Things change all of the time when it comes to patient care, so have an alternative plan.
- Make a list of tasks and cross off items accomplished as you do them.

- Utilize your critical thinking skills when planning your time management.
- Delegate appropriately. (See Chapter 12 on delegation.)
- Hone and develop good critical thinking skills.

Critical Thinking Skills

Critical thinking skills consist of being able to analyze and evaluate issues, situations, and notions to form a judgment that connects evidence or fact with common sense. Critical thinking can be described as your ability to make reflective or reasonable choices or decisions. Gaberson and Oermann (1999) refer to critical thinking as a process in problem solving. It may require you to reflect upon concrete reality or intangible information.

Critical thinking skills, in addition to analysis, depend upon reasoning and evaluation. Critical thinking skills are an important part of management skills. Critical thinkers gather information from a variety of places that may include observation, personal or professional experience, and formal education and then use this information and apply it to make decisions about the known and unknown. Critical thinking is a complex and ongoing process and actually is not a skill whose ideas can be taught or memorized. It is a reflective process. It requires you to be open and thoughtful without prejudicial preconceptions (Porter O'Grady & Malloch, 2007).

In nursing, we are required to use our critical thinking skills on a daily basis. We are called upon to use problem-solving skills, and without the ability to think critically we may not make the best choices. According to Paul and Elder (2003), there are eight elements in the process of critical thinking:

1. The purpose of the thinking
2. The actual problem to be resolved
3. The assumptions upon which the thinking is based
4. How one analyzes his or her own point of view and other points of view
5. The data or evidence
6. Theories upon which the thinking is based
7. How the data is weighed
8. The consequence of the reasoning

A person with good critical thinking skills must be an independent thinker, must be a self-directed learner, and must be able to reevaluate and self-correct decisions made (Paul & Elder, 2003).

A person with good critical thinking skills does the following:

- Raises critical questions
- Gathers relevant information
- Keeps an open mind when pondering an issue, looks at all sides of an issue
- Communicates well with others in determining solutions to problems (Paul & Elder, 2003)
- Is a *very* good listener

Listening skills are a very important part of communication. It does no good to think through something without listening and clarifying ideas and by asking critical questions. Being a good listener is the first step in becoming a good critical thinker. You must also be in touch with the impact of critical decisions that are made, by your own values, societal demands, and personal bias.

Summary

Good time management is how effectively and efficiently we use our time. How we manage time in our personal and work lives affects what we accomplish. It is important to be in touch with how you handle your time. To be in touch with this, you must first begin to understand yourself; you need to understand your physical and emotional needs because they affect how you work.

An important component of time management is how we utilize our critical thinking skills. Time management, being able to prioritize, and the ability to think critically are important aspects of successful career development.

QUESTIONS

1. The nurse manager on a busy medical unit is feeling overwhelmed with work and feels this may be related to a lack of good time management. To begin to work on time management skills, the nurse should first
   a. arrange for a 3-week vacation in Hawaii
   b. ask nurses from other units to share some of the workload
   c. begin to attempt to understand herself and how she works
   d. ask the nurse educator to evaluate the unit

2. Which step can improve time management?
    a. Plan one's day
    b. Be prepared for change
    c. Make a list of tasks for the day
    d. All of the above

3. Critical thinking skills are
    a. one's ability to make reflective or reasonable choices or decisions
    b. getting the work done on time
    c. the ability to delegate the work to others
    d. one's ability to get the work done correctly in a relaxed manner

4. Good critical thinkers
    a. can be trusted to find solutions to all situations
    b. always make the correct decision
    c. are always good leaders
    d. are able to analyze and evaluate situations

5. Critical thinking is one's ability to
    a. make reasonable choices or decisions about a situation
    b. lead a group into a successful experience
    c. move forward in one's choices to success
    d. find solutions to every problem encountered in a situation

References

Gaberson, K. A., & Oermann, M. H. (1999). *Clinical teaching strategies in nursing education*. New York: Springer.

Murray, J. S. (2008). No more nurse abuse. *American Nurse Today, 3*(7), 17–19.

Oermann, M. H., & Gaberson, K. A. (2006). *Evaluation and testing in nursing education* (2nd ed.). New York: Springer.

Paul, R., & Elder L. (2003). The miniature guide to critical thinking: Concepts and tools. *Foundation for Critical Thinking*. Retrieved November 4, 2008, from http://www.criticalthinking.org/files/Concepts_Tools.pdf

Porter O'Grady, T., & Malloch, K. (2007). *Quantum leadership: A resource for health care innovation* (2nd ed.). Sudbury, MA: Jones and Bartlett.

Schein, E. H. (1996). *Organizational culture and leadership* (2nd ed.). San Francisco: Jossey–Bass.

Smith, M., Jaffe-Gill, E., Segal, J., & Segal, R. (2007). Preventing burnout. *HelpGuide.org*. Retrieved November 4, 2008, from http://www.helpguide.org/mental/burnout_signs_symptoms.htm

Spector, R. E. (2004). *Cultural diversity in health and illness* (6th ed.). Upper Saddle River, NJ: Prentice Hall.

Chapter 10

Your First Job: Ready, Set, Go: You Have Graduated, Now What?

Marilyn Klainberg

OUTLINE

Licensure and the NCLEX

After graduation from a nursing program, to practice nursing and to become licensed as a registered professional nurse you must take and pass the National Council Licensure Examination–Registered Nurse (NCLEX). All states and territories in the United States require nursing school graduates to take the NCLEX to practice as a licensed professional nurse. The NCLEX is a standardized examination that aims to measure test takers' knowledge and capabilities of practicing safely at an entry level.

The NCLEX is a computerized adaptive test (CAT). The CAT tests new graduates at an entry-level nursing competency. CAT testing uses item response theory, which is different from classical test theory (Oermann & Heinrich, 2004). The CAT decreases test length and improves reliability (Gershon & Bergstrom, 1991). Each test taker is compared with passing standards to determine whether the individual passed or failed the examination (Julian, Wendt, Way, & Zara, 2001). The CAT is designed to measure mastery of a subject and may vary in length for each test taker. It adapts to the test taker's knowledge and skills. CAT adjusts the questions based on the test taker's response. If the test taker answers a question correctly, the level of difficulty of the examination increases (Bushweller, 2000). With each correct response, the number of questions is then decreased. Therefore, not all questions on the CAT are the same, and neither do all test takers have the same number of questions to answer (Oermann & Heinrich, 2004). The NCLEX CAT can take up to 4 hours to complete. The test is given only in English.

All questions developed for the NCLEX are validated by practicing nurses, educators, and regulators from throughout the country. The content of the NCLEX is reviewed and edited every three years. For the most part, the examination is a multiple-choice examination, but during the past few years fill-in-the-blank questions and graphic response questions, which require the student to identify a response to a graphic image, have been added.

To become licensed as a registered nurse by all of the Boards of Nursing in the United States, candidates are required to pass the NCLEX, which is managed through the National Council of State Boards of Nursing (NCSBN). To find your board of nursing go to the following Web site: https://www.ncsbn.org/boards.htm. The NCSBN is a not-for-profit organization whose membership is made of the Boards of Nursing of all 50 states, the District of Columbia, and territories of the United States.

Passing scores may vary from state to state. Reciprocity is granted to nurses who move from one state to another in that they may receive a license to practice in their new state by application without having to retake the licensing examination. Military nurses and nurses employed by the Veterans Administration are not required to reapply for a new license even if they are working in another state. Presently, many states either already have or will have collaborative agreements to allow nurses to work without requiring an additional license. This is referred to as compact agreements.

Preparation for Taking the NCLEX-RN Examination

Begin studying for the NCLEX-RN as soon as you graduate. There are several computer programs that you can use to prepare for your examination, or you can enroll in one of the commercial NCLEX-RN preparation courses available. Whichever you do, practice by answering as many test questions as you can. Practice answering test questions on the computer because that can increase your comfort level with taking the examination online and reading questions from a computer screen.

Next, you must send in an application to the board of licensure (your state's Board of Nurses). The forms are available on the Internet or you may request to have them mailed to you. Complete the forms and return them with certified checks. Your school must send in proof of your graduation from an approved nursing program.

Next schedule to take the exam with Pearson VUE. The National Council of State Boards of Nursing has collaborated with Pearson VUE to deliver the NCLEX. Pearson VUE is the official provider of the NCLEX-RN examination. You will be sent an authorization to test and a time to take the NCLEX-RN (NCLEXinfo.com, 2008).

You are required to bring two forms of identification to be allowed to take the NCLEX-RN. Be prepared to take the NCLEX-RN as soon as you can. The longer you wait after graduation, the poorer your chances of passing the NCLEX-RN. If you initially fail the exam, you can retake the NCLEX-RN, but there is a fee for each additional examination.

Temporary Permits

In most states and territories, temporary, limited permits are available for new graduates who are waiting to take the NCLEX-RN. This is dependent upon the policies of the individual states and places of employment. You *must* apply for a temporary permit through your state's Board of Nursing. To acquire a permit to practice as an RN, you must be a graduate of an approved school of nursing and must be under the supervision of a professional nurse who is registered and has permission of the agency by which she or he is employed. A limited permit is good for one year.

Requirements for a License as a Registered Professional Nurse

To practice as a registered professional nurse in most states in the United States you must fulfill the following requirements:

- Be of good moral character
- Graduate from a nursing program (either with a degree in professional nursing or a diploma in nursing)
- Be at least 18 years of age
- Meet educational requirements

- Complete coursework or training in the identification and reporting of child abuse that is offered by an approved provider
- Pass the NCLEX-RN

Fees

Fees are charged for your original and continuing licenses and a fee is charged to take the NCLEX. These fees change from state to state. You are also charged a fee for limited permits. Fees are subject to change. The fee is due when your application is received. If fees are increased retroactively, you will be billed for the difference.

Do not send cash to pay for fees. And remember to make your personal check or money order payable to your state's Education Department. Your canceled check is your receipt.

Verifying Education Credentials from Non-U.S. Programs

Registered professional nurses who have completed their RN education outside of the United States must have their education credentials verified by the Commission on Graduates of Foreign Nursing Schools (CGFNS International, 2008).

Contact CGFNS at:
The Commission on Graduates of Foreign Nursing Schools (CGFNS)
PO Box 8628
Philadelphia, PA 19101-8628
Phone: (215) 349-8767

Choosing Your First Job

You've graduated and passed the NCLEX—*now what?*

Choosing your first job is important. The job market is vast, and choosing where you want to be in 10 years may not be on your mind right now, but do consider the fact that you may not want to remain in the area you first choose. Your initial job goal may change as well as your needs. My first job was exactly what I thought I wanted; however, after a little more than a year I realized that the job did not meet my professional goals and personal needs. I needed to change and grow in my career goals. So, the benefit of being a nurse generalist kicked in. I tried several areas, from medical surgical nursing to obstetrical nursing. Then, by chance and simply because of need, I answered an advertisement to become a community health nurse in an outpatient clinic. I found that I enjoyed this and thought I found what I like to do! I went back for my master's degree in community health and tried teaching. I fell in love with teaching and have been a nurse educator and university administrator ever since. That being said, the following are some tips to acquiring your first job.

First, explore what is available in the area you wish to become employed. Then, after selecting several places where you would like to be employed, find out about each agency; read its mission and philosophy statement to determine whether there is a match between your goals and the goals of the agency. Does the hospital have Magnet status? (See Box 10-1.)

As you choose the hospital/health agency you wish to work in, and the position you would like, also consider the opportunities available for your further education, the support of nursing leadership of the roles and responsibilities of the professional nurse, and the opportunities you would have to participate in nursing governance.

Oh, the places you'll go!

—Geisel, *Oh, the Places You'll Go!*

Most new graduates consider bedside nursing as their only option. Bedside nursing is a great choice, but be aware that nursing offers many opportunities for you to plan your career path and your future. You may initially choose an

---

Box 10-1 Magnet Status

Magnet status refers to hospitals that have been identified by the American Nurses Credentialing Center (ANCC), an affiliate of the American Nurses Association, as meeting the standards of providing quality patient care. These standards measure the strength and quality of their nursing.

"A Magnet hospital is stated to be one where nursing delivers excellent patient out-comes, where nurses have a high level of job satisfaction, and where there is a low staff nurse turnover rate and appropriate grievance resolution" (Center for Nursing Advocacy, 2008).

Source: Center for Nursing Advocacy. (2008). What is Magnet status and how's that whole thing going? Retrieved November 4, 2008, from http://www.nursingadvocacy.org/faq/magnet.html

area, and as your career grows you might change to another career within nursing. Remember, you will always take what you learn from each experience and utilize it in the next experience.

Initially, when new graduates think about a first work experience, they consider areas that they have become familiar with during their education, such as working on a medical surgical unit, a pediatric unit, in psychiatry, obstetrics and gynecology, the emergency department, critical care units, or the operating room. However, other areas, such as home care, epidemiology, public health, long-term care, geriatric nursing, palliative/hospice nursing, infection control nursing, nursing in jails with incarcerated populations, forensic nursing, rehabilitation nursing, chemical dependency nursing, occupational nursing, school nursing, technology nursing, military nursing, and more, are available.

You must also think of becoming a lifelong learner and plan initially to pursue continuing education and then higher education. Higher education in nursing is considered advanced practice nursing, which will open doors to a variety of areas such as being a nurse educator, an academic nurse, a nurse researcher, a nurse administrator, a nurse practitioner in a specialty area, a nurse–midwife, a nurse anesthetist, and other roles we have not yet thought of in nursing. You may also choose to get your doctorate in nursing. Each step in your career path enhances the next. The American Nurses Association is now lobbying to make all advanced practice nurses independent practitioners. It has not yet occurred, but this is being considered. This is just at the beginning of your future! See Box 10-2 and Box 10-3 to read how two nurses navigated their career paths.

Box 10-2 Career Choices and Chances

Dawn F. Kilts

As I revisit my professional nursing career, I realize how the choices I made about my education and the positions I have taken have made my progress to a position of leadership, in this case as dean of a major New York school of nursing, an inevitable one for me. In the mid-1960s, I was determined to go to college to be a nurse. Everyone around me told me to go to a diploma program, but I desperately wanted to be the first person in my family to graduate from college. In addition, for some reason still unknown to me, I believed that nursing should be considered a learned profession, and I wanted to be part of

that. I was very lucky to choose an excellent university with a progressive nursing program. My dean later became the Executive Director of the ANA, and she was a subtle force in setting standards for us. As students, it was always expected that we would be a changing force in nursing.

I had worked as a nursing assistant in the ICU of the community hospital in my hometown in upstate New York throughout college. Coincidentally, the night charge nurse of the ICU retired just as I graduated from college. I was offered her job. And, with the hubris of youth and my usual gusto, I took it.

I was working under a permit for several months. I survived, the patients survived, and I learned a lot about management, leadership, and taking responsibilities. One of the funny things I remember is that it was the custom at that time to stand up when the nursing supervisor or a physician came in the room. I never did. I waited every night to be disciplined but never was. After a while, most of the nurses on night shift stopped. I have always had difficulty doing things purely because that's the way they have always been done.

Soon after this I moved to New York City and took a job at a leading cancer hospital. I learned a lot and saw state-of-the-art treatment while I worked there. In retrospect, I find that the longest enduring lesson I learned there was how not to be a good manager. I left that position and took a position as an Assistant Director of Nursing in charge of in-service education at large long-term care facility. Again, this was a bit of a stretch for someone with my limited nursing experience. I loved the job and feel I did a good job. However, I was not destined to stay in a comfortable position. The Director of Nursing became ill and soon resigned, and I became second in command, often running the nursing department by myself. It was challenging, and I had many days when I wanted to run away. I learned patience and persistence there, but I also learned what an adrenaline rush "being the boss" is. I think that was when my future was written.

I moved back to upstate New York for two years after that while my husband (I had gotten married just before moving to New York City) got his master's degree. Luckily, I had

married someone who had assumed I would have whatever career I wanted and has stood by my professional choices for 40 years—not a small thing in those days. I taught in a diploma school during this time and gained my love of teaching. While teaching there I realized I wanted to teach, but on the baccalaureate level. When I returned to New York City, I immediately started my master's degree in nursing at an exciting school where I really learned what it was to think creatively and independently. My years in graduate school were a heady experience. I was surrounded by nursing scholars, leaders, and thinkers. I loved every minute I spent there. I believe that one of the most important things we can do is to surround ourselves with terrific role models and just soak in everything we can. I worked in an inner-city emergency room during the days and went to school at night. Those were very good years.

As I was finishing my master's, I became an adjunct assistant professor at the school where I still work. Upon graduation, I became a full-time faculty member. Immediately, I began the PhD program in nursing at the same school. Somehow, I still haven't gotten around to finishing my dissertation. In fact, I have also completed all the course work for a PhD in education. I have, however, become a certified adult nurse practitioner along the way. My university career has been a very interesting one as I have stayed at the same place for 34 years. Up until the time I became dean seven years ago, I have always had a part-time practice position at the same time. I was a manager in an ER, Assistant Director of Nursing evenings and nights on weekends, co-authored a leading nursing text, and was an adult nurse practitioner at a shelter for homeless addicted men. These jobs not only helped me maintain contact with the current practice setting but also have helped to maintain my sanity. They were an opportunity to do what I had started out to do many years before: be a nurse giving care to patients.

During my years at the university, I have had several different positions in and out of nursing. I have been a faculty member (tenured, full professor), head of the program when we were just a department, director of a campus-wide grant for innovative teaching, director of the graduate programs, and now finally, dean. Ironically, the only position I have held there that I didn't want to take is the one I have now—dean. The higher administration had been pursuing me for 13 years to be dean, but I had avoided it because I liked what I was doing and I felt the dean should have an earned doctorate. I almost lost the chance to do the job I now love more than any I have ever had because I didn't want to face the pressure of not having the same credentials as those around me. I knew I could do it and those around thought I could do it, but I didn't want to move out of my comfort zone. I finally took the position when my provost challenged me by saying that I should put my money where my mouth is. I had always been vocal about what changes I wanted for the School of Nursing, so now was my time to make those changes. My years as dean have been everything I ever have wanted in a job and I almost missed that opportunity because I didn't want to take a chance.

Box 10-3 The Journey

Tara A. Cortes

I started my career as a nurse just after I graduated from Villanova University. I came to the "Big Apple" from a small town in Pennsylvania to work at a prestigious medical center that had a rich heritage in its own diploma school of nursing. After six months at the bedside, I realized I could not be a "charge nurse" or a "team leader" because I did not wear that hospital's "cap." I left for another prestigious medical center where after two years as a bedside nurse in the cardiothoracic ICU, I became the night supervisor for all the critical care areas.

By attending graduate school part-time while working full-time, I completed my master's degree in nursing and decided to take a position as an assistant professor at Hunter College Bellevue School of Nursing in New York City. Simultaneously, I enrolled in the doctoral program in nursing at New York University and completed my PhD in 1976. I was a tenured faculty member at Hunter College for 21 years, and during that time I headed the undergraduate program, was associate dean, and taught in the graduate program.

After 21 years, I felt it was time to do something different and I left my tenured position and took a job as the Director of Research and Information Systems in a large academic medical center in New York. After nine months, there was a large reduction in staff and I and my department were eliminated. I was laid off! I always say that this became the opportunity that shaped the road I have come to travel. After three months, I was appointed as the chief nursing officer at Rockefeller University Hospital. This experience became my internship and residency to nursing and hospital administration. While at Rockefeller, I redesigned the pharmacy and radiology services, reduced the operating budget by 10%, and implemented a model of care using advanced practice nurses. After five years, I was recruited to Mount Sinai Medical Center in New York as the Director of Medicine and Adult Ambulatory Care.

Mount Sinai provided me with an opportunity to work in a very complex system where I grew the role of advanced practice nurses, created a care continuum in geriatrics, and tackled the quickly growing phenomenon of emergency room overcrowding. While at Mount Sinai, I was selected as a Robert Wood Johnson Executive Nurse Fellow, which enabled me to enhance my skills and knowledge and hone my leadership ability. After five years at Mount Sinai, I was recruited to Bridgeport Hospital as the Senior Vice President for Patient Care Services and Chief Nursing Officer.

At Bridgeport Hospital, I created an environment that empowered nurse managers as the CEOs of their units, while managing budget constraints in the ever-changing healthcare system. I was appointed a clinical professor at Yale University School of Nursing—a position I still retain today. When I left Bridgeport Hospital, the nurse managers had a luncheon for me and thanked me for "giving them professionalism."

After three years at Bridgeport Hospital, I received a call from a search firm asking me of my interest in the position of president and chief executive officer at Lighthouse International. Not knowing much about this organization in New York City, I asked to see the specifications of the job. I saw it was everything I had ever done—patient services, research, education, and advocacy all under one roof! I threw my hat in the ring, was one of 16 candidates, and became the new head of Lighthouse International. In the three years I have been here, I have turned around the fiscal position of the organization, changed the paradigm from a social charity to health care, attained financial stability, and developed new programs to meet the needs of the impending epidemic of vision loss in this country related to the aging of America and diabetes. We have created partnerships with other vision organizations nationally and around the globe as we develop a global network structure to affect vision loss.

I serve on the Villanova University Board of Trustees, the New York State Executive Board for the Blind and Visually Handicapped, the board of the International Association for the Prevention of Blindness, and the National Advisory Committee for the RWJ Executive Nurse Fellowship Program.

It has been a wonderful journey, and I always marvel at all the opportunities that I have had because I am a nurse. The breadth of knowledge and the skills of risk taking and decision making can take us from the bedside to the boardroom without ever losing the values of who we are.

Applying for Employment

Send a letter of interest concerning employment (your cover letter) and a copy of your résumé. You may do this regardless of whether you are responding to an advertisement for employment. However, if you are responding to a position that has been advertised or posted on a Web site, read the criteria for employment and refer to your qualifications or interests related to what is contained in the position advertisement.

Résumé Preparation

Prepare your résumé thoughtfully. It represents you and is a tool to sell yourself for the job you want. Several Web sites and computer programs can help you to organize your résumé. Your résumé should be only one page, *unless* you are requested to submit a curriculum vita (CV). A CV is usually long because it is the complete sum of your work and education during your life. Most employers (except for universities and colleges) prefer a résumé. Unless requested, do not send a CV, send a résumé.

Persons reading your résumé should find it clear. It should be prepared on a good stock paper, either off-white or light gray, and should be easy to read. The best font is 12-point size and usually Times New Roman. You can use one of several formats. Most word processing programs have a template for a résumé or you can choose to create one yourself. Many Web sites and books are available on creating your résumé.

Several items must appear on your résumé. There should be a header that gives your contact information: name, address, phone number where you can be reached (preferably one with an answering machine), cell phone number, and e-mail address. Make sure that the telephone number you place in this section has a professional response recorded on it—no cute music or sayings; simply note whose phone is being answered. Your e-mail address should also be professional; no cute names or nicknames. Imagine asking a potential boss to send an e-mail message to bubbleslamour@server.com. Your e-mail address should also reflect your professional persona, so MarySmith@server.com would be more appropriate.

Your recent education should be listed next in chronological order. You do not need to include your high school or elementary school in this section. Year of graduation or completion should accompany your higher education programs. List them all. If you did not graduate, simply put the dates of attendance. Your work history comes next. Your potential employer wants to see that you have a good work record, not only where you worked. If your work history is not related to the health field and you worked for several years in one job, the potential employer will see that you have good, employable work qualities. Professional organizations are listed next and then volunteer positions. Each section should have dates of membership or employment (as appropriate). Each should have its own section that is clearly marked. Figure 10-1 is a list of the items that you should include on your résumé and the order in which they should be set. Figure 10-2 is a sample cover letter.

Portfolio

A portfolio is a purposeful collection of materials that exhibits an individual's work history. It provides evidence of progress and achievements in one or more of the areas in which the individual has worked. The portfolio is simply an alternate method of judging the value of one's work. Although not everything is presented in a portfolio, it should represent a collection of one's best work. It ought to be a sample of work experiences and documents that represent growth and development. A portfolio can be presented electronically or in a folder. It should contain copies of a driver's license, résumé, cer-

---

Figure 10-1 Sample Blank Résumé

Your Name
Street Address
City, State, Zip Code
Phone Number
E-mail Address

Education

Honors

Work Experience

Related Work Experience

Volunteer Experience

Skills (such as second language, computer skills)

Professional Membership

Certification (such as CPR)

Figure 10-2 Sample Cover Letter

Your Address
Date

Name of recipient or contact person
Title
Organization
Address

Dear (*last name and correct title of the contact person*):

I am applying for (*name of the position for which you are applying*). If you heard about this position in an advertisement, state which one and when. If you are sending this out without having seen an advertisement, ask if there is an available opening (if you want a specific area of work, state that here).

Note that a résumé is enclosed.

Tell why you want the position and why you want to work in this institution. If you have any related experiences, include them here.

State your appreciation for this person's consideration of your employment and for taking the time to read this cover letter. Ask for an interview. Refer to your address, e-mail address, and phone number listed above as your contact information.

Sincerely yours,

Your name

tifications (such as CPR, PICC Line, etc.), diplomas, honors, membership in organizations (including an indication of membership—such as a membership card—and any leadership or membership participation), and documentation of any continuing education courses taken.

Portfolios are often used to assess student work and may be requested by employers when applying for a job. Portfolios explore student work, courses taken, actual exhibits of work, and self-reflection. They sometimes also include instructor notes on student work, such as student papers, logs, journals, or group projects.

Interviewing

Your interview is an important part of acquiring your job. First impressions are important. Be calm and be prepared! Before you go for your interview, think about how and what you want to present to the interviewer. Be assertive about your goals, but do not be aggressive. Have an idea of what you want to do, but be ready to think about an alternate experience.

Know about the agency with which you are interviewing. This is extremely important. Go to the agency's Web site or ask for materials to be sent to you prior to your interview. Look at the mission and philosophy of the agency or institution you are applying to and determine whether this is a good match for you. It is impressive to the person interviewing you if, as a professional, you know something about where you have chosen to work. The interviewer is not only looking at whether you are going to be a good employee, but whether you will be someone who will stay with the institution. Often, your retention is determined by what you know about the agency before you begin your employment.

Be prepared to present your work history, even if it is not in the healthcare profession. Talk about your most recent job, especially if it is in the healthcare field. You may also present information about your internship experience. Be prepared to present your strengths and weaknesses. *Never* say that your weakness is that you work too hard! Think about what might be considered a weakness and present it in a positive

manner. You might say, "I am slow at doing some tasks at the bedside, such as *(fill in the blank)*, but know with experience I will improve and get faster at doing this." Know that as a novice nurse you will not be expected to have the skills or the speed at some tasks as an experienced nurse who has been working for many years.

When you receive an appointment for an interview, take the time to plan what you will wear and most important how you will get to the interview. Do a trial run to the interview site on a day and at a time similar to the time of your interview appointment so that you can get an idea of how long the trip will take and the best way to get to the interview. Do it at a similar time of day so that you can account for the traffic and congestion on the roads or public transportation schedules.

Always plan on delays on the day you go for your interview. Leave early and leave enough time for such possible delays. It is better to arrive early for your interview than late. Bring two copies of your résumé with you, even if you have sent one to the agency in advance. Do not chew gum during the interview! Take a deep breath before going into your interview and try to remain calm and relaxed, but not so relaxed that you slouch in your chair. Give a good firm handshake. Keep good eye contact with your interviewer.

DRESSING FOR THE INTERVIEW

Dress conservatively for your interview. Dress for success!

Men should wear a dark suit or sports jacket, shirt (preferably a plain white or light colored one—*not* a sports shirt), a tie, and trousers (not jeans). Hair should be neat and jewelry limited to a watch and wedding band (if applicable). No earrings or nose or tongue jewelry.

Women should wear a dark, simple suit (pants suits are acceptable) or dress. Wear low-heeled shoes. Hair should be neat and worn close to the head, as it would be worn on the job. If your hair is long, put it up in a simple style. Jewelry should be limited to a watch, wedding band (if applicable), and if you wear earrings, they should be small and simple. No facial or tongue jewelry should be worn for the interview.

Behavioral Interviews

Many facilities are adopting behavioral interviewing techniques to find the best match for the job. A behavioral interview is similar to other types of interviews, except that it is more focused on the candidate's previous experience. Unlike a one-to-one interview, a behavioral interview includes an interviewing team of several staff members who ask specific questions. The interviewers are usually staff from a specific unit and a staff member who does not work in that unit but who knows the area or specialty. The questions they ask will be consistent with questions asked of other persons interviewing for a position at the agency.

The interview team will reflect on issues of motivation, delegation experience, communication, and motivation for the job. They will also be interested in your performance and accountability.

WHAT YOU SHOULD KNOW ABOUT BEHAVIORAL INTERVIEWS

Behavioral interviewing is based on the notion that previous job behaviors or experiences determine how well you will do in a new, similar work setting. Based upon research, it is believed that a behavioral interview is a better way to make hiring decisions and increase retention (McKay, 2008).

To prepare yourself for a behavioral interview, think about your past experiences with patients and their families, co-workers, and your manager, and share concrete experiences that describe why these behaviors were important. Prepare a wide range of stories that describe specific examples of your competencies. Also, to prepare for your interview be familiar with the standards of care and the nursing code of ethics.

THE BEHAVIORAL INTERVIEWING PROCESS

The interviewers have a set of questions to ask you. Answers to these questions are scored based on your responses (total score is 100%). After the interview, there is a post conference where the interviewers discuss the candidate and the answer scores given by the interviewers. The final score is totaled. The higher the score, the greater the possibility that the candidate will be hired.

BEHAVIORAL INTERVIEW QUESTIONS

Behavioral interview questions have no right or wrong answers and they allow the candidate to respond to real-life situations or events. The interviewers give the applicant an opportunity to talk about specific examples from their personal experiences or demonstrate their ability to solve problems. The interviewee must know and anticipate specific answers to questions. Most questions will start with "What if . . . ?" or "What has been your experience with . . . ?" or "What has been the most challenging or rewarding or difficult situation(s) when . . . ?"

Remember to listen carefully to the questions and if you are not sure of what is being asked, request clarification. When you respond, take a moment to clarify and organize your thoughts. Speak clearly.

When your interview is complete, the group leader will usually stand, offer you a handshake, and thank you for coming. That is your cue to leave.

To complete your interview, when you arrive at home, write a note of thanks for the interview and send it to the leader of the interview team.

WHAT SHOULD YOU ASK?

Request materials or visit the Web site of an agency at which you think you might be interested in employment. After you have collected information about the agency, become familiar with the mission and philosophy of the institution to see whether they match your goals and philosophy. The Web site or written materials might have further information about employment benefits or perquisites (perks). You may also inquire about benefits when you apply for the job. You may want to know whether the institution pays for continuing education or provides it. Will the institution pay and support you in getting an advanced degree? What are its policies on overtime and is it mandatory? What is the staffing ratio on each unit? Staffing is an important issue and involves the number registered nurses, licensed practical nurses, unlicensed assistive personnel, and others who provide care to patients. The acuity of care needed by each patient is important to determine the numbers of staff needed to provide excellent patient care.

Does the agency or institution have a pension plan or offer health insurance? And if so, what is your share in the cost? You may ask about the salary range, but do not ask about the exact salary until after you get the position!

Mandatory Overtime

Because of the nursing shortage, many hospitals and institutions require mandatory overtime. The American Nurses Association has been lobbying against this because it is an unsafe practice. Nurses working double shifts or nurses who do mandatory overtime are more prone to accidents and making medication errors. Furthermore, many nurses have children, elderly parents, and a spouse or a partner who needs their care and attention. Being conflicted over their responsibility to work and their family has caused tremendous stress on the nurses required to do mandatory overtime. Some states have made mandatory overtime illegal.

When you are interviewing for a job, be sure to inquire whether they have a mandatory overtime policy.

Box 10-4 Climbing the Ladder

Theodora T. Grauer

It has been a 50-year journey since I graduated from the Bellevue School of Nursing as a diploma nurse and arrived at my present position, that of Dean of the School of Health Professions at the C. W. Post Campus of Long Island University. Over these many years, I have had many positions and have completed my master's and doctoral degrees. I've been married for 43 years to the same wonderful man, and we raised three wonderful sons. Along the way, I learned a lot about navigating the professional world as well as a busy home life. In terms of professional activities, I gained many insights along the way—

some garnered from mistakes made, some from helpful mentors, and some just out of experience. Here are the principles that guided me along the way as I "climbed the ladder" through the university system:

- If an interesting job offer appears, take it. If you don't completely understand the job, believe me, you will quickly learn on the job—everyone faces a learning curve, some steeper than others.
- Use colleagues for assistance and advice.
- Be ready at all times for advancement by staying abreast of professional issues as well as issues specific to your subject if you are teaching or the area you are administering.
- Make yourself known; be a helpful colleague.
- Don't wait until you are fully prepared to take a position because with each position the learning curve is swifter.

Be Lucky and Plucky!

Shortly after graduating from Bellevue, I worked evenings on pediatric surgery and the pediatric emergency room while working toward completing my BS degree from Hunter College. Almost immediately upon receiving my degree, I was appointed ward instructor (WI) on this unit. The city of New York required the bachelor's degree for this position. I was soon promoted to clinical instructor, which involved teaching all pediatric didactic courses and being in charge of all ward instructors. The pediatric units consisted of pediatric surgery and ER, acutely ill infants under two, communicable diseases, and pediatric urology.

In December 1964, I got married. I continued to work at Bellevue until one week before my eldest son was born in May 1966. In December of that year, my husband was drafted into the Army, and we went to Fort Sam Houston for his basic training. We were then stationed in Aberdeen, Maryland, during which time I had another baby boy (1967). My husband was discharged in December 1968. He got a job as a general surgeon and I stayed home with two little boys under the age of three. We were living in Syosset, New York, and in fact are still there, only now the nest is empty. I tried to get a part-time job at Syosset Hospital, but at that time part-time nurses were not valued. I took an intensive Lamaze preparation course and then developed my own private practice of Lamaze and ran a busy practice for the next 12 years.

My third son was born in 1971. In 1978, I started an MS program in Community Health with Pediatrics as the main emphasis. I accepted a job at Adelphi University teaching pediatrics and obstetrics and taking students through various clinical experiences. In 1982, I started the doctoral program at Adelphi and that same year I accepted a position at the C. W. Post Campus of Long Island University as a faculty member in the Nursing Department. Following the granting of my PhD (1987), I became chairperson of the Nursing Department.

In 1998, I accepted an offer to be dean of the School of Heath Professions and Nursing without having a real idea of what the job entailed. This school consists of five disciplines:

radiologic technology (undergraduate), nursing (RN completion program and several graduate programs—NP, CNS, and Ed), biomedical sciences (undergraduate including clinical laboratory sciences, forensic science, and graduate programs in immunology, hematology, microbiology, medical chemistry, and medical microbiology as well as a joint program with the Department of Surgery at North Shore University Hospital in cardiovascular perfusion), and nutrition (graduate, dietetic internship, and master's degree).

At this point in time, I am still in the dean's position, still learning, enjoying my work, and hoping to continue in this position for quite a while.

Good luck to all of you reading this!

You Got the Job, but Now You Ask, What Was I Thinking?

After getting your dream job, it is not unusual, after a few months or a year, for a new graduate to think, "Is this what I really wanted?" Most new nurses go through the shock of finding that their first job is not just what they envisioned it would be. It is important to be in touch with your feelings and perhaps discuss this with your nurse manager or someone in the human resources area of the institution where you are working. This may be a temporary reality shock, or you may, in fact, want to discover a different area of interest in nursing. You may also return to your school and request career counseling. You may wish to contact a friend or a former professor for some ideas.

Career change within nursing is very possible. On the other hand, once acknowledging that you are not happy you may still wish to stay at your job and work out what is causing you to feel displeased. Sometimes it is not choosing the right area or simply not getting sufficient support or feeling isolated. Discussing your feelings with your nurse manager often can help you feel more relaxed and grow accustomed to the job.

Issues on the Job

Working in a healthcare environment brings with it a great many stressors. Some of these are caused by the physical demands on the nurse's body; others are emotional. Physical issues can be related to heavy lifting of patients, moving equipment, and exposure to disease or infection. Emotional stress is related to working with very ill patients, patients' families, and dealing with death and dying.

Collective bargaining agreements, state regulations, and standards set by professional organizations deal with many of these concerns. Issues of safety and workplace environment safety are legally controlled by government agencies such as the Occupational Safety and Health Administration (OSHA), which is part of the U.S. Department of Labor. The Occupational Safety and Health Administration's goal is to ensure that employees have a safe and healthy workplace environment. It works with employers and employees to create safe working environments (Occupational Safety and Health Administration, 2007). The National Institute for Occupational Safety and Health (NIOSH) is a research agency that focuses on occupational health and safety. NIOSH works closely with OSHA but is not a part of the U.S. Department of Labor. If workers feel that their workplace is unsafe, they can contact OSHA for investigation of the problem. Safety concerns such as needle sticks, injury, exposure to chemicals, and ventilation are issues that have been and are addressed by OSHA. OSHA is now pressing for an end to workplace violence. Figure 10-3 lists workplace safety concerns for nurses.

Workplace Abuse

Workplace abuse is defined as "any behavior that humiliates, degrades, or disrespects another, including intimidating behaviors, such as condescending language, exploding in angry outbursts, using threatening body language, and making physical contact" (Murray, 2008) in the workplace. These attacks and behaviors have not only a physical but also an emotional effect that can leave victims intimidated. Many suffer physically, even if the attack is not one in which physical contact has occurred (Murray, 2008). Such physical or emotional abuse makes the recipient feel powerless and may cause recurrent anxieties or actual physical reactions, such as sleeplessness.

An increase in workplace violence and conflict is of great concern because it has invaded the workplace of nursing. It has become a growing issue at hospitals and clinics. As these facilities have become more short staffed, patients and their families become frustrated with the care they or their loved ones are receiving and often act out violently.

Although workplace abuse is often thought of as a physical assault or abuse from a superior, peer, a patient, or their family, workplace abuse can occur when a person for whom you work is the attacker, and this can be physical or emotional aggression. Employees may feel even more intimidated and not want to report this type of incident because they are afraid of reprisals or even of losing their employment.

If you are confronted with workplace violence and physical abuse, it is important to stay calm and move from the situation and contact security. If you are dealing with nonphysical abuse, it is important to report the abuse to your supervisor or a higher authority. Conflicts between employees and managers resulting from working in a high-stress profession, drug and alcohol abuse, access to and prevalence of weapons in society, limitless access to hospitals and clinics, an increase of gangs, and long waits in emergency departments and clinics are all reasons for workplace conflict.

Many healthcare facilities have begun to develop policies regarding workplace abuse incidents and are developing intervention teams and policies. Unions are also beginning to address this as an important issue to deal with. However, this puts nurses at risk. Legislation has been enacted in some states in an attempt to prevent workplace violence. The New York State legislature recently passed a bill that will make an assault on a nurse a felony. The bill is now awaiting passage by the New York State Assembly (Jaiswal & Dyckoff, 2008). Protecting nurses from violence while at work not only protects the nurse, but patients. It is important that

---

Figure 10-3 Workplace Safety and Health for Nurses

- Infection as an occupational hazard
- Exposure to hazardous chemical agents
- Injuries
- Workplace violence

workplace violence at any level be reported and properly addressed.

Summary

After graduation from a nursing program, to practice nursing and to become licensed as a registered professional nurse you must take and pass the National Council Licensure Examination–Registered Nurse (NCLEX). This chapter explains this process. The chapter discusses applying for and getting your first job and workplace issues and concerns for the nurse.

QUESTIONS

1. When you begin your search for employment, you should first
   a. find out about transportation to and from the workplace
   b. read the mission and philosophy statement of the agency
   c. ask about the salary
   d. ask about the benefits

2. A nurse approaches a patient's room and hears one of the family members of a patient yelling and threatening to hit the nurse manager. The nurse should first
   a. run in and defend the nurse manager
   b. tell the family member that she is being inappropriate
   c. notify security to come to the patient's room immediately
   d. notify the supervisor of the unit to contact security

3. A behavioral interview is
   a. rarely used when nurses go for a job interview
   b. a focused interview concerned with your former experiences
   c. concerned with your understanding of the workplace mission
   d. always done at nursing interviews

4. The American Nurses Association is lobbying against mandatory overtime. Nurses know that it
   a. is necessary because of the nursing shortage
   b. creates improved situations in hospitals for patient care
   c. is unsafe for nurses and patients
   d. is not approved by unions because nurses are not paid for overtime

5. The term *staffing* refers to
   a. the number of persons, professional and assistive, who provide care for the patient
   b. the acuity of care needed
   c. how many registered professional nurses provide care on a unit for the patients
   d. workload responsibility

References

Bushweller, K. (2000). *Throw away the no. 2 pencils—here comes computerized testing.* The School Technology Authority. Retrieved December 5, 2008, from www.electronic-school.com/2000/06/0600f1.html

CGFNS International. (2008). Who we are/what we do. Retrieved August 13, 2008, from http://www.cgfns.org/sections/about/

Gershon, R. C., & Bergstrom, B. (1991). *Individual differences in computer adaptive testing: Anxiety, computer literacy and satisfaction.* Paper presented at the Annual Meeting of the National Council on Measurements in Education. Retrieved December 5, 2008, from http://eric.ed.gov:80/ERICDocs/data/ericdocs2sql/content_storage_01/0000019b/80/14/bb/f3.pdf

Jaiswal, M., & Dyckoff, D. (2008, July). When violence knocks at the hospital door. Retrieved December 5, 2008, from http://include.nurse.com/apps/pbcs.dll/article?AID=/20080714/NY02/107140135

Julian, E., Wendt, A., Way, D., & Zara, A. (2001). Moving a national licensure examination to computer. *Nurse Educator, 26*(6), 264–267.

McKay, D. R. (2008). What is a behavioral interview? *About.com: Career planning.* Retrieved November 4, 2008, from http://careerplanning.about.com/od/jobinterviews/a/beh_int_lng.htm

Murray, J. S. (2008, July). No more nurse abuse. *American Nurse Today, 3*(7), 17–19.

National Council of State Boards of Nursing. (2008). Boards of nursing. Retrieved August 20, 2008, from https://www.ncsbn.org/boards.htm

NCLEXinfo.com. (2008). NCLEX format. NCLEX Test Review. Retrieved August 15, 2008, from http://www.nclexinfo.com/nclex_format.htm

Occupational Safety and Health Administration. (2007). OSHA facts—August 2008. Retrieved August 20, 2008, from http://www.osha.gov/as/opa/oshafacts.html

Oermann, M. H., & Heinrich, K. T. (2004). *Annual review of nursing education* (2nd ed.). New York: Springer.

Chapter 11

Trends and Issues in Health Care

Marilyn Klainberg

OUTLINE

Technology and Education
   Fast-Track Education
Health and Technology
Provision of Health Care and Technology
Dealing with Disasters

Biological Matters
Environmental Issues
Impact of Culture on the Provision of
   Health Care

A *trend* is a tendency toward something usually new, but the word *trend* does not always refer to what is actually new but can refer to how we utilize things in a new or innovative way. For example, the use of television and the Internet. Both have been around for a long time, but how we utilize them today has evolved and changed over the years. Technology has changed nursing education in the classroom as well as outside the classroom. Students can do research and read assigned articles online, from home, in their pajamas, in the middle of the night, and by visiting most library resources online. With the growth in technology, these resources are increasing.

Technology and Education

The movement toward distance learning as an approach to higher education has become a trend. The notion of distance education is not new, but the latest or up-to-the-minute way we utilize technology is. The relationship of technology to how we are exposed to distance education is recent. Using the Internet for distance education has rapidly evolved and creates opportunities for distance education to serve persons at greater distances and more quickly. In the past, if you took a distance education course, you would receive materials by mail (snail mail), and then return materials to the faculty member by mail. You would be required to use a local library for resources or to purchase the research or reading materials sent to you. Use of the Internet has sped up the process and the communication. Today you can visit a virtual classroom or simply take courses online. Some institutions provide entire educational degrees in this way. Many schools of nursing now offer entire baccalaureate programs or individual courses and make advanced degrees available to students online.

Using this technology, you can do virtual science projects, take examinations, and use programs such as Wimba to participate in virtual classrooms. Wimba is a commercial product that uses technology that facilitates communication between students and faculty in synchronous online courses. Merging software products such as Wimba, which allow interactive discussions online simply by using a speaker and a headset, with programs such as Blackboard, Web CT, or Moodle provides various platforms for nursing or other disciplines to offer baccalaureate, continuing education, and advanced degrees online. To provide clinical experiences, baccalaureate online programs additionally use local preceptors.

In the classroom, using technology to record classes and upload them to a computer for students to download on their iPod is available and being utilized. Students can hear their lecturer while they are at the beach or in the car.

Clickers are used in the classroom to enhance student participation. *Clickers* are remote personal response systems used in the classroom to engage students and increase full student participation through group responses. The use of clickers also provides the faculty member with information about student knowledge (Educause Learning Initiative, 2005).

Personal digital assistants (PDAs) provide technical and pharmacological information for students by making access to current information available in PDA programs or over the Internet.

Online testing that provides immediate feedback and, in some programs, the ability to predict outcomes on the NCLEX, enhances and improves education. Laptop computers give students the mobility to work and navigate the learning environment. Nurses in hospitals or working for home care agencies use computers to record their nursing notes. They can use laptops for the collection of patient data and for accessing laboratory work, nutrition information, and activities of daily living.

Advances in simulation technology have made simulators such as SimMan available. This technology is being used to prepare students in providing patient care in nursing laboratories and in hospitals for new nursing graduates.

Fast-Track Education

Another trend in nursing education has been driven by need. Many schools of nursing are providing 1-year programs for college or university graduates who have decided to change their major to nursing or persons who wish to make a career change. The 1-year programs are designed to recognize prior educational work and include the necessary components of a nursing curriculum for licensure.

Although not totally new, there has been an increase in nurses who have graduated from associate degree programs and return to attain the baccalaureate degree. They also take the option of enrolling in associate degree and master's degree programs.

Health and Technology

As technology has improved, it has entered our lives in ways that may not only affect the provision of health care but that have implications for future healthcare needs. The use of cell phones by the young is one of the issues in question. How does cell phone use affect the physiology of the brain of a young child? In one way, having a cell phone might make children safer because parents can know where children are, but we do not know the consequences of cell phone use on the developing brain. It is furthermore not clear how the use of computer games and other technology affects children. We do know that there is a rise in obesity and hypertension among children. Is this a result of sedentary play, using computers, watching television, or something else? These issues affect the future provision of health care and prevention within the nursing practice role.

Provision of Health Care and Technology

Technology in the healthcare setting has changed how we manage, provide, and implement patient care. The use of technology to some extent is found in most hospitals in the United States (Malloch, 2007). This includes the use of computers, electronic records (e-records), and personal digital assistants (PDAs). These devices help to reduce errors and improve patient safety.

PDAs provide a good solution with which to manage the constant flow of information regarding new and complicated pharmaceuticals and treatments. These small, pocket-sized wonders are used in many healthcare settings by student nurses, physicians, and bedside nurses. PDAs can access a drug database with information concerning medications and their interactions; acute care references; specialty nursing information, such as procedures and nursing assessment information; and much more. The information

on PDAs is updated and maintained each time they are connected to a computer.

Other technological advancements that have improved bedside nursing include technology to check patient identification before administering medication, medical robots that assess clients, and the ability to transfer current records rapidly through departments within the hospital or other areas of the healthcare agency. This technology maintains patient records that can be called up easily for patients who have been discharged but return to emergency departments or urgent care centers for additional care.

Electronic records create an easy and rapid method of storage for client records. Electronic records reduce the number of unnecessary treatments or medication errors and are used by the Continuous Quality Improvement team (CQI) for assessment to improve the quality of care. Security is a risk to patient confidentiality, but these systems are protected, requiring strict attention to access of information.

Dealing with Disasters

Disasters are emergencies of great severity that often arise unexpectedly and that cause great damage or death to persons and destruction of property. These can be natural disasters such as earthquakes, tornadoes, floods, and weather-related or imposed disasters such as terrorist attacks. Are disasters new? No, but how we address the planning and the implementation of prevention programs is new.

Disaster preparedness became of greater concern for nursing and other healthcare education programs as a result of events such as the terrorist attacks on New York City and Washington, DC, on September 11, 2001, and natural disasters such as Hurricane Andrew in Florida and Hurricane Katrina in New Orleans in August

2005. Of particular concern to healthcare providers is how prepared communities are for disasters and how services and care are provided to them. There is a growing concern related not only to dealing with the consequences of the aftermath of disasters, but with prevention and preparedness. This includes preemptive education, evacuation to prevent loss of life, and dealing with physical destruction and the impact of infection, morbidity, and mortality following a disaster.

Public health professionals are responsible for the health of a community during disasters. This is true of local, state, and the federal governments. Concerns include issues related to the water supply and waste disposal, food supply, vector control, sanitation, and the prevention of injuries (related to physical and mental health) and death (Landesman, 2001).

We are more aware today about not only our personal preparedness, but also the role preparedness plays for the healthcare professional. For most who work in hospitals, professional preparedness is not completely new but has been enhanced. For example, for many years nurses have been educated on how to respond to fire in the institution, but more recently, issues such as natural disaster and nonnatural disaster training for terrorist attacks have entered our vocabulary.

Communities are also looking into preparedness and prevention as well as dealing with the aftereffects of a disaster. Nurses are asked to be prepared and trained so that they can function as leaders in the event of a disaster, in their agencies and outside in the community. Nurses are being asked to become participants in Disaster Medical Assistance Teams (DMATs). Along with the National Guard, police, emergency response teams, and other federal, state, and local programs, DMATs have a new role in disaster preparedness. DMATs consist of self-sustaining, trained civilian physicians, nurses, and other health professional volunteers who become available to provide triage and continuing medical care within hours of activation in response to a disaster (Landesman, 2001). Each disaster requires different responses, and specific training for the healthcare provider is important. DMATs provide support to local response teams.

Nurses and other healthcare providers are also called upon to teach the community about personal preparedness. This entails a plan for keeping oneself physically and mentally ready for a disaster. There are now courses and many books that expand on information related to disaster management. Graduate programs have been designed and are implemented for healthcare providers interested in working in the area of disaster management. In the area of Information Technology, new software programs and databases on disaster recovery, also called event recovery, are available. Nurse knowledge about these programs, and nurse participation in writing them as nursing informatics specialists, is a new and growing area of nursing practice.

Personal preparedness is very important for members of the DMAT. If DMAT nurses are not prepared, then they will have little to provide others. Personal preparation gives nurses the opportunity to attend to patient needs sooner. Professional preparedness requires the nurses to understand the disaster plan at their workplace and determine how that plan fits into the community disaster plan. Communities and community organizations vary in their level of preparedness. Nurses should be familiar with written disaster plans if they exist, and if they do not exist, nurses should help to implement one.

Biological Matters

Issues such as limited availability of organs for the number of transplants needed have created the need to find new ways to find organs for transplant. This has created a place for xenotransplantation (the transplantation of living cells or organs). Transplanting organs from live donors, such as happens in kidney transplants, has been available for a long time, but new to the scene and somewhat controversial are partial liver transplants from live donors to recipients who are in need. Other issues have to do with organs that are made available for sale outside of the United States. Concern about the marketing of organs outside of the United States exists. The selling of organs, particularly in developing nations, is also of great concern, not only because of ethical issues, but for other reasons such as the spread of disease.

Issues such as stem cell research, both embryonic and adult (but particularly embryonic stem cell research), are controversial and remain a national debate. The Human Genome Project, an international project, was proposed in 1990. A *genome* is the entire set of DNA in an organism. These genes carry information required by all organisms. Genomes are studied for reasons such as disease prevention, the effects of chemicals on living species, and genetic therapy. Thus far, the Human Genome Project scientists have identified approximately 20,000 to 25,000 genes in human deoxyribonucleic acid (DNA) (Human Genome Project Information, 2008). Concerns related to privacy include use of the genetic information by insurers and other sources such as educational institutions to interfere with the care a person receives or which school they attend. Another concern is the possible impact or issue raised of genetic differences among people. Would known genetic differences affect where people are permitted to live or which career they may have? Additionally, issues and information that influence decisions concerning reproduction are also controversial

and, for some, outweigh the benefits of information obtained from DNA. Presently, genetic testing is being used to advise prospective parents about genetic possibilities that will affect the health of a newborn. The upside of this is that genetic testing will have a profound effect upon healthcare needs of an individual and can be personalized to meet individual needs.

Environmental Issues

As we become more aware of environmental issues, we need to address them as part of our commitment to the provision of health care. As nurses, we need to explore steps to decrease the impact of the hospital equipment and waste upon the environment. Nurses can lead the way by creating or joining Nursing Green Teams (NGTs) to explore ways to improve the environment within the institutions in which we work (Carpenter, 2008).

Nurses need to explore issues such as recycling batteries, paper waste, and the impact of plastic bottles for intravenous therapies as opposed to glass. We know that institutions separate blood products from other waste materials for disposal, and most separate plastic products and paper for recycling, but do they use unbleached paper products such as paper plates and paper towels in the hospital? Institutions should develop policies concerning conservation of supplies. Think about what you do when a patient leaves the hospital. Do you send along items in their bedside stand such as bedpans or wash basins for use at home, or do you discard them? If there are unused, unopened adhesive bandages and sterile dressings, can they be reused?

Another issue is the need to discover whether the institution is using energy-saving lightbulbs. Is the food that patients are fed healthy and is it local? Does the agency attempt to purchase fresh food from within a 500-mile radius? The use of local fresh and natural food products increases the benefits to the patient and decreases the cost on the environment related to trucking food long distances, which is a waste of fuel. Less trucking additionally benefits the larger community by decreasing pollutants in the air.

Being a paperless environment is important to a green environment because it not only saves space, but trees and ink. Does the agency recycle ink cartridges?

The NGT should also explore whether the air in the institution is fresh and whether the cleansers used in the hospital are environmentally friendly, nontoxic, and safe for the environment in which you and your patients breathe—or are you and your patients inhaling fumes from cleansers and disinfectants (Carpenter, 2008)?

Impact of Culture on the Provision of Health Care

Culture refers to the attitudes, beliefs, and behaviors of a group. These social or ethnic beliefs and behaviors affect individuals' health beliefs and values. It was believed for a long time that the United States was a melting pot of cultures. However, American society can be thought of as a big salad, made up of delicious and unique flavors. Each individual part of the salad adds to the whole. Therefore, people in the United States, while maintaining their own uniqueness and diversity of cultures, religions, and history, make up one country.

We must not forget that diversity influences the needs of individuals and the health care they receive. A recent surge in the diversity in health care and of the American society simply seems new, but it is not because this has been a nation of immigrants since the 1600s.

Initially, three areas of concern related to cultural diversity in health care come to mind. One concern has to do with meeting the cultural needs of patients, another is the impact of an increase of cultural diversity among members of the professional staff, and the third is the needs of undocumented individuals.

Because of the nursing shortage, many institutions are bringing in nurses from other countries to meet the decline in numbers of nurses in the United States. Although this seems to be a current trend, in the 1980s during a nursing shortage in the United States, foreign nurses were recruited to work in the United States. Many of these nurses stayed, and some returned to their home countries. Recruiting nurses from other countries is an ethical dilemma because some of the countries from which we are recruiting nurses are also experiencing a nursing shortage.

Concerns related to bringing nurses from other countries with different cultures raises issues related to communication and cultural sensitivity, for the nurse and for the patients they will be treating. Nurses arriving from other countries and cultures often have difficulty adjusting to language (this is true even if they come from English-speaking countries, and it has to do with the use of slang, idioms, jargon, and expressions). Time orientation and attitudes to space (personal space and distance) may also arise from cultural differences.

Relationships between nurse and physician and nurse and the patient's family members are often quite different in diverse cultures. The foreign nurse will need support in expanding these roles in a new country. Understanding cultural differences in attitudes toward birth, death, pain, and beliefs about disease is also important for the foreign nurse and multicultural patient populations.

Nurses from other countries need to be welcomed and oriented to the hospital or agency in which they will be working, as well as to the culture of this society. Many go through culture shock. For example, some may find it difficult to find food that they are comfortable eating, and others are unaccustomed to living conditions. Some lack a full understanding of how the healthcare system in the United States operates. They may be skilled in patient care but unaccustomed to the customs of the new overriding culture in which they are now practicing. They too may need to become sensitive to a variety of cultures to which they were not accustomed in their country of origin. Nurses need to be in touch with their own unique and diverse culture and must attempt to look for similarities among cultures, not differences.

Cultural care of the patient must reflect the patient's cultural diversity. *Cultural care* refers to professional health care that is "culturally sensitive, culturally appropriate and culturally competent" (Spector, 2004, p. 8). This means that the provider delivers care with some understanding or knowledge of the health traditions of the group or person for whom care is being given, that this care is the best possible care available, and that the care incorporates understanding and knowledge of the patient's attitudes and beliefs (Spector, 2004). When caring for patients, the nurse might want to do a cultural assessment. Suggested questions for a cultural assessment include those in Figure 11-1.

Figure 11-1 Suggested Cultural Assessment Questions

1. Where were you born?
2. Where were you raised? If not in the United States, how old were you when you came to this country?
3. Were you raised by your biological parents? (If adopted, do you have any information about your cultural history?)
4. Where were your parents/caregivers born? If they were first-generation inhabitants, when did they come to the United States?
5. Where were your grandparents born?
6. What language/languages do you speak? Can you read and write in your native language? Can you read and write in English?
7. What is your religion? What is your degree of involvement in your religion?
8. Is your spouse/partner the same religion as you?
9. Is your spouse/partner from your county of birth?
10. Do most of your friends come from the same background as you do?
11. Do you celebrate religious or ethnic holidays? Which ones?
12. Where were you educated?
13. What are the foods you like to eat on a regular basis?

Source: Taken from: Klainberg, M., Holzemer, S., Leonard, M., & Arnold, J. (1998). *Community health nursing: An alliance for health.* New York: McGraw-Hill.

Another issue is the care of undocumented persons who encounter the healthcare system. These persons are often very ill when they come into the healthcare system because they do not come into the system until late for fear that they will be deported or arrested. To allow the nurse to assist these patients, the nurse may wish to attempt cultural brokering. *Cultural brokering* is the term used to describe the process of getting someone of a similar culture or who speaks the patient's language to act as an intermediary or middleperson to help the nurse connect with the patient (Rankin & Stallings, 2001).

Concerned with issues related to providing appropriate cultural care, the Office of Minority Health in 1997 developed national standards for cultural and linguistic health care of diverse populations (Spector, 2004). These standards are available at http://www.omhrc.gov/templates/browse.aspx?lvl=2&lvlID=15.

It is important to note that all individuals being treated in the healthcare system are entitled to interpreters if needed. This includes those who speak diverse languages and sign language.

Summary

This chapter explores current issues in health care of which nurses should be aware. Issues and trends change from time to time, and this chapter touches upon only some current issues, such as cultural diversity, the environment, disasters, technology, and educational issues.

QUESTIONS

1. The professional nurse who is a part of a DMAT team realizes that the role of the nurse is important and
   a. that if DMAT nurses are not personally prepared themselves, they will have little to provide others
   b. that they must travel to meet the needs of a disaster
   c. that communities must all be prepared at the same level
   d. being a member of the DMAT team guarantees that nurses will be able to provide care to others

2. A *genome* is the entire DNA in an organism. The nurse working for a research project knows that genomes are studied to improve knowledge of which of the following?
   a. How genes carry information required by all organisms
   b. Disease prevention
   c. Genetic therapy
   d. All of the above

3. Scarcity of organs has created which of the following situations?
   a. Prevention of organ transplants throughout the United States
   b. Eradication of live donor transplants in the United States

  c. Organs are being sold illegally outside of the United States

  d. International prevention of organ transplant sales

4. A licensed professional nurse at a county hospital is part of a group of healthcare professionals concerned with environmental issues at the hospital. The nurse is aware that

  a. the hospital is exempt from recycling

  b. getting rid of supplies is of no concern for this team

  c. it is important to explore the use of glass instead of plastic bottles for intravenous therapies

  d. bed pans and other used supplies should not be sent home with patients upon discharge

5. Mrs. W., a patient at a diabetic clinic, tells the nurse that she cannot eat any of the foods on the food list she received last week. The nurse reviews the list with the patient, and the nurse

  a. realizes the patient is being noncompliant

  b. asks Mrs W. about her preferences and if she has a plan that she prefers to follow

  c. knows Mrs. W. will not follow any diet

  d. asks Mrs W. her food preferences and if she has any dietary restrictions related to her religion

References

Carpenter, H. (2008). Environment, health, and safety. Nursing green teams: Volunteer today. *American Nursing Today*, 3(5). Retrieved December 5, 2008, from http://www.nursingworld.org/MainMenu Categories/ANAMarketplace/ANAPeriodicals/ AmericanNurseToday/Archive/2008/May08ANT/ EnvironmentHealthandSafetyMay08.aspx

Educause Learning Initiative. (2005). 7 things you should know about clickers. Retrieved on November 4, 2008, from http://net.educause.edu/ir/library/pdf/ ELI7002.pdf

Human Genome Project Information. (2008). Home page. Retrieved August 27, 2008, from http:// www.ornl.gov/sci/techresources/Human_Genome/ home.shtml

Klainberg, M., Holzemer, S., Leonard, M., & Arnold, J. (1998). *Community health nursing: An alliance for health*. New York: McGraw-Hill.

Landesman, L. Y. (2001). *Public health management of disasters: The practical guide*. Washington, DC: American Public Health Association.

Malloch, K. (2007). The electronic health record: An essential tool for advancing patient safety, *Nursing Outlook, 55*(3), 159–161.

Rankin, S. H., & Stallings, K. D. (2001). *Patient education: Principles and practices*. New York: Lippincott.

Spector, R. E. (2004). *Cultural diversity in health and illness*. Upper Saddle River, NJ: Prentice Hall.

Veenema, T. G. (2001). *Disaster nursing and emergency preparedness for chemical, biological, and radiological terrorism and other hazards*. New York: Springer.

Unit Three

Leadership, Policies, and Management

Chapter 12

Delegation

Christine Coughlin

OUTLINE

Why Delegation?
The Organization Structure for Safe Delegation
Communication Is the Key to Effective
   Delegation
   Barriers to Communication

Organizational Commitment to Education
Accountability
The Responsibility of the Organization
   and the RN

Delegation is the process of assigning to others tasks or work that they are capable and competent to perform. The National Council of the State Boards of Nursing (NCSBN) and the American Nurses Association (ANA) issued statements defining delegation as the process for a nurse to direct another person to perform nursing tasks and activities. Both organizations stress that the nurse still maintains accountability (ANA & NCSBN, 2005). In actuality, there are two types of accountability, individual and organizational.

The key to successful delegation, whether you are the chief nursing officer or a staff nurse, is understanding that delegation is a process. Delegation is a process that requires assessment,

implementation, evaluation, monitoring, and feedback. If one of the steps is missing, the delegation of a task or assignment will likely fail. The NCSBN clearly states this process in outlining *The Five Rights of Delegation*:

Right task

Right circumstance

Right person

Right directions and communication

Right supervision and evaluation
(NCSBN, 1995)

The process of delegation is dynamic; it does not end but requires continued surveillance. An important responsibility of leaders in healthcare organizations is continually overseeing that the staff nurses are delegating nursing tasks to competent unlicensed personnel. Nurse leaders hold the responsibility of providing the structure in their organization that allows the delegation of nursing tasks to occur safely. Not only does the structure have to be evident, the communication to staff regarding the structure has to be very clear. The nurse leaders with input from all levels of nursing have the responsibility to design a structure that ensures that the process of delegation is centered on patient safety.

Why Delegation?

How we delegate work to others has always been important, but changes in the healthcare environment make delegation of patient care extremely important in today's world. What has changed? The answer is everything. We are facing an ever-growing nursing shortage, an aging population, escalating healthcare expenses, and public demand for patient safety and quality care. In addition to legal issues (discussed in Chapter 15), the nursing profession has become more complex with the increased use of technology, which requires increased skilled nursing time. Technology has enabled us to monitor our patients more closely with just-in-time information. Decisions regarding patient care are quicker and lengths of hospital stays are shorter. Patients in the hospital are sicker and need education and preparation to go home. Professional registered nurses spend more time educating patients and families. These trends and demographic changes have caused healthcare leaders to look at delivery of care models and respond to the needs and demands of patients. The use of delegation is one of the responses to these trends in health care.

The Organization Structure for Safe Delegation

The outcry for patient safety and the emphasis on quality care place greater importance on the role of the nurse leader in healthcare institutions. Chief nursing officers are accountable for designing an infrastructure for safe, effective, quality care delivery. The structure needs to demonstrate that there are systems established to assess, monitor, verify, and communicate ongoing competence requirements in areas related to delegation.

The structure of the care delivery model informs nurses, physicians, patients, and the public about how and by whom care will be delivered. One of the earliest decisions in designing a care delivery model is deciding which tasks must be done by the registered nurse (RN) and which tasks can be delegated to unlicensed assistive personnel (UAP). The role of the UAP is assisting the nurse in providing direct patient care in compliance with national standards and the state nurse practice act (Kleinman & Saccomano, 2006). Each nurse has the responsibility of knowing his or her state's nurse practice act.

ANA has consistently emphasized that the nurse may delegate specific aspects of care but does not delegate the nursing process. In the joint statement issued by the ANA and the NCSBN, it is acknowledged that most state nurse practice acts authorize nurses to delegate (ANA & NCSBN, 2005). The nurse leader of an organization is responsible to see that the organization's policies are in compliance with the state nurse practice act. Delegation must be in the scope of practice for the licensed nurse to delegate to a UAP. The nurse leader of the organization is responsible for the delivery of care model that stipulates what can be delegated and to whom tasks are delegated.

Only tasks not involving ongoing assessment or interpretation can be delegated to the UAP. The NCBSN, as part of the 2005 joint ANA and NCBSN statement on delegation, has produced a decision tree that clearly states the steps for the delegation of tasks to the UAP. The decision tree has four steps. The first step is the assessment and planning phase. Under the guidance of the state's regulations, tasks are selected that are consistent with patient safety. These tasks should be tasks that are the same for each patient and do not involve change from one patient to the next. An example might be the task of gathering the daily weights of patients or routine vital signs. The task should be within the range of the functions of the UAP. In no way should the task compromise a patient's well-being. The UAP must also demonstrate the competency and have the knowledge to perform the task (ANA & NCSBN, 2005).

Once the decision for delegation of appropriate tasks has been made, the organization must support the decision with educational programs, appropriate staffing, and methods of evaluation to determine the ongoing competencies of the staff. The competencies are twofold. One is the competency of the unlicensed personnel to accomplish the task, and the other is the ability of the registered nurse to delegate. From my personal experience as a chief nurse, testing the ability of the UAP is the easier work. It has been my experience that the nurses frequently lack understanding of the delegation process and fail to remain accountable for the patient's care or have no faith in the delegation of tasks to assistive personnel and repeat the tasks themselves. I have had more than one nurse tell me they always retake the vital signs.

Communication Is the Key to Effective Delegation

Delegation depends on effective communication and is a two-way process. The UAP must be able to ask questions and verify the assignment. There needs to be a meeting of the minds so that the RN and the UAP both have the same clear understanding of the assignment. Not only are communication and directions important, but the nurse needs to be absolutely certain the UAP can explain the directions clearly and that there is no confusion about any aspect of the task. This requires active listening skills. Listening to the UAP describe the delegated tasks assures the nurse that the assignment has been mutually understood.

The UAP needs to know when to call for the input of the RN. The RN needs to know when the UAP is not clear on the assignment or is embarrassed to ask for clarification. The communication needs to be patient centered; both have the quality of care for the patient as the most important parameter. The UAP should understand when to report information about a patient immediately and not wait until the end of the work shift. Communication needs to be ongoing throughout the shift.

At the end of the work shift when the nurse is evaluating the care of the patient is the time to review the assignment with the UAP. The nurse should find out if the assignment was good for the UAP. Was it the right amount of work or was the UAP overwhelmed? Was it rewarding or fulfilling for the UAP? Following up and seeking feedback promotes open communication and good teamwork. It also helps in evaluating the UAP.

Barriers to Communication

The nurse needs to understand that the communication needs to be professional and not be interpreted as condescending. The RN needs to convey his or her willingness to support the UAP. If this fails to happen, a barrier to effective communication and understanding can result.

The communication process becomes more complicated when working with a diverse workforce. Cultural norms vary with regard to delegation. Delegating to persons from a different culture might cause some misunderstandings. Different cultures have different values and expectations regarding eye contact, body language, and the concept of time. It is important to understand the cultural differences and how they affect communication and mutual understanding (Hansten & Washburn, 1998).

Cultural competency becomes important in the communication process. Leininger (2006) describes in detail cultural care. Her model can be used in dealing with all people, not just patients. It is based on knowledge, attitudes, behaviors, and diverse cultural experiences. To be culturally competent means showing respect for the values and beliefs of others. Research has indicated that cultural awareness is based on knowledge and therefore closely linked to education (Schim, Doorenbos, & Borse, 2005). A responsible organizational structure provides the education in delegation that includes culturally competent communication. A responsible nurse masters cultural competence to overcome potential barriers to quality patient care.

Organizational Commitment to Education

The organizational structure supporting the education of nurses on the five rights of delegation, as listed in Table 12-1, and the responsibility cannot be overemphasized.

The fifth right of delegation, right supervision and evaluation, needs to be fully explored with the registered nurses (NCSBN, 1995). The NCSBN divided this into two separate steps, supervision and evaluation. The third step in the decision tree is surveillance and supervision. This step addresses the monitoring and supervision of the UAP's performance by the RN. It emphasizes the nurse's responsibility for patient care. The fourth NCSBN step is evaluation and feedback. It is essential to receive feedback from the UAP to ascertain that the UAP fully understood the task. Does the person know when to report unexpected outcomes? Does he or she clearly understand the task? Understand the value and importance of the task? Understand

---

Table 12-1 Five Rights of Delegation

First Right of Delegation	Right Task, appropriate in specific care situations
Second Right of Delegation	Right Circumstance
Third Right of Delegation	Right Person, the competencies match patient needs
Fourth Right of Delegation	Right Direction or Communication
Fifth Right of Delegation	Right Supervision and evaluation fully explored with registered professional nurse

that he or she is contributing to patient outcomes? If not, you are liable to receive a report at the end of the shift that every patient had a respiratory rate of 20! The communication between the nurse and the UAP must flow in both directions to establish clear understanding. Evaluation and feedback is an important step in the process. Delegation done well promotes team building and safe, efficient patient care.

Accountability

In delegating to the UAP, the registered nurse does not give up the responsibility of assessing the patient. RNs delegate certain tasks while maintaining accountability for complete patient care. Research has identified that one of the reasons for missed nursing care was ineffective delegation. Nurses failed to follow up on tasks given to assistive personnel. The nurses failed to retain accountability (Kalisch, 2006).

The accountability for delegation in the end rests with the chief nursing leader of the healthcare organization. The structure must support the ongoing education, monitoring, and evaluation of the care delivery model including the aspect of delegation (ANA & NCSBN, 2005). The education of the staff is ongoing as the nurse grows from novice to expert. As the nurse becomes more confident and skilled, delegation skills should also grow. The evaluation process of the registered nurse should include appraisal of delegation skills and opportunities for improving those skills. Evaluation time is an opportunity to review theories and principles of delegation.

During the orientation phase of a new nurse's employment is a valuable time to help the registered nurse acquire the knowledge and the skill to delegate effectively. The nursing education needs to be structured so that there are ongoing opportunities to enforce the delegation theory and apply the principles of delegation. Once the orientee no longer has a preceptor, he or she will be responsible to delegate to others. Preceptors must help orientees understand that they need to become comfortable with the delegation process (Baltimore, 2004). Therefore, education needs to be an ongoing aspect of staff development. In this way, the novice nurse gains confidence in delegation as professional growth occurs.

The initial education about delegation theories and skills starts in the schools of nursing. Education leaders are responsible for initiating the education of delegation in the curriculum. This should be both didactic learning and practice in the clinical setting. The skill of delegation and the understanding of the complete process should be woven throughout every clinical course. The professional role of the nurse as stipulated by the state nurse practice act in most states includes the aspect of delegation of nursing tasks to others.

The Responsibility of the Organization and the RN

The organization is responsible for creating and documenting the policies that guide delegation. Which tasks may the nurse delegate and for which patients? It may be appropriate to delegate vital signs, but certainly not for every patient. It may be appropriate for the UAP to assist a stable patient to ambulate but not to assist an unstable patient or to assist a patient who is getting out of bed for the first time after surgery. The RN has the final judgment for analyzing the decision of whether or not to delegate. These aspects of what can be delegated need to be clearly defined in the organization's policy manual.

According to the joint statement on delegation, the organization is accountable for providing the resources that support the delegation process (ANA & NCSBN, 2005). The resources include educational resources, adequate staffing, and documentation of staff competencies. The staff registered nurses have the right to have access to view the competencies of the UAP to ensure that the tasks they are delegating are performed by competent staff members. The organization needs to have policies that ensure competencies are maintained and periodically evaluated. The ANA and the NCSBN include in their organization-related principles statement the need for nurses to have input and active participation in the development of policies on delegation and the educational needs of the UAP personnel. They specifically mention that staff nurses, managers, and administrators need to be included in the process of providing input and developing these policies (ANA & NCSBN, 2005).

UAPs have the responsibility of working only within their defined scope of work. They are responsible for completing the required training and maintaining the competencies required or for reporting to the RN when they are deficient. Every member of the team has the responsibility of providing safe, quality care.

Summary

Delegation is a professional right and responsibility (ANA & NCSBN, 2005). Our healthcare environment demands that nurses practice safely and efficiently in delivering quality patient care. Practicing nurses need to feel confident that they understand the process of delegation. Educators have the responsibility of educating healthcare personnel in all aspects of the delegation process. Nurse administrators have the responsibility of providing the infrastructure that ensures safe delegation. Nurses have the responsibility of delegating appropriate tasks to UAPs so that the nurses are free to perform RN-level tasks. Good communication promotes good teamwork and safe, quality patient care. Delegation requires communication, communication, communication!

QUESTIONS

1. A patient requires her blood pressure to be taken every hour. The patient is otherwise in a stable condition. The nurse delegates this to the unlicensed assistive personnel (UAP). The nurse knows that
   a. in delegating to the UAP, the registered nurse does not give up the responsibility of assessing the patient
   b. the UAP will do an excellent job
   c. in delegating to the UAP, the registered nurse can now take on other patients
   d. this is a simple task and there is no need to worry

2. Research has identified that one of the reasons for missed nursing care is
   a. nurses taking too much time at coffee breaks
   b. new nurses cannot complete their tasks
   c. ineffective delegation
   d. ineffective nurse managers

3. How the UAP accomplishes a task is measured by
   a. the competency of the UAP and how the registered nurse delegates the task
   b. testing the UAP and letting the person choose the tasks he or she wants to do
   c. how experienced the nurse is in testing the UAP for a competency
   d. how compliant the UAP is with the work assigned

4. It is the responsibility of the nurse who is delegating tasks to the unlicensed assistive personnel to
   a. never permit direct patient care by the UAP
   b. be aware of the national standards of care
   c. know the state's nurse practice act and be sure the UAP is aware of his or her limitations in compliance with national standards
   d. be aware of the role of the UAP in compliance with both national standards and the state nurse practice act

5. For delegation at all levels to be successful and provide outstanding patient care, the nurse knows
   a. this is an ongoing process
   b. it must be supported by the institution and the staff
   c. monitoring and evaluation are important in the process
   d. All of the above

References

American Nurses Association and National Council of State Boards of Nursing. (2005). Joint statement on delegation. Retrieved March 18, 2008, from http://www.ncsbn.org/Joint_statement.pdf

Baltimore, J. (2004). The hospital clinical preceptor: Essential preparation for success. *Journal of Continuing Education in Nursing, 35*(3), 133–140.

Hansten, R., & Washburn, M. (1998). *Clinical delegation skills.* Baltimore: Aspen.

Kalisch, B. (2006). Missed nursing care. *Journal of Nursing Care Quality, 21*(4), 306–313.

Kleinman, C., & Saccomano, S. (2006). Registered nurses and unlicensed assistive personnel: An uneasy alliance. *Journal of Continuing Education in Nursing, 37*(4), 162–170.

Kummeth, P., de Ruiter, H., & Capelle, S. (2001). Developing a nursing assistant model: Having the right person perform the right job. *MedSurg Nursing, 10*(5), 255–263.

Leininger, M. (2006). Cultural care theory and uses in nursing administration [Revised reprint]. In Leininger, M., & McFarland (Eds.), *Cultural care diversity and universality: A worldwide nursing theory* (2nd ed., pp. 365–381). Sudbury, MA: Jones and Bartlett.

National Council State Boards of Nursing. (1995). Concepts and decision-making process. National Council position paper. (1995). Retrieved May 15, 2008, from https://www.ncsbn.org/323.htm

Schim, S., Doorenbos, A., & Borse, N. (2005). Cultural competence among Ontario and Michigan health-care providers. *Journal of Nursing Scholarship, 37*(4), 354–360.

Chapter 13

Financial Management

Patrick R. Coonan

OUTLINE

The backbone of any hospital is its ability to maintain financial solvency. Nurses have a significant role in making this happen. As the largest group of healthcare providers in any organization, nurses have an obligation to assist in the growth and financial stability of the organization. To understand how the finances of institutions work, it is important to understand some basic financial concepts. In this chapter, we outline the tools of financial management, basic budget concepts, types of hospitals and organizational structure, where the money comes from, the nurse's role in financial management, and health policy related to finance.

Costs, Revenues, Charges, Expenses

Health care is an expensive business. So, to understand the expenses of the business, it is imperative to understand the costs and cost centers. *Cost center* refers to those departments or group of departments that incur costs but do not produce revenue. For example, engineering and housekeeping are cost centers. *Revenue centers* are those departments that generate revenue by providing direct services to patients. This does not imply that a department that does not produce revenue directly is unimportant.

Departments that provide support services are necessary to the function of those departments that do provide direct services to patients.

Providing a good plan for controlling expenses for the coming year requires an understanding of the nature of costs. Costs are generally collected for service units or units of service. The *service unit* is a basic measure of the item being produced by the organization, such as clinic visits, discharged patients, patient days, home care visits, and hours of operations. Most measurements of costs relate to the volume of service units. Within one healthcare organization, a number of different types of service units may exist. A basic cost issue is the distinction between fixed and variable costs. The total cost of running a unit or department can be divided into those costs that are fixed and those that are variable. More of this is discussed under expenses.

If a nurse were to ask what it cost to treat patients on a unit, finance people would probably tell you that it depends. Costs are not unique numbers that are always the same. The cost to treat a patient depends on several factors, one of which is the volume of patients for whom care is being provided. In trying to understand costs, is important to understand that fixed costs do not change in total; the cost per patient or patient day does change as volume changes. With greater volume, there is a larger number of patients to spread out the fixed costs. Let's say that fixed costs may be $1000. If we had to take care of five patients, our fixed cost per patient would be $200, but if we had to take care of 10 patients, our cost per patient would be only $100. Therefore, it is beneficial to be able to spread fixed costs over more patients.

Revenue is the inflow of assets in exchange for services or products that are sold. Revenue is not necessarily cash. In accounting, revenue is

recorded at the time it is earned so that it might be considered accounts receivable. It is an increase to the asset side of the balance sheet resulting from earnings. In healthcare organizations, revenue is often the amount that is charged for services, and it does not consider what portion of charges, if any, will not be paid due to such factors as bad debt or charity.

Revenue is also one of the primary portions of the operating budget. In healthcare organizations, the sources of actual revenue include patient room and nursing charges, medications, diagnostic services, medical supplies, procedures (such as surgery, outpatient procedures, and other ancillary testing), treatments (such as physical therapy), and use of equipment (such as specialty beds or hypothermia units). The charges associated with each of these items become the actual revenue recorded for the patient. Other sources of revenue for healthcare organizations may include the cafeteria, office space rental, seminar fees, and other non-healthcare-related items.

A *charge* is the amount of money that has been set for a product or service as its price. It is what the facility providing a service or product has determined as the value. The charge is the anticipated revenue from the service or product, without consideration of what will become cash. The charge is usually the cost of the service/ product plus a margin or profit. Charges can be determined by many factors. These include the original cost for the product and the costs associated with providing the service. The mix of patients that receive the service or use a product also may influence the charge. Competition is another factor in the determination of the charge.

Expenses are the services or products consumed in operating the organization. Expenses may be categorized as those necessary for operations (operating expenses) of the healthcare organization. These operating expenses include such things as salaries, supplies, equipment repair, minor equipment, insurance, and other contract fees. Expenses related to the purchase of major equipment are called *capital expenses*. These are expenses for equipment or a project that has a lifetime greater than a preset time and that cost over a predetermined amount. The predetermined time frame in cost varies from facility to facility. Expenses may be categorized by their relationship to fluctuations in volume. For example, in a hospital setting the salary expenses on a nursing unit should vary with the census. If there are more patients to be cared for, there will be a need for more nurses and therefore salary expenses will rise. This is called a *variable expense*. Other variable expense items include office, medical, and sterile supplies. *Fixed expenses* are those expenses that do not change in response to any volume change. Some examples of fixed expenses include the manager's salary and possibly clerical salaries. Expenses may also be categorized by how they are assigned. *Direct expenses* are costs that are assigned directly to the department that incurred them. These include salaries, supplies, and possibly some equipment. *Indirect expenses* are those that are difficult to assign and are allocated to a specific department based on some calculation or proration. Examples of this type of expense may be the cost of utilities, security services, and interest expenses.

Budgets

The process of budgeting has become more important because of rising healthcare costs and the emphasis on cost containment. Budgetary projections guide decision making by managers at every level in healthcare organizations. Bud-

get documents need to be organized, comprehensive, and related to the organization's strategic plan, and nurses should be aware of the relationship of the unit operational plans to the strategic plan of the organization and of the importance of the nurse's unique contribution and program responsibility because nurses influence the performance of the entire healthcare organization. The budget is a formalized plan setting direction for the unit within the strategic plan of the facility. As an operational plan, the budget is one of the most widely employed methods for managerial planning and control. Although the budget does not in and of itself determine or control operations, it is the most powerful management tool used to ensure organizational goal achievement when coupled with management action. The budget defines the standard by which operational performance can be evaluated. As a plan, it is the statement of management's knowledge, experience, and goals expressed in quantitative and financial terms.

Budgets are useful for two managerial functions: planning and control. Budgetary planning involves establishing goals and objectives in quantitative terms and identifying the resources and performance levels that are required. Budgetary control involves the ongoing process of comparing actual performance results against those plans and making corrections or modifications during the budget cycle. The responsibility for strategic planning rests at the highest level of an organization's management hierarchy, that being the governing board and the chief executive officer. Together they determine organizational mission and goals and develop strategies that will be undertaken to achieve these goals, while determining which people will be responsible for specific sections of the plan. Strategic planning focuses attention on the future to position resources and take actions that support adaptation and change. Planning and control for the organization in its entirety is accomplished by integrating all unit, program, and departmental operational budgets. Budgets developed by nurse managers on units serve as one of the many operational plans supporting the organization's long-term strategy and goals.

Different types of budgets support hospital operations in health care, whereas 50% or more of an entire budget is made up of personnel. This is why the personnel budget can be one of the most important operational components in maintaining the financial viability of healthcare organizations. Nurses devote more time and energy to planning and controlling the personnel budget than to any other aspect of the operating budget. The personnel budget accounts for the largest expense in nursing budgets. Because nursing is more labor intensive in many units, such as intensive care, the personnel budget becomes a significant challenge to the nurse manager. The challenge is to schedule appropriate hours of care for quality patient outcomes according to available skills, hours, mix, and preferences of staff. A thorough understanding of the components to be considered and the variables that affect the personnel budget enables nurse managers to proceed with confidence.

Unit personnel budgets are constructed from knowledge of the personnel resources needed to accomplish the work of the unit and the corresponding costs. Fiscal year objectives may refer to the quantity of work, such as patient-days or census, as well as to those factors more programmatic in nature, such as personnel, skill mix, or staff orientation. The quality of work in patient outcomes and productivity must be identified with the process. Objectives have an impact on the number of full-time equivalent

positions (FTEs) and their associated costs. An FTE is made up of any combination of hours that equals one full-time position. The specific unit objectives and the assumptions about how the unit works will affect the personnel budget. Personnel budgets are built based on assumptions that reflect quantity of activity, programs, structure, and functions. The resulting budget is a plan indicating personnel and dollar requirements needed to achieve objectives and is a statement of financial outcomes or targets to be met.

In addition to the personnel budget, there is generally an overall operating budget for each unit in an institution. This budget is called the operating budget and is an essential financial function in every healthcare organization. The budgeting practicalities of providing adequate supplies, ordering minor equipment, arranging for repairs and maintenance, and allowing staff opportunities to attend training and education programs confront every nurse manager who is responsible for budgets, and the budget is where it is accounted for.

The third type of budget is called the capital budget. The capital budget includes durable fixed and movable assets with the price above a specified amount at an estimated life of greater than one year. The physical plant, land, and major equipment fall into the category of capital assets. To develop an accurate capital budget it is important to know where the organization is going in the next several years. As a patient diagnosis determines the plan of care with expected outcomes, the strategic plan sets direction for the future and the financial plan offers the time line for disbursement of funds in a healthcare organization. Capital budgeting is the practice of planning and decision making for capital assets. This includes determining future assets and financial feasibility, evaluating asset operations, and integrating capital expenditures with long-range financial plans. Capital budgeting includes planning for disbursement of funds needed for land acquisition, plant development or expansion, and capital equipment expenditures.

The financial pressures faced by healthcare organizations in recent years have resulted in significant budget cuts. Nurses have had to find ways to make do with less revenue. A major concern in this environment is that quality patient care is likely to suffer. This concern has been borne out by evidence of problems with quality of care that are landmarked in two significant reports from the Institute of Medicine (Kohn, Corrigan, & Donaldson, 2000; Committee on Quality of Health Care in America, 2001). These reports from the federally sponsored agency gained the attention of politicians, policymakers, and the American public. The result has been a strong refocusing of attention from cost control to a dual focus on conserving financial resources while placing strong emphasis on quality and outcomes of healthcare services. Budgeting helps managers focus on the results that departments and organizations achieve. This process is called *performance* or *outcomes budgeting*. This technique evaluates the activities of a cost center in terms of what the center accomplishes as well as the cost of that accomplishment. It is an approach to budgeting specifically designed to evaluate multiple outcomes of costs rather than a single budget output, such as the number of patient-days or clinic visits. Performance budgeting provides a mechanism for gaining a better understanding of the relationships between financial resources and the level and quality of results. Traditional budgets focus primarily on the resources used by a department or cost center. Performance budgeting shifts the focus from the resources the unit plans to use to the various goals it is trying to accomplish.

Hospital Organization

Hospitals in the United States exist for the purpose of providing health care and all must have a mission statement. This mission statement reflects the values, purposes, benefits, and priorities the hospital plans to contribute to the community. It shares beliefs and values and often mentions the scope of services offered. Developing a mission statement is complex and political and requires planning and coordination with the governing body, medical staff, and administrative team. A clear mission statement facilitates planning, marketing, development of services, and public relations of the hospital. Some mission statements also identify beliefs about the employees. In addition to the hospital mission statement, typically hospitals will also list their vision and their values. A hospital's vision is where it sees itself now and in the future, and its values are things that it believes in that are important to the delivery of quality health care.

Hospitals in the United States are divided into two major groups, not for profit and for profit. They are further subdivided by two major types of ownership, public and private. Not-for-profit hospitals include both public and private institutions. Public hospitals are supported by tax dollars appropriated by federal, state, or local governments. Private not-for-profit hospitals are usually owned by corporations or private groups. These hospitals are established for the common good rather than for individual gain and are granted broad federal, state, and local tax exemptions. For-profit hospitals are owned by private corporations or groups. They can declare dividends and distribute profits to individuals. An understanding of the breakdown of hospital organization is essential for nurses to know. The five most common types of hospital organization in the United States are community, investor-owned corporation, university medical center, urban public, and government.

Community hospitals provide personal health care in a manner that uses available resources most effectively for the community's benefit. Community hospitals are the most common type of hospital in our country and generally provide personal and public health for the community; they are concerned with the environmental health care in the area and serve as an economic corner post for many communities as a large employer. Community hospitals located in rural or urban areas may be an investor-owned corporation. The positive benefits of a for-profit hospital are that it provides a new effort toward innovation, is more responsive to the needs and desires of patients and physicians, uses approaches to management that are financially sound and more business oriented, and provides an important source of new capital for health services. There are demands against the model that have value as well. These arguments are that it is incongruent with the traditional mission and values of healthcare institutions, is a threat to the autonomy and ideals of the medical profession, and does not provide medical care to people who cannot pay. There have been no studies done to support the fear that for-profit health care is incompatible with quality of care.

University medical centers are primarily located in large urban areas on the campus of the university. The priorities in university medical centers are research, physician training, and patient care. The mission of the teaching hospital is very complex. Characteristics of teaching hospitals include a marked increase in the number of health professions students and increases in biomedical research and research training opportunities. They are expensive to maintain, and the costs continue to escalate secondary to the education involved. Research is essential; however, it is not a moneymaking program. They are expected to provide state-of-the-art technology while providing services to the community. Many teaching hospitals are now facing increasingly threatening and unstable environments. Challenges such as increased pressure to accept indigent patients and decreased financial support for medical education are among the major threats to university-owned or academic health centers.

Public hospitals provide most of the care for uninsured patients. Although they serve Americans at all income levels, caring for the uninsured and the indigent is the fundamental mission of an urban public hospital. These hospitals, interestingly enough, are only a small minority of nonfederal public hospitals in the United States. Similar to public hospitals, the federal healthcare system encompasses extensive and diverse services provided in both military and civilian facilities. A federal healthcare system provides military health care, public health care, and veterans' services. A centralized bureaucratic structure common to the federal healthcare system is often cited as a differentiating factor between public and private delivery models. However, many private hospitals are also structured along bureaucratic lines. The distinguishing difference from a financial perspective is that federal agencies are subject to policies and budget ceilings established annually by Congress. Funds appropriated to each department within the federal healthcare system are then allocated to programs within that department. The federal deficit and pressure to control healthcare costs are national problems that affect both public and private healthcare providers.

Sources of Healthcare Funding

With the increased emphasis on cost containment in health care, how providers are paid for the services they deliver has become an ongoing issue. Prior to 1983, hospitals and physicians were reimbursed by third-party payers (private, nongovernmental) for the actual cost of the services provided. When the prospective payment system (PPS) was implemented in 1983, payment for services for Medicare patients took a radical step toward cost containment. In this system, pay is a predetermined fee according to a diagnosis-related group (DRG) and was intended to be payment in full for the service.

Healthcare providers have seen a move toward increased cost containment by private payers as a result of the changes in the Medicare system. Private payers rely on strategies that restrict or limit the type of insurance plan available, contracting with selected providers, or restricting services to certain hospitals or settings. Copayments and deductibles in insurance coverage forced consumers to be selective in utilizing healthcare services and to make discriminate choices. Unfortunately, this has led to a decrease in utilization of services for less acute illness and an exacerbation of chronic health needs that are more costly to treat. Another concern of this limitation by insurers is that a form of rationing of healthcare services based on ability to pay may lead to a two-class system of health care. Greater than 90% of insured

patients are no longer covered by "traditional" health insurance. Health maintenance organizations (HMOs; organizations that integrate the financing and delivery of health care into one organization), preferred provider organizations (PPOs; organizations that provide discounted provider services to insurance carriers and employers), and managed care (cost, quality, and access) have all been established to offer alternatives to the high cost of health care.

Medicare (public/governmental) is a federal health insurance program for people ages 65 and older, people under age 65 with certain disabilities, and people of all ages with end-stage renal disease. Medicare has Part A hospital insurance. This hospital insurance helps cover inpatient care in hospitals, including critical access hospitals and skilled nursing facilities (not custodial or long-term care). It also helps cover hospice care and some home health care. Beneficiaries must meet certain conditions to get these benefits. Medicare also has Part B insurance. Most people pay a monthly premium for Part B. This insurance helps cover doctor services and outpatient care. It also covers some other medical services that Part A does not cover, such as some of the services of physical and occupational therapists and some home health care. Part B helps pay for these covered services and supplies that are medically necessary. Medicare also has prescription drug coverage that most people pay a monthly premium for. Everyone with Medicare can now get prescription drug coverage that will help lower prescription drug costs and help protect against higher costs in the future. Medicare prescription drug coverage is insurance. Private companies provide coverage. Beneficiaries choose the drug plan and pay a monthly premium.

Medicaid is another federal program. Medicaid is available only to certain low-income individuals and families who fit into an eligibility group that is recognized by federal and state law. Medicaid does not pay money to the covered person. Instead, it sends payments directly to the healthcare providers. Depending on the state's rules, participants may also be asked to pay a small part of the cost (copayment) for some medical services. Medicaid is a state-administered program, and each state sets its own guidelines regarding eligibility and services. Many groups of people are covered by Medicaid. Even within these groups, though, certain requirements must be met. These may include age, whether the participant is pregnant, disabled, blind, or aged; the participant's income and resources (such as bank accounts, real property, or other items that can be sold for cash); and whether they are a US citizen or a lawfully admitted immigrant. The rules for counting income and resources vary from state to state and from group to group. There are special rules for those who live in nursing homes and for disabled children living at home. Children may be eligible for coverage if they are US citizens or lawfully admitted immigrants, even if the parent is not (however, there is a 5-year limit that applies to lawful permanent residents). Eligibility for children is based on the child's status, not the parent's.

Medicaid does not provide medical assistance for all poor persons. Even under the broadest provisions of the federal statute (except for emergency services for certain persons), the Medicaid program does not provide healthcare services, even for very poor persons, unless they are in one of the designated eligibility groups. Low income is only one test for Medicaid eligibility. Assets and resources are also tested against established thresholds. Categorically needy persons who are eligible for Medicaid may

or may not also receive cash assistance from the Temporary Assistance for Needy Families (TANF) program or from the Supplemental Security Income (SSI) program. Medically needy persons who would be categorically eligible except for income or assets may become eligible for Medicaid solely because of excessive medical expenses.

The Nurse's Role in Financial Management

Nurses are a key part of a hospital's revenue cycle (the delivery of services, billing, and collecting for the service), yet their input usually is not sought during the development of organizational business plans. That oversight should change in the near future as hospitals face increasing costs in coming years and need to make their organizations as efficient as possible. All parties need to be involved in strategic financial planning. Sharing information between the nursing staff and finance can be a big improvement in the creation of annual budgets and business plans. Nurses often feel "caught in the middle" in the financial tug-of-war between hospital administrators, physicians, and the needs of patients and families. Nevertheless, most nurses, even those in leadership positions, do not have the advanced management or financial training that could help a hospital's finance team during the budgeting process. It is important that chief financial officers help educate nurses and bring them into the decision-making process as well as have nurses learn as much as they can about the financial operations of their organization.

Nurses can be a great help in developing new product lines or offering new services. Nurses know vendors as well as their clinical colleagues in other local hospitals. They are great resources for market research. It is important that nursing managers understand the impact of overall hospital profitability. In many cases, chief nursing officers are unaware of the importance of a hospital's liquidity position, and CFOs should make nurses aware that "profitability is everyone's problem."

Nurses and nursing managers may not have much budgeting experience, but they can still be helpful in developing realistic budgets. Nurse leaders need to know who makes decisions on purchasing hospital-wide. The CFO has to educate nurses on all aspects of capital budgets and must explain the impact of something like return on investment (ROI). To get nurses more involved in issues related to hospital finance, CFOs should develop a process for nursing input. Hospitals should develop a "patient throughput team" as well as include nurses in discussions about reducing supply costs. CFOs also need to invest money into leadership education for nurses to help manage nurse retention. Nursing and finance need to work together on nurse retention. Nurses feel beaten up by productivity tools, and there is a real difference in thought between nurses and CFOs on budgeting for productivity. Nurses need to understand their importance in making a hospital run. They are key players in financial success for programming, efficiency, and customer service.

Hospital CFOs will have difficulty changing external factors associated with cost increases, but by focusing on internal issues such as improving relations with nursing, they can augment both quality and the institution's bottom line. Nursing leaders may not be accustomed to talking with CFOs about business development issues, but disasters can happen if they are not included in these discussions.

The Key Financial Statements of the Organization

Three financial statements are crucial to understanding the finances of an organization. These are the balance sheet, or the statement of financial position; income statement; and the statement of cash flows. Statement of financial position, more commonly referred to as a balance sheet, indicates a financial position of an organization at a particular point in time. It illustrates the basic accounting equation Assets = Liabilities + Equity on a specific date. That date is the end of the accounting period. The accounting period ends at the end of the organization's financial year. Most organizations also have internal accounting periods, often monthly for internal information purposes and quarterly for external purposes. Most organizations end the year at the end of the calendar year. The basic components of the balance sheet consist of assets and liabilities. The first asset subgroup is current assets, and the first liabilities subgroup is current liabilities. Current assets generally become cash within a year. Current liabilities are obligations that must be paid within a year. These items get first attention by being at the top of the balance sheet. The balance sheet goes on to list long-term assets. These are usually broken into fixed assets, investments, and intangibles. Fixed assets represent the organization's property, plant, and equipment. Investments are primarily securities purchased with the intent to hold onto them as a long-term investment. In addition to current liabilities, organizations typically also have obligations that are due more than a year from the balance sheet date. Such liabilities are termed long-term liabilities.

The income statement compares the organization's revenues to its expenses. Revenues are the monies the organization has received or is entitled to receive in exchange for the goods or services it has provided. Expenses are the costs incurred to generate revenues. Net income is simply the difference between revenues and expenses. Unlike the balance sheet, which is a photograph of the organization's financial position at a point in time, the income statement tells what happened to the organization over a period of time. This is usually a month, a quarter, or a year. The income statement is frequently used as a tool for the presentation of changes in retained earnings from year to year.

The balance sheet and income statement are the traditional financial statements that have been required in annual reports for many years. In contrast, the statement of cash flows has only been required since the late 1980s. This statement has been added to the annual report in response to demands for better information about the organization's cash inflows and outflows. The current assets section of the balance sheet of the organization shows how much cash the organization has at the end of each accounting period. This can be compared from year to year to see how much the cash balance has changed, but that gives little information about how or why it has changed. This results in erroneous interpretations of financial statement information. For example, an organization experiencing a liquidity crisis (inadequate cash to meet its currently due obligations) may sell off a profitable part of its business. The immediate cash injection from the sale may result in a substantial cash balance at year-end. On the balance sheet, this may make the organization appear to be liquid and stable. However, selling off the profitable portion of the business may have pushed the organization even closer to bankruptcy. There is a need to show how the organization obtained any cash. Organizations

typically need to maintain cash in the bank to meet their payroll obligations. Although these three statements may sound complicated, they are rather simple and easy to read. It is more important that you understand that these are three simple statements that you can use to evaluate the status of any company or corporation.

Health Policy Related to Finance

Information about healthcare economics and financing quickly becomes outdated, particularly in this time of rapidly changing policies to address rising costs and demand. In terms of budgeting, future trends indicating growing concerns about costs and access indicate increased focus on the ability of health professionals to manage and control resources. As a result, budgeting skills are expected to increase in importance throughout the healthcare professions. Recent corporate financial scandals in health care and non-healthcare-related industries have placed an increased focus on fiscal responsibility. Healthcare institutions are expected to face more comprehensive and intense financial review, with increased regulation of accounting practices. Skills in reviewing and analyzing financial reports will be increasingly helpful to health professionals who want to critically examine and understand financial operations of their organization and work setting.

As shown in Table 13-1, Roberts and Clyde (1993) have developed eight policy questions that may be used as a framework for tracking future trends in health care and relating these trends to health economics and financing. The table also includes possible trends for the immediate future.

In the table, cost is listed as the first question because it is usually the most relevant to

Table 13-1 Policy

Policy Question	Future Trends
Cost	Ongoing need for improved cost measures; rising costs; cost concerns influence all policy questions
Quality	Increased application of quality management concepts and techniques; improved outcome measures; increased emphasis on outcomes research and tracking
Access	Parity vs. disparity; design of entitlement programs; demise of charity care
Universality	Debates about expanding coverage or national health coverage
Equity	Controversy about healthcare rationing and priority setting
Efficiency	Increased emphasis on productivity; increased application of other industry models; computerization
Choice	Willingness to pay for choice; demand for choice vs. limited resources
Prevention	Increased concerns about bioterrorism; better methods disease detection; outcomes research

future trends in health economics and finance compared with those being related to any healthcare trend or policy. It is essential to think about the impact of policies, plans, and decisions affecting the cost and changes in the cost of healthcare goods and services. Cost control is also a fundamental expectation of healthcare consumers and providers. One implication is that budgeting skills will become increasingly important for persons working in healthcare fields.

Quality and access are the next policy questions posed by Roberts and Clyde (1993). These are also fundamental expectations of healthcare consumers and providers. Problems in analyzing these issues include difficulties in measuring both quality and access. However, resource allocation decisions based on health economics and financing are likely to affect both the quality of care available and access to health care. Increased application of quality management concepts and techniques is likely in health care, with improved clinical outcomes measures linked to costs of care, as a result of increased emphasis on outcomes research and tracking.

Summary

Understanding the components of finance in your organization is important to your ability to function effectively within that organization. As a nurse, you have an integrated role in making the organization successful through your work. You handle supplies and equipment as well as caring for patients and their recovery and/or treatment. These practices all affect the cost of the patient's visits and eventually the financial solvency of the healthcare organization.

Knowing the basics of financial management in healthcare organizations will make you a better team player because you will understand the language and be able to participate in conversations regarding finance. The nurses closest to the patient have a large impact on the financial success or failure of the organization, and you will want to add to the organization's success.

QUESTIONS

1. To function effectively in hospitals, nurses need to become part of
   a. the hospitality committee
   b. financial planning
   c. the education team
   d. deficit spending

2. If nurses and nursing managers do not have much budgeting experience, they
   a. can still be helpful in developing realistic budgets
   b. should not participate in financial areas
   c. can still help plan parties for the units
   d. would be of no use in developing a realistic budget

3. Medicaid reimburses medical expenses by sending payments directly to the
   a. persons receiving services
   b. healthcare provider
   c. bank account of the recipient of care
   d. family of the recipient of services

4. There are three financial statements that are crucial to understanding the finances of an organization. These are
   a. the balance sheet, the income statement, and the statement of cash flows
   b. the statement of cash flow, the credit line, and the debit line
   c. where the money is deposited, the income sheets, and the debit line
   d. the statement of cash flow, the credit record, and the debit information

5. Medicare (public/government) is a federal health insurance program for
   a. people age 65 or older
   b. people under age 65 with certain disabilities
   c. people of all ages with end-stage renal disease
   d. All of the above

References

Committee on Quality of Health Care in America, Institute of Medicine. (2001). *Crossing the quality chasm: A new health system for the 21st century.* Washington, DC: National Academy Press.

Kohn, L. T., Corrigan, J. M., & Donaldson, M. S. (Eds.). (2000). *To err is human: Building a safer health system.* Washington, DC: National Academy Press.

Roberts, M. J., & Clyde, A. T. (1993). *Your money or your life: The health care crisis explained.* New York: Doubleday.

Health Policy

David M.
Keepnews

Health-related actions and decisions (policies) made by government bodies, such as legislatures, government agencies, and the courts, have a broad impact on health status and health care beyond the level of individual clients, clinicians, and healthcare organizations. Actions taken by some international bodies such as the World Health Organization or the World Bank can also have an impact on health and health care, particularly by influencing decisions made by national governments. All of theses local, statewide, national, and global actions and decisions—as well as the process by which they are developed and efforts to influence them—are generally referred to as *health policy*.

In some cases, health policy can also include decisions made by some private entities. For example, decisions by employers to reduce healthcare coverage, or actions taken by health plans to raise their premiums, may have a negative impact on individuals' access to healthcare services. For the purposes of providing an initial understanding of health policy, this chapter focuses primarily on health-related public policy—that is, actions and decisions by government.

What Do You Need to Know About Health Policy?

Sometimes, nurses and nursing students who have not previously had the opportunity to learn about health policy may see this area as too complex or believe that it should be left to "experts" to address. It is true that some nurses choose to focus greater time and attention on health policy issues, and some continue their education to become experts and specialists in this area (Keepnews, 2005). But all nurses and nursing students should develop at least a basic understanding of health policy and the impact that policy changes have on them and their patients. This is an important dimension of advocacy for patients and the nursing profession (Malone, 2005). Achieving a basic level of competence in this area is a realistic and achievable goal for *all* nurses and nursing students.

The Healthcare System: Issues of Access, Cost, and Quality

Providing the best care possible for individuals, families, and communities requires nursing interventions and strategies at a number of levels. Each nurse, of course, brings her or his own education, experience, skills, and compassion to each patient encounter. Each healthcare organization develops and adopts policies and protocols to guide nurses and other clinical staff in providing care. Guidelines from accrediting organizations such as The Joint Commission set standards for healthcare organizations and systems in organizing and planning patient care.

At the level of the healthcare system itself, the ways in which care is organized, structured, and paid for also have a significant effect on nursing practice. In particular, federal, state, and local government policies have a profound impact on whether, how, and where patients receive care; what staff nurses and advanced practice nurses can do for their patients; how nursing services are paid for; and what requirements (if any) apply to nurse staffing levels and other aspect of nurses' working conditions.

The healthcare system in the United States is complex and faces several challenges. These are often grouped into problems of access, cost, and quality.

Access

Access to healthcare services depends on a number of factors. One is whether an individual has health insurance. Insured individuals may be covered by private health insurance or government-sponsored plans, including Medicare (a federal health insurance program for the aged, the permanently disabled, and individuals with end-stage renal disease) and Medicaid (a joint federal-state program for many low-income individuals and families). However, millions of individuals lack any health insurance at all. The number of uninsured has grown significantly over the course of many years. In 2007, the number of uninsured was estimated to be 45.7 million (US Census Bureau, 2008). Most of the uninsured are individuals (and their families) who work in jobs that do not provide insurance but who do not qualify for government-sponsored programs. The uninsured are much less likely to have access to a regular source of healthcare services; on average, their health status is worse than the insured population (Institute of Medicine, 2004).

Although health insurance is a critically important aspect of access to care, even patients with insurance may face barriers to obtaining needed care. Patients in rural areas, for example, may reside a long distance from available healthcare providers. In some areas, patients may have difficulty locating providers who accept Medicaid or some other sources of payment.

Cost

The cost of health care in the United States is considerable. In 2006, US healthcare spending represented 16% of the gross domestic product—a total of $2.1 trillion, or $7,026 per person. (Catlin, Cowan, Hatman, & Hefler, 2008). Increasing healthcare costs have been attributed to a number of factors, including the growth of new technologies and new drugs; an increased demand for access to high-cost technologies, drugs, and services; an aging population; the growing prevalence of chronic diseases; lack of planning; insufficient emphasis on health promotion and primary care; and duplication and inefficiency in the healthcare system. There likely are multiple explanations for this steady increase in healthcare costs. Most efforts to control healthcare costs have been only briefly successful, if at all.

Quality

Quality of care has become an increasing focus of concern over the past two decades. Despite high healthcare spending, the United States ranks below many other countries in key measures of health status (Commonwealth Fund Commission on a High Performance Health System, 2008). Studies of healthcare error have pointed to large numbers of preventable injuries and deaths among hospitalized patients (Kohn, Corrigan, & Donaldson, 2000). Healthcare ser-vices are often poorly coordinated, and many have criticized the healthcare system's emphasis on high-tech, highly specialized care at the expense of primary care and prevention-oriented services. A growing interest in evaluating healthcare quality by health services researchers has helped reveal shortcomings in healthcare outcomes (along with efforts to improve quality). These include evidence of inequality, or disparities, in access to services, health status, and outcomes for minority populations (Smedley, Stith, & Nelson, 2003).

Relationships Among Access, Cost, and Quality

Of course, issues of access, cost, and quality are closely related. Attempts to fix problems in one area are likely to have an impact on the others. For example, increased healthcare costs have contributed to rising health insurance premiums, which have driven many employers to shift some of the costs of insurance to their employees—through increases in the share of premiums that employees pay, or in out-of-pocket costs such as copayments and deductibles. Many employers have reduced coverage for their retirees, and some have dropped coverage altogether. All of this, of course, in turn contributes to problems with access—in some cases because of loss of coverage, and in other cases because increased out-of-pocket cost or reduced benefits make healthcare services less affordable for many people.

On the other hand, efforts to control costs may have an impact on healthcare quality if they lead to decreased health insurance benefits, diminished availability of services, or reduction in numbers of providers available to deliver services. In the 1990s, for example, many hospitals sought to adjust to decreased insurance payment levels by reducing their use of professional staff, including registered nurses. Subsequent research supported what many nurses warned at that time—that nurse staffing is closely tied to positive patient outcomes, and that reducing nurse staffing endangered patient safety and quality of care.

Changing Health Policy

How are health policy decisions made? How can nurses have an impact on health policy—how can they make their voices heard effectively?

The Structure of Government

Before addressing these questions, it is helpful to briefly examine how government is structured. In the United States, government is organized into three branches: the legislative branch, the executive branch, and the judicial branch. Each has an important role to play in healthcare policy, and nurses have opportunities to try to influence the decision-making processes of each of them.

Legislative Branch

At the federal level, the legislative branch of government is the US Congress. Congress is made up of two houses (or chambers)—the US House of Representatives and the US Senate. The House is composed of 435 members elected from districts in each state. The number of districts in each state is based on the size of the state's population, so larger states have more congressional districts while smaller states have fewer. California, for example, currently has the most congressional districts (and thus the most members of the US House of Representatives) at 53, while Alaska has only one. The US Senate is made up of 100 members. Two US Senators are elected

from each state, regardless of the size of the state's population. The Senate is sometimes referred to as the upper house (or chamber) of Congress, while the House of Representatives is sometimes called the lower house (or chamber).

Most state legislatures follow a similar structure, with the two houses known by different names in different states. For example, the lower house may be known as the State Assembly in some states and the House of Representatives in others. (The sole exception to this two-chamber structure is Nebraska, in which the state legislature is made up of only one chamber.)

The legislative branch of government sets policy by debating and voting on legislation (or laws). A new piece of legislation, especially when it has been proposed but has not yet been adopted, is often referred to as a *bill*.

Executive Branch

The chief executive of the United States is the president. The chief executive of a state is the governor. One important role that the president and governors play with regard to health policy is the power to approve or to reject (*veto*) legislation that has been approved by the legislative branch. At the federal level, once Congress has voted to adopt a new law, it is sent to the president, who can then either sign it into law, veto it, or do nothing, in which case the bill becomes law after 10 days. If the president vetoes a new law, Congress can vote to override his veto, but doing so requires a two-thirds vote (instead of a simple majority), which is often difficult to obtain.

For example, in 2007, Congress passed legislation expanding the State Children's Health Insurance Program, which helps provide health insurance for otherwise uninsured children of lower-income families. President George W.

Bush vetoed this legislation. Although a majority of Congress opposed the veto, supporters were unable to achieve the two-thirds majority necessary to override the veto (Pear & Stolberg, 2007). (Subsequently, compromise legislation on children's health insurance was passed, which the president then signed into law.) In 2008, Congress passed legislation that, among other things, reversed reductions in Medicare reimbursement for physicians, advanced practice nurses, and other clinicians. President Bush vetoed this legislation. This time, however, supporters of the legislation were able to achieve a two-thirds majority, and the president's veto was overridden—which meant that the legislation was enacted despite the veto (Stout, 2008).

In addition to the power to sign or veto legislation, another way in which the president and the state governors exercise important influence on health policy is through their authority over a large array of government agencies, often referred to as *administrative agencies* or *executive agencies*. The US president appoints the heads of large federal agencies that administer significant government programs related to health care, such as the US Department of Health and Human Services (DHHS). Within DHHS are a number of agencies such as the Centers for Medicare and Medicaid Services (CMS), which operates the Medicare, Medicaid, and State Children's Health Insurance (SCHIP) programs; the Agency for Healthcare Research and Quality (AHRQ), which funds and operates initiatives related to healthcare quality and patient safety; and the Health Resources and Services Administration (HRSA),which, among other duties, administers programs to provide financial support for basic and graduate nursing education. Many other federal agencies administer significant programs related to health care and nurs-

ing. For example, the Veterans Administration operates hospital and other healthcare services for veterans; the Department of Defense provides and funds healthcare services for active-duty service members and their families. The top leadership of these agencies—such as the Secretary of Health and Human Services, who heads DHHS—is appointed by the president and generally implement the president's policies.

These government agencies implement the laws that are passed by the legislative branch. However, it is important to understand that this often involves a great deal of authority to set policy.

In general, the relationship between state governors and state government agencies is similar to the relationship between the US president and federal government agencies, as discussed. The names, functions, and structure of these state agencies differ from state to state. For example, the agency that oversees hospital quality may be known as the Department of Health in one state, the Department of Public Health in another, and the Department of Health Services in another. Generally, the practice of nursing, medicine, and other health professions are regulated at the state level, so state government agencies have an important role to play in this process.

Judicial Branch

The court system comprises the judicial branch of government. Two parallel court systems—state and federal—interpret and apply laws, including state and federal legislation. The courts also have the authority to strike down laws or regulations under certain circumstances—for example, if a federal court finds that a law passed by Congress violates the US Constitution. The courts are also sometimes called upon to determine whether a regulation issued by a government agency is consistent with relevant state or federal laws.

There are many ways in which nurses can help to change health policy by having an impact on decision makers, including legislators and government agency officials. As individuals, nurses can express their opinions to elected and appointed officials by writing letters and making telephone calls—for example, to urge a state legislator or member of Congress to vote in favor of proposed legislation. Nurses can also get directly involved by contributing to and campaigning for candidates they support—and, of course, voting for those candidates.

Nurses can significantly increase their impact on health policy, however, by joining and becoming active members of their professional organizations. In the United States, organized groups wield considerable influence in the policy-making process. This is true not just for nurses, but for a wide variety of groups that are affected by changes in health policy. Organizations representing almost every interest and perspective imaginable seek to make themselves heard on issues of importance to them. These are often called *interest groups*, sometimes referred to as *stakeholder groups*, *constituency groups*, or by similar names. These are groups that represent the interests of their constituents or members.

In health care, interest groups include organizations representing health professionals, such as the American Nurses Association, the American Medical Association, American Psychological Association, American Pharmacists Association, National Association of Social Workers, and many, many others. Healthcare interest groups also include organizations representing healthcare institutions and agencies, including the American Hospital Association, the National Association for Home Care and Hospice, and the American Health Care Association (which represents long-term care providers), and groups representing other industries, such as the Health Industry Manufacturers Association, the Pharmaceutical Research and Manufacturers Association, and America's Health Insurance Plans (which represents the health insurance industry).

There are also groups that represent consumers, such as the AARP, which, as part of its broader agenda of representing the interests of older Americans, addresses many issues related to health care. (Many nurses are also active members and leaders of AARP.) Several organizations focus on specific diseases or conditions and, as part of their mission, seek to represent consumers affected by those diseases or conditions, as well as providers and researchers who focus their efforts on them. These organizations are sometimes referred to as disease-specific organizations or as voluntary organizations. Prominent examples include the American Cancer Society, the American Heart Association, and the American Diabetes Association. The March of Dimes focuses on promoting children's health by preventing prematurity and birth defects.

Within many health professions and industries, there are also organizations representing more specific or specialized groups. For example, while the American Medical Association (AMA) seeks to speak on behalf of physicians, there are also many organizations that represent physicians practicing in various specialties and subspecialties. The American Hospital Association (AHA) represents US hospitals, but there are also organizations that represent specific types of hospitals, including public hospitals, for-profit hospitals, Catholic hospitals, psychiatric hospitals, and others.

Similarly, although the American Nurses Association (ANA) serves as the professional association representing nursing as a whole, there are a large number of other organizations representing nurses in different specialty areas (such as the American Association of Critical-Care Nurses, the Association of periOperative Registered Nurses, Emergency Nurses Association, Oncology Nurses Society, American Psychiatric Nurses Association, and the Association of Nurses in AIDS Care, to name a few examples) and roles (such as the American Organization of Nurse Executives). Two large organizations also focus on nursing education (the American Association of Colleges of Nursing and the National League for Nursing). Several organizations represent minority nurses, including the National Black Nurses Association, National Association of Hispanic Nurses, Philippine Nurses Association of America, Asian American/Pacific Islander Nurses Association, and National Alaska Native/American Indian Nurses Association. A list of many nursing organizations is located at the Web site of the Nursing Organizations Alliance (see http://www.nursing-alliance.org/member.cfm).

There are also several labor unions whose membership consists primarily or exclusively of nurses (such as the United American Nurses and the California Nurses Association/National Nurses Organizing Committee) or whose membership includes large numbers of nurses (such as the Service Employees International Union and the American Federation of Teachers),which devote varying degrees of attention to nursing issues.

Organizations generally determine their positions and priorities on policy issues based on the interests of their members or constituents. Most of them have a process through which members (or their representatives) guide the organization's policy directions, while also providing a means for its leaders to respond quickly to changing issues and circumstances.

Many of ANA's policy positions, for example, are adopted by its House of Delegates (HOD), a decision-making body consisting of representatives elected by members. The HOD meets only once every two years, so between meetings the ANA Board of Directors (BOD), which is elected by the HOD, makes decisions on behalf of the organization. The ANA's decisions are also facilitated by the ANA Congress on Nursing Practice and Economics (CNPE), which makes recommendations to the HOD and Board of Directors on current and emerging practice and policy issues. The CNPE includes members elected by the ANA HOD and also representatives of those nursing specialty organizations that are organizational affiliates of ANA.

Different interest groups may find themselves in agreement on some issues and in conflict over others. For example, in many states, nursing organizations have supported proposals to ease restrictions on the scope of practice and independence of advanced practice nurses, while many medical organizations have opposed such proposals. On the other hand, medical and nursing organizations often agree on other important issues, such as opposing reductions in Medicare payment to providers.

Even among groups that have common interests and professional identities, there may be differences of opinion on some issues—depending in part on differing perspectives, strategies, or interpretations of the impact of certain legislation or policy proposals. For example, on the issue of ensuring safe staffing levels in hospitals, some nursing organizations and unions (including the California Nurses Association, Service Employees International Union, and the United

American Nurses) have strongly favored legislation to establish mandatory staffing ratios that would set the maximum numbers of patients that each nurse can be assigned. (Thus far, such legislation has been enacted only in California.) Other nursing groups (including the American Nurses Association and many of its state affiliates) oppose mandatory staffing ratios and instead favor legislation requiring hospitals to establish committees to determine staffing levels for patient care units within each hospital. Such legislation has been enacted in Oregon, Washington State, and Illinois.

Although the large variety of groups representing nurses in different roles, specialties, and subspecialties may be viewed as a reflection of nurses' diverse clinical and functional interests and needs, it may also be seen as representing an ongoing fragmentation of the profession, making it more difficult to speak with one voice. This fragmentation can weaken nursing's effectiveness in shaping policy, especially if policymakers hear conflicting messages from multiple groups speaking on behalf of nursing.

Different strategies can be employed to decrease this fragmentation or to reduce its negative impact on nursing's effectiveness in shaping policy. One mechanism through which major national nursing organizations coordinate some of their policy efforts is the Tri-Council for Nursing, which consists of ANA, the National League for Nursing, the American Association of Colleges of Nursing, and the American Organization of Nurse Executives. Also, in recent years, the ANA has modified its structure to seek to involve other nursing organizations in its work. Many nursing specialty organizations are ANA organizational affiliates, which are represented at ANA HOD meetings and on the ANA CNPE. (A current list of ANA organizational affiliates can be found at http://www. nursingworld.org/FunctionalMenuCategories/A boutANA/WhoWeAre/AffiliatedOrganizations _1/OrgAffiliates.aspx.) Many nursing organizations also work together in various *coalitions*. Coalitions are structures that are formed to provide a means for different groups to collaborate on specific issues.

Shaping Policy

Nursing organizations have become increasingly active in advocating on behalf of the profession and our patients. Activities designed to influence Congress or the state legislatures are often referred to as *lobbying*. Many nursing organizations such as the ANA utilize professional lobbyists who devote their time to advocating on behalf of the organization—meeting with elected officials, explaining the organization's positions supporting or opposing legislation, and helping to analyze and explain proposed legislation and its impact on the profession.

Although professional lobbyists play an important role in policy advocacy, nursing organizations have increasingly emphasized the importance of involving their members—individual nurses—in advocating on behalf of the profession. For example, ANA or a nursing specialty organization might send out an e-mail message urging members to call or write their members of Congress to urge them to vote for more funding for nursing education. Advocacy activities by members of an organization are often referred to as *grassroots lobbying*.

POLITICAL ACTION COMMITTEES

As part of their advocacy strategies, many interest groups have created *political action committees* (PACs). PACs provide an organized means for members to endorse candidates, campaign for them, and contribute money to support them. PACs have sometimes been criticized as a way for large and powerful industry groups and corporations to exert influence on the political process. However, PACs are also a way for individuals with common interests to pool their resources to have a more powerful political voice. Thus, for example, many individual ANA members generally contribute modest amounts to the ANA Political Action Committee (ANA-PAC). The ANA-PAC endorses and contributes money to candidates who are supportive of nursing's policy agenda, thus helping to maximize nursing's impact on the policy process in a manner that small contributions by individual nurses cannot. Decisions to support candidates are made by the ANA-PAC Board of Trustees, which is appointed by the ANA Board of Directors.

While the ANA-PAC is the oldest and largest federal nursing-related PAC, a few other national nursing organizations (including the American Association of Nurse Anesthetists, the American College of Nurse-Midwives, the American Academy of Nurse Practitioners, the American College of Nurse Practitioners, and the United American Nurses) have also established PACs. Other healthcare organizations, including the American Hospital Association and the American Medical Association, have their own PACs. Most unions have PACs as well. (Although many PACs include the phrase *political action committee* as part of their name, not all do. Many union PACs, for example, have traditionally been known by the name "Committees on Political Education," or COPE.)

In addition to federal PACs, which support and contribute to federal election campaigns (i.e., president, US Senate, and US House of Representatives), which are regulated under federal law, each state has its own law and rules governing election campaign financing and contributions. Thus, many state-based healthcare organizations (including state nurses associations, hospital associations, medical societies, etc.) have their own state PACs, which endorse and contribute money to candidates for state offices (such as governor, state legislators, and other elected officials).

Supporting political activity through their national and state professional associations is an important way for nurses to have an impact on the political process. Nurses can also be active as individuals in supporting and contributing to election campaigns for federal, state, and local offices. Many nurses have gained important policy-related experience by becoming active in political campaigns. This can also be a good way to help ensure that other political activists—as well as political candidates and elected officials—are aware of nursing issues and concerns. Many nurses, often building on a record of political activity, have themselves run for and won election to political office. Many nurses serve as state legislators, city council members, and in other state and local elected offices. Currently, three nurses—Lois Capps, RN (D-CA); Eddie Bernice Jefferson, RN (D-TX); and Carolyn McCarthy, LPN (D-NY)—serve as members of the US House of Representatives.

Helping to elect political candidates is one important way for nurses to have an impact on health policy. But nurses also need to make their voices heard on policy issues, including proposed legislation and regulations.

Many nursing organizations also organize events to bring nurses together to help lobby on pending legislation. For example, most state nurses associations hold a Lobby Day (different names may be used in different states) on which nurses and nursing students from around the state will travel to the state capitol, gather to hear about the current status of several important bills under consideration in the state legislature, and then go in groups to visit their legislators to urge them to support nursing's positions on those bills.

Reforming the Healthcare System

Given the problems faced by our healthcare system, many people have called for making major changes in the system. Proposed changes in the system are generally referred to as *healthcare reform*, or *health system reform*. But there are many different approaches to reforming the system, and many different ideas about what needs to be changed, so simply hearing an elected official, candidate, or healthcare organization declare support for healthcare reform may not tell you what kinds of changes they favor.

Currently, access to care is the primary focus of many health reform advocates. Many proposals for increasing access focus specifically on access to health insurance and on how to cover the tens of millions of uninsured Americans. Notably, access to health insurance is a problem that the United States has grappled with for decades, but which is much less of an issue in other industrialized countries. In those other countries, the government pays for healthcare services for its citizens—either by providing services through government-operated providers (such as in the United Kingdom) or through government-sponsored health insurance (such as in Canada). In the United States, systems in which government provides health insurance for everyone are often referred to as *single-payer* sys-

tems because the government is the sole source of payment for healthcare services (in contrast to the current US system in which people are covered by one of many private insurance plans or public programs), or, in the case of the uninsured, by no plan or program at all.

Over the years (starting as far back as the 1920s), many people in the United States have supported proposals for such a system, so far without success. Instead, the United States has followed a different approach.

Until the 1930s, healthcare services were generally paid for either by an individual paying a physician or hospital for services or through support provided to hospitals by charitable foundations. In the 1930s, as the United States went through the period of the Great Depression, many people were unable to pay for healthcare services themselves, and the availability of support from charitable organizations was greatly reduced. Without reliable, consistent sources of funding, hospitals faced great financial uncertainty. A response to this problem came with the development of the early Blue Cross plans— hospital insurance plans that were sponsored by state hospital associations. Subscribers paid a regular fee (premium) to these plans, in exchange for which the plan would pay the hospital for the cost of the subscribers' hospital care if and when it was needed. Later, state medical societies developed a similar approach by sponsoring insurance plans—the early Blue Shield plans— that paid for physician care.

Although a few employers provided health insurance as a benefit of employment, for the most part such insurance was purchased directly by individuals for themselves and their families. This remained true until the late 1940s. At that time, US industry was growing rapidly as World War II came to an end. Large employers needed to attract workers but were prevented from raising wages because a government-imposed wage–price freeze, which had been instituted to help focus economic resources on the war effort, was still in effect. Instead, employers offered increased benefits packages as a way to recruit employees. Health insurance was one of these benefits.

This approach to healthcare payment brought coverage to large numbers of Americans, but of course it still left many people out: workers whose employers did not provide insurance; older Americans who were no longer working; and other individuals who did not work because of disability or other circumstances.

Many people continued to advocate a single-payer (government-sponsored) national health insurance program that would cover all Americans. Beginning in 1946, President Harry S. Truman proposed such a program. Among its fiercest opponents was the American Medical Association (AMA), which viewed it as a threat to physicians' autonomy—that is, they feared that government involvement in paying for healthcare services might lead to government interference in medical practice. (In part reflecting the political tenor of the times, opponents of President Truman's plan charged that it was a step toward "socialism" and would institute "Soviet-style medicine" in the United States.) The AMA was very vocal in its opposition and had its members pay an additional fee above their regular dues to help finance a campaign against President Truman's proposal. AMA created a special fund of more than $4 million to finance this campaign (Corning, 1969) and played a major role in defeating Truman's healthcare proposal.

By the late 1950s, the plight of uninsured older Americans drew increasing attention.

Single-payer advocates (including, at that time, some large and influential groups, including labor unions) also recognized that achieving a system of government-sponsored insurance for all Americans was politically unlikely, at least for the time being. Thus many groups and individuals threw their support behind a proposal to provide health insurance to Americans age 65 and older. This proposal, to be based on expanding the Social Security system of income support for older Americans, later came to be known as Medicare.

The Medicare proposal initially faced opposition from the American Medical Association and the American Hospital Association. The American Nurses Association (ANA), on the other hand, voted to support it—in fact, ANA was the first health professional organization to come out in support of Medicare. This was a particularly bold move for nursing to make at the time—such a degree of political independence, taking a position at odds with AMA and AHA, was unprecedented and controversial (Editorial: Taking a stand, 1959; Keepnews, 2007).

Proposals to establish the national health insurance program for the elderly were defeated in Congress in 1957 and 1959. Finally, in 1965, a compromise was worked out among major interest groups, and Congress passed legislation for the following three programs (which continue through today):

Medicare Part A. Also known as hospital insurance, Medicare Part A covers the costs of hospital care (as well as some other types of institution- or agency-based care, including, under specified circumstances, skilled nursing facility care and home health care) for individuals age 65 and older (later expanding to include the permanently disabled and patients with end-stage renal disease).

Medicare Part B. Also known as supplemental medical insurance, Medicare Part B covers the costs of physician services (and, more recently, services of some other clinicians, including advanced practice nurses).

Medicaid. Medicaid is a joint federal and state program that covers services for many poor patients. Medicaid is administered by the states with federal funding (generally at 50% or more).

Although these programs have provided coverage for millions of Americans who would otherwise be uninsured, they cannot plug all gaps in insurance coverage. Neither can they address the more recent erosion of employer-provided insurance.

Many people remain firmly convinced that only a government-sponsored program of health insurance coverage for all Americans (a single-payer system) can ensure that everyone will be insured. Although proposals to establish a single-payer system have been voiced by many groups and individuals and by some political leaders, the long history of defeat faced by previous proposals has convinced others that such a system may be a worthy goal but that it is not achievable.

In the early 1990s, concern with the growing number of uninsured helped to galvanize interest in healthcare reform, particularly as many Americans feared that their own coverage might be vulnerable. During his successful 1992 campaign for president, Bill Clinton emphasized his support for health reform. In 1993, President Clinton proposed a plan for reorganizing health care. While proposing universal coverage, it

supported achieving this goal through a combination of private and public plans and programs. The Clinton plan included far-ranging proposals to address healthcare costs and quality in addition to its proposals for expanding access to insurance coverage. The plan also contained proposals for expanding availability of primary care services, including increased utilization of advanced practice nurses.

Although ANA and many other groups supported the Clinton proposal, many organizations (including AMA) were either opposed or equivocal. By the end of 1994, Congress failed to enact the Clinton plan or any health reform legislation, and the prospects for enacting health reform at any time soon had become dim. The focus for most health reform advocates shifted to state-based reform efforts as well as initiatives to adopt *incremental* reforms. The idea behind incremental reform is that even if wide-scale change is not immediately achievable, smaller reforms may at least lead to some improvements and, optimally, could eventually add up to more comprehensive reform. Following defeat of the Clinton plan, early efforts at incremental reform included improved health insurance portability and expanded coverage for uninsured children (through the State Children's Health Insurance Program, SCHIP).

Despite many proposals and efforts aimed at reducing the number of uninsured Americans, their ranks have grown. A renewed focus on covering the uninsured has led to new proposals for health reform. Most proposals seek to build on the current system while expanding public programs and increasing the availability and affordability of private health insurance.

A significant current issue related to reducing the numbers of uninsured Americans is whether there should be an *individual mandate* to carry health insurance. This means that all individuals would be required to have insurance—either through their employers, through a government program (if they qualify), or by purchasing a plan from a private insurer. Massachusetts enacted a healthcare plan that included such an individual mandate, along with an expanded public program and measures designed to ensure affordable private insurance, in 2006. Similar approaches have been included in other state and federal health reform proposals.

Supporters of individual insurance mandates argue that this approach is necessary to achieve universal coverage, and many suggest that it is consistent with existing policy approaches in other areas, such as requiring drivers to carry automobile insurance. Opponents argue that individual mandates are unfair, that ensuring truly affordable coverage for lower-income individuals and families is unlikely, and that penalizing them for failing to secure coverage punishes those who can least afford it. Many also argue that guaranteeing access to healthcare coverage should be a social responsibility carried out by government and that individual mandates shift that responsibility to individuals instead.

Other proposals for reducing the number of uninsured Americans have included permitting individuals younger than age 65 to purchase Medicare coverage. Single-payer advocates have focused their recent efforts on proposals to expand the current Medicare program so that it covers all Americans—in other words, to transform Medicare into a system of universal coverage.

Nursing and Health Reform

In 1991, the ANA and the National League for Nursing endorsed a common platform for healthcare reform, *Nursing's Agenda for Health Care Reform* (ANA, 1991). *Nursing's Agenda* calls for establishing universal access to a core of essential services, to be provided through a combination of public and private plans. It calls for "a restructured health care system that will focus on the consumers and their health, with services to be delivered in familiar, convenient sites, such as schools, workplaces, and homes" (ANA, 1991, p. 2). *Nursing's Agenda* also calls for "a shift from the predominant focus on illness and cure to an orientation toward wellness and care" (ANA, 1991, p. 2). It also calls for expanding the use of nurses, including advanced practice nurses, to increase access to primary and preventive services and to decrease costs.

Nursing's Agenda drew widespread support within the nursing profession and was eventually endorsed by 60 nursing organizations. It was the basis for efforts by ANA and other groups to promote health reform goals and also served as a means to assess other reform proposals. As noted earlier, ANA supported President Clinton's health reform proposals; this was based in large part on the conclusion that his proposals were consistent with the principles of *Nursing's Agenda*.

ANA has revised and updated *Nursing's Agenda* twice since the defeat of health reform in the 1990s. The most current version, called *Health System Reform Agenda*, was issued in 2008 (ANA, 2008).

Many nursing organizations have strongly supported single-payer approaches to health reform. These include some ANA state affiliates such as the New York State Nurses Association and other groups including the California Nurses Association and the United American Nurses. At its 1999 House of Delegates meeting, ANA adopted a motion to (1) endorse the single-payer mechanism as the most desirable

---

Box 14-1 Personal Message from a Contemporary Nurse Leader

Polly Bednash

Growing up in rural Texas when I did, there were few professional career paths open to women. But I was not going to let that stop me. Nursing was a choice I made when my best friend decided to become a nurse. I followed her lead and enrolled in Texas Woman's University, where I graduated with a Bachelor of Science in Nursing degree. Nursing turned out to be exactly the right choice for me and has provided me with multiple opportunities for growth and change over the years. I have been constantly challenged, both intellectually and personally, with choice and growth opportunities always present within the nursing field.

Following my service with the Army Nurse Corps, which including work as a staff nurse in Vung Tau, Vietnam, I pursued a Master of Science in Nursing from the Catholic University of America in the mid-1970s and began my long career as a nurse educator. While teaching in the nursing program at George Mason University in Virginia, I had the opportunity to also serve as a nurse practitioner at the Ft. Belvoir Family Practice Residency Program, where I saw patients, taught in the family practice program, and provided consultation to the residents/staff at this practice site. In this work, I was able to bring new insights to my teaching and enlighten students about the rich rewards and challenges of a nursing career. All of the work was intermingled and

allowed me to see common themes in all the expressions of nursing and bring excitement to the students who were learning the science, and art, of nursing.

It is important to acknowledge that becoming a nurse educator did not take me away from nursing. Instead, it helped me to focus on the science of the profession and provided me with another wonderful challenge, the opportunity to teach a new generation of nurses every year. The students were constantly teaching me, too, as they looked with fresh eyes at our field and our patterns of practice. Work as a nurse educator is a very rewarding way to express being a professional nurse, and work as a faculty is absolutely vital to creating the future for nursing.

While pursuing a doctorate in higher education policy and law at the University of Maryland, I interned in the Government Affairs department at the American Association of Colleges of Nursing (AACN). This chance placement led to my appointment as AACN's Director of Governmental Relations in 1986. My work in this capacity again focused on nursing education and practice. AACN's mission spans two major domains: health and education. In the area of governmental affairs, I was able to bring life to the policy process through informed discussion about the real work of nursing practice and education. Although I was forced to give up my patient care work with this position, I was able to affect nursing by helping shape nursing policy. Working with staff on Capitol Hill and with the members of our organization, I was able to help advance both funding and practice opportunities. Nursing continued to provide me with challenging opportunities, not on an individual level, but on a greater level.

Appointed to the role of AACN Executive Director in 1989, I made it my primary goal to work with my staff to achieve the mission and objectives established by our board and members. Our focus on baccalaureate and graduate nursing education means we believe that a well-educated nursing workforce is vital to the health of the nation. AACN also champions the important research conducted in our schools of nursing, which creates the science that shapes nursing practice and leads to innovation. We are committed to creating the best of nursing for the present and the future, and all of our work and our collaborations are directed toward this goal.

Over the course of my career, I have been blessed to have accomplished a number of my personal goals, including my graduate studies, my experience as a Robert Wood Johnson Faculty Fellow in Primary Care, my experience in the military, and my work here at AACN. One thing I have learned is that setbacks happen for a reason. In those times when I have sought particular work or opportunities and have not achieved them, I realized later that the opportunities that opened up instead had greater value than what I originally sought. I did not originally see myself as a nurse; I wanted to be an actress! I think I made the better choice when I enrolled in nursing school and am proud that I was smart enough to take this path.

My greatest reward in my current position as the chief executive officer and executive director of AACN is the chance I have to work with nursing leaders in this country and abroad who are committed to preparing the best educated nursing workforce possible. I am grateful to have the opportunity to work with a staff of smart and committed individuals who are also good colleagues. I am happy to come to work every day and find each day a gift and a reward. This is the best career I could ever have chosen, and I am in the place that fits best with my life goals.

For those of you new to the nursing profession, I encourage you to identify your professional goals early in your career and then work, in a systematic and balanced way, to achieve them. Understand where you want to end up in terms of your career and the education you need to get there, and remember that you have a long time to get it all done. You can't do it all at once, but you should be continuously learning, challenging yourself, and finding personal reward in your career and family life. Find joy in your work, and you will find the right places to compromise and move ahead.

option for financing a reformed healthcare system, and (2) continue to advocate for other measures to increase access to quality health care for all (ANA, 1999). For the most part, however, ANA has not emphasized its support for single-payer health care since that time.

Summary

As the challenges facing the healthcare system become increasingly apparent, debate and discussion continue regarding the best way to achieve a healthcare system that provides access to quality, affordable care to all Americans. The opportunities for nurses to make themselves heard on health policy issues that directly affect them and their patients will continue to grow. Recognizing and understanding major policy issues are essential for the nursing profession. By remaining aware of these issues and committing to utilizing the tools to help change policy, nurses can have a major impact on the future of our healthcare system.

QUESTIONS

1. Mr. J, an 80-year-old man, needs to schedule a visit with his physician for treatment of a medical problem. Because he has Medicare Part B, he knows
   a. He will probably have to pay some of the costs of his visit himself.
   b. Medicare Part B will cover all of the costs of his visit to the physician
   c. Medicaid would cover all of his expenses
   d. He will have to pay the entire cost of his visit himself.

2. At the federal level, the legislative branch is made up of the
   a. Supreme Court and the US Congress
   b. House of Representatives and the president of the United States
   c. US Congress, which is composed of the Senate and the House of Representatives
   d. All of the above

3. Political action committees (PACs) create and provide a
   a. place to discuss professional issues
   b. way for members of a professional organization to endorse candidates and contribute to their campaigns
   c. way to fund your professional association's work
   d. None of the above

4. Challenges facing the healthcare system are often grouped into issues of
   a. professionalism, continued competence, and licensure
   b. veracity, fidelity, and autonomy
   c. access, cost, and quality
   d. risk, benefit, and alternatives

5. One of the factors that led to the current system of employer-provided health insurance was
   a. employers offering benefits such as health insurance in order to recruit workers at the end of World War II, since they were not allowed to increase wages
   b. the development of Medicare and Medicaid
   c. the spread of managed care
   d. widespread concern about error-related death and injury

References

American Nurses Association (1991). *Nursing's agenda for health care reform*. Washington, DC: Author.

American Nurses Association (1999, June 19). Nursing's preference for single-payer model of health finance and organization. *ANA House of Delegates*.

American Nurses Association. (2008). Health system reform agenda. Retrieved August 7, 2008, from http://www.nursingworld.org/MainMenu Categories/HealthcareandPolicyIssues/HSR/ ANAsHealthSystemReformAgenda.aspx

Catlin, A., Cowan, C., Hatman, M., & Hefler, S. (2008). National health spending in 2006: A year of change for prescription drugs. *Health Affairs*, 27(1), 14–29.

Commonwealth Fund Commission on a High Performance Health System. (2008). Why not the best? Results from the National Scorecard on U.S. health system performance. Retrieved November 17, 2008, from http://www.commonwealthfund.org/usr_doc/Why_ Not_the_Best_national_scorecard_2008.pdf? section=4039

Corning, P. A. (1969). The evolution of Medicare. Retrieved August 7, 2008, from http://www. ssa.gov/history/corning.html

Editorial: Taking a stand. (1959). *American Journal of Nursing*, 59(9), 1245.

Institute of Medicine. (2004). *Insuring America's health— principles and recommendations*. Washington, DC: National Academies Press.

Keepnews, D. M. (2005). Health policy: A nursing specialty? *Policy, Politics & Nursing Practice*, 6(4), 275–276.

Keepnews, D. (2007). Meeting the challenge of health reform. *Policy, Politics & Nursing Practice*, 8(3), 156–157.

Kohn, L., Corrigan, J., & Donaldson, M. (Eds.). (2000). *To err is human: Building a safer health system*. Washington, DC: National Academy Press.

Malone, R. E. (2005). Assessing the policy environment. *Policy, Politics, & Nursing Practice*, 6(2), 135–143.

Pear, R., & Stolberg, S. G. (2007, October 19). House sustains president's veto on child health. *New York Times*. Retrieved August 7, 2008, from http:// www.nytimes.com/2007/10/19/washington/19 health.html

Smedley, B. D., Stith, A. Y., & Nelson, A. R. (Eds.), Committee on Understanding and Eliminating Racial and Ethnic Disparities in Health Care. (2003). *Unequal treatment: Confronting racial and ethnic disparities in health care*. Washington, DC: National Academies Press.

Starr, P. (1984). *The social transformation of American medicine*. New York: Basic Books.

Stout, D. (2008, July 16). Congress overrides Bush's veto on Medicare. *New York Times*. Retrieved August 7, 2008, from http://www.nytimes.com/2008/07/16/ washington/16medic.html?fta=y

US Census Bureau. (2008). Household income rises, poverty rate unchanged, number of uninsured down. Press Release August 26, 2008. Retrieved December 1, 2008 from http://www.census.gov/ Press-Release/www/releases/archives/income_ wealth/012528.html

Preparation for Leadership: Legal and Regulatory Considerations for Safe Patient Care

Jerelyn Peixoto
Weiss

OUTLINE

Systems That Facilitate the Most Effective
Management of Healthcare Personnel
The Safety Nurse
Competency Programs

The Importance of Understanding and
Meeting Patients' Expectations
How Documentation Can Be the Most
Effective for Nurse Managers

This chapter on legal and regulatory considerations is for nurses new to leadership positions to prepare them to maintain, promote, and facilitate the highest standards of care to meet today's patient care practice challenges. The current quality performance climate and trends for system-wide standardization of all healthcare practice is reviewed. Insights into how to anticipate and then lay the groundwork for consistent, safe patient care are presented. Examples of the most frequent and common nursing malpractice cases, liability-laden incidents, and everyday practice obstacles in a variety of areas of nursing practice are presented. Proven methods for resolution and anticipatory guidance are offered to avoid potential liability and regulatory compliance risks.

The information presented can assist new nurse leaders to organize more efficiently how they approach monitoring day-to-day nursing practice, motivate the healthcare team to provide the safest care, manage staff members effectively, and implement productive actions to achieve the safest patient outcomes.

Developing Protocols

The importance of developing protocols, guidelines, and job descriptions that are correlated with the necessary skill and procedure competencies is discussed to assist new nurse leaders as they begin their leadership careers. The protocols presented here include leadership considerations that encompass nursing standards of care in a variety of specialty settings. Legal and risk management concepts, governmental regulatory compliance requirements, and state health department criteria that can be applied to everyday clinical and administrative situations are also presented. Rather than describing isolated laws and general standards of care affecting nursing practice, real examples of situations that face nurses in a variety of inpatient and outpatient settings are presented to illuminate the ways in which applicable laws, regulations, and nursing standards of care can guide safe, effective nursing practice and nursing leadership every day.

A variety of practice situations and settings are included in the discussion from acute inpatient care to community health nursing and care of the elderly in extended care facilities. The specialties presented here include acute medical care; surgical care, including pre- and postoperative care; pediatric acute care; emergency care; perinatal nursing; elder care; psychiatric nursing; and community health nursing care.

Even though presenting actual malpractice cases that illustrate the very worst nursing practice leading to the most detrimental patient care outcomes may seem like a negative instructional approach, analysis of the cases that finally go to trial presents a number of significant insights. For example, actual cases provide an account of nursing practice from a nonnursing perspective.

The cases provide nurses with the opportunity to analyze what went wrong and why. The outcome of case analysis can lead to the formulation of a plan for nursing practice that avoids those very points at which the quality of nursing practice broke down (Murchison, Nichols, & Hanson, 1982).

Often these cases document the black and white, cut and dry, very obvious breaches of nursing standards that make the reader wonder how that avalanche of poor decision making and those omissions of careful planning and vigilance for safe patient care ever did occur. Interestingly, in the *Journal of Nursing Management*, Rosemary Luquire points out, "Experience has shown that frequently malpractice actions are preceded by a clearly identifiable trail of substandard performance" (Luquire, 1989, p. 57). Also, analysis of hospital incident reports has revealed that most incidents occur between 8:00 A.M. and 11:00 A.M., one of the most demanding and busiest times in the healthcare team's day (Poteet, 1983).

The cases that are published are the worst-case scenarios, and unfortunately they can occur. At the same time, day after day nurses have to deal with the gray areas of practice, those daily events that may not injure a patient but, if magnified by lack of adequate staffing, lack of competent nursing oversight, lack of complete and concise oral and written communication between and by the healthcare team, as well as a lack of an established safety-focused plan of care, could lead to detrimental consequences.

The intention here is to present pertinent information from actual cases and from the most common everyday practices to help alert the reader to situations that may present the potential for negative outcomes in order to prevent those outcomes from occurring. Methods for developing safe patient care systems that facilitate productive work environments for staff are illustrated.

A Decade's Perspective on Efforts in the Healthcare Service Industry to Provide Safe Patient Care

Nurses and the practice of nursing do not exist in a vacuum. To place the profession's practice challenges into a national perspective, it is important to step back and view the status of the entire healthcare service industry before homing in on nursing practice and the discussion of methods for providing systematic, consistently safe patient care.

In 1999, the Institute of Medicine's (IOM) report *To Err Is Human* analyzed a wide range of patient safety problems and the need for improvement. In 2001, the IOM developed a second report entitled *Crossing the Quality Chasm* that called for fundamental change and that proposed a national initiative to provide strategic direction for redesigning the healthcare system of the 21st century. Both reports stressed that the resolution for the frequent occurrence of negative outcomes from healthcare provider mishaps wasn't a matter of placing blame on individual providers, but that these outcomes occurred because of poorly designed systems or lack of systems for providing consistency, standardization, and methodical recurring checks and balances to prevent or catch potential human errors before they resulted in morbidity or mortality.

In July 2002, The Joint Commission implemented standardized performance measures that were designed to track the performance of accredited hospitals and encourage improvement in the quality of health care. For many hospitals that complied, the results were promising (Williams, Schmaltz, Morton, Koss, & Loeb, 2005).

However, in 2003, the *New England Journal of Medicine* published a report that described how clinicians failed to provide appropriate care in nearly half of all cases (Bates & Gawande). In 2004, the National Commission on Quality Assurance stated that "1,000 Americans or more die each week because the healthcare system regularly fails to deliver appropriate care" (Brook, 2007, p. 124).

At the end of 2005, the *New England Journal of Medicine* reported that more than 3000 US hospitals showed consistent performance improvements in implementation of The Joint Commission's 2002 standardized performance measures. The diagnostic areas reflecting the improvements in the process of care were acute myocardial infarction, heart failure, and pneumonia (Williams et al., 2005).

However, despite the national alert for hospitals to work assertively to prevent risk and initiate incentives on a grand scale to improve patient care and success in some medical conditions, errors remain and consistent progress throughout the nation has not been attained as planned.

In July 2005, the Centers for Medicare and Medicaid Services (CMS) developed a quality improvement road map (The Centers for Medicare and Medicaid Services). The vision is that every person will have the right care every time. To encourage the realization of that vision, CMS has developed five strategies for improving care. The most potent of the five strategies is the following: "To pay in a way that expresses commitment to supporting providers for doing the right thing—improving quality and avoid-

ing unnecessary costs—rather than directing more resources to less effective care." The federal Medicare program began denying Medicare payments to hospitals for certain medical errors in 2007. Hospitals cannot bill the beneficiary for any charges associated with the hospital-acquired complication. In New York State, after the Department of Health revealed the 2006–2007 preventable errors data reported by New York State hospitals, the continuing error rate was so widespread that the state's Medicaid program initiated withholding of medical reimbursement to those hospitals with preventable errors in 2008 (Edelman, 2008). The errors are real and horrific and, more importantly, do not show overall improvement, as documented in Table 15-1.

The Medicare fee withholding strategy for preventable errors became a reality in New York State beginning October 1, 2008. The New York State Health Department reported that the Medicaid program, the state payment source for medical care provided to the underserved populations, began refusing to pay hospitals for botched care and treatment to fix the damage. Insurance companies such as Cigna and Empire are planning to follow suit (Edelman, 2008). Unfortunately, this path of denying payment to hospitals by insurance companies will cause a bigger financial burden for hospitals. Will it make a difference? Hopefully, one difference will be the continued development of effective systems of care that incorporate consistent checks and balances to prevent errors and create safe healthcare environments.

Shannon Brownlee (2007) views the healthcare industry's problems from another perspective in her book titled *Overtreated: Why Too Much Medicine Is Making Us Sicker and Poorer.* Besides shattering the myth that most medicine is based

Table 15-1 Preventable Errors Reported by New York State Hospitals in 2006–2007

Event (examples)	2006	2007
Deaths from medication errors	9	9
Permanent harm from medication errors	13	17
Surgery performed on wrong patient or wrong body part	20	22
Wrong invasive procedure performed outside the operation room, such as ER	95	106
Objects such as surgical tools left inside the patient's body (illustrative of this error, the *New York Post* on April 27, 2008, pictured an abdominal X-ray showing forceps left in the abdominal cavity following surgery)	129	122
Equipment malfunction causing death or serious injury	2	5
Suicides and attempted suicides while under care	16	10
Rapes while under care	0	8
Total	284	299

Source: Edelman, 2008.

on sound science, she offers many viable suggestions for moving toward a more efficient, effective system, so patients are the biggest winners of all.

Brownlee suggests that the use of patient decision aids will result in more effective use of medicine. *Patient decision aids* are mechanisms that strengthen the patient's role in choosing a particular treatment or test. Patients, she maintains, don't always understand the competing risks and benefits in elective procedures, and doctors don't always recognize how different patients can be and what patients value most when it comes to medical treatment.

Her book promotes a reshifting of priorities in the provision of medical care, and she stresses the need for more primary care doctors and fewer specialists, with emphasis placed on prevention and health education. The use of nurses as "health coaches" is outlined to save health insurance companies millions of dollars. For example, patients with multiple or terminal illnesses, who are the most costly to treat and typically take up only 1–2% of the average patient population while accounting for 30% of the costs, can best be served by nurses making home visits and daily phone follow-up calls to help patients control pain and other symptoms and stay out of the hospital. At Franklin Health, a company based in Upper Saddle River, New Jersey, this type of low-tech but intensive service costs insurers an average of $6,000 to $8,000 per patient—but saves them $14,000 to $18,000 per patient in medical bills (Brownlee, 2007). Most importantly, Brownlee conveys a message of hope and ways of controlling costs while improving the quality of US medicine.

Regulatory Influences

In their book titled *Nurse Management Demystified*, Irene McEachen and James Keogh differentiate the authoritative influence between federal and state regulations (2007). Federal regulations generally focus on public health, welfare, Medicare and Medicaid, social services, and bioterrorism and include rules that cover the administrative aspects of a healthcare facility, such as accounting, labor, and wages. However, now the federal government is using its accounting leverage to make a difference in the care that is provided because, from a cost–benefit perspective, the type of care that is provided is directly related to the generated expenses to provide that care. By instituting safety-focused systems and processes to standardize how medical care is provided, the federal government is striving to produce more healthy outcomes, save lives, and reduce costs.

State governments focus on protecting the public by licensing healthcare professionals and healthcare facilities. Nursing is a regulated profession. The goal of nursing regulation is to protect the public from harm that could be caused by an unqualified, incompetent, or unfit practitioner. The earliest nursing registry laws were passed in the 1900s. They afforded title protection and legally recognized nursing, set education standards, and established a mechanism for examination. In 1938, New York was the first state to mandate licensure and define nursing practice; other states followed suit after World War II. Through the 1950s and into the 1970s, all US jurisdictions established mandated licensure for registered nurses and licensed practical nurses (LPNs) (Flook, 2003).

Nurse practice acts define the legal practice of nursing, the scope of practice in each state. The practice acts constitute the legislative basis for the regulation and control of nursing education and practice. Individual state laws dictate the scope of nursing practice, which can vary from state to state. Denise Flook notes that an act may include the following elements:

- Standards of nursing practice
- Standards of professional conduct
- Professional nurse reporting requirements
- Disciplinary procedures
- Delegation and supervisory roles and criteria
- Continuing education requirements
- Name and address notification requirements
- Process and requirements for licensure and licensure renewal
- Advanced practice parameters
- Structure and authority of the Board of Nursing (Flook, 2003)

Healthcare Facility Regulation

Through the certificate of need process, states determine the number and types of healthcare facilities that are adequate and appropriate for any given community, as well as regulate safe practices and environmental safety standards for healthcare facilities. The certificate of need process, which was once voluntary, is now mandated by the federal government and affects a multitude of healthcare institutions, including but not limited to hospitals, adult care facilities, diagnostic and treatment centers, residential healthcare facilities, certified home health agencies, long-term home healthcare programs, hospices, certain health programs associated with mental health care, and the care of individuals with developmental disabilities (New York State Department of Health, 2007).

Healthcare facilities generally fall into two categories: privately operated and publicly operated. Privately operated healthcare facilities can be for-profit or not-for-profit and provide health care in return for a profit or for the sole purpose of providing health care to the community, respectively. A not-for-profit healthcare facility is expected to generate a surplus of funds and to reinvest those funds into providing additional services to the community (McEachen & Keogh, 2007).

The healthcare industry is one of the most regulated industries in the United States. Its revenue is strongly influenced by guidelines established by Medicare, Medicaid, and medical insurers. Healthcare facilities must be accredited by an accrediting organization that establishes standards for providing health care in order to receive either public or insurance third-party reimbursement. The Joint Commission is the most prominent accrediting body in the United States. The Joint Commission is an independent organization; however, only institutions that receive a passing grade from The Joint Commission are accredited, which enables them to receive reimbursement from the federal and state governments and private insurers. The Joint Commission's Web site and key resource references for preparing for accreditation are listed in the references at the end of this chapter.

Sources of Law

A general explanation of the historical basis for constitutional, common, statutory, and administrative laws in the United States will provide an outline of our country's legal system and the context for nursing malpractice case law.

There are four sources of law in the United States: constitutional law, common law, statutes, and administrative law. The US Constitution defines the judiciary's power to decide cases or controversies concerning particular subjects.

The Constitution guarantees to the people certain basic fundamental liberties. Constitutional law defines the relationship between governmental authority and individual freedoms. Constitutional law generally deals with issues such as freedom of religion, freedom of speech, the right to assemble, and anti-discrimination. All powers not granted explicitly to the federal government by the Constitution are retained by the state governments or the people of the country. The state's power to govern includes laws necessary to preserve the public order, the public's health, safety, welfare, and morals (Northrop & Kelly, 1987).

Common law is law made by a judge as opposed to a law created by the legislature or a regulation created by an agency. Common law relies on the doctrine of *stare decisis* (to stand by that which was decided), or precedent. This doctrine follows English law and holds that prior decisions should not be disturbed where the same points arise in litigation. The American courts have not looked at *stare decisis* as an absolute, and judges have overruled earlier decisions when they believed the prior decision was mistaken (Northrop & Kelly, 1987).

Statutory law is enacted by the legislative branch. The federal and state governments have codified laws relevant to health care. In the federal system, these statutes are published in the United States Code; in the states, the statues are published under the particular state's code. Some examples of healthcare-related statutes are nurse practice acts (state statutes) and the Health Insurance Portability and Accountability Act (HIPAA: a federal statute).

Administrative law is established by those agencies that have been authorized to put into operation regulations that will implement a particular statute. For example, state boards of nursing are generally authorized by nurse practice acts to put into operation or to implement specific regulations governing practice (e.g., educational requirements, licensing requirements, and disciplinary actions).

Defining Negligence and Professional Malpractice

Negligence and professional malpractice fall under the common law category in the specific area of law known as tort law. *Tort law*, unlike criminal law, which is defined as a violation or intentional act against the state and, if proven, results in punishment or rehabilitation, is an unintentional act, an accident, or an omission to act that causes another individual injury or financial damages. The law attempts to make the injured individual whole again. Negligence includes specific classifications such as personal injury, abandonment, intentional infliction of emotional distress, fraud/misrepresentation, and professional malpractice.

Ordinary negligence is defined as a deviation from or failure to follow the standard of care that a reasonable person would use in a particular set of circumstances. Professional malpractice related to nursing, also referred to as professional negligence, constitutes a deviation from a professional standard of care relating to the act of nursing when the nurse performing the act in question fails to follow the acceptable standard of nursing practice at the time of the act. To quote Dr. Rose Constantino: "The law doesn't expect nurses to be perfect; it only requires that they be *reasonable*. This means that as trained professionals, nurses are expected to follow the standards of care enunciated by their profession" (Constantino, 2003,

p. 24). Professional malpractice requires expert testimony at trial to explain the technical aspects of the case to the judge or jury.

There are four essential elements of negligence: duty, breach of duty, causation (the breach of duty must have been the cause of the injury), and damages or injury. All of the elements must be present to succeed when bringing a malpractice case.

Duty concerns an established relationship between a nurse and a patient, and that relationship is established when a nurse accepts responsibility for care and treatment of an individual. A case exemplifying this is *Lunsford v. Board of Nurse Examiners*.

In this case, the patient, Donald Floyd, was brought by a friend, Miss Farrell, to the Willacy County Hospital with complaints of chest pain accompanied by numbness and pain radiating down his left arm. Miss Farrell left Mr. Floyd in the hospital waiting room and went in search of medical assistance. Within the facility, she spoke with a physician who subsequently referred her to seek help from the RN on duty, Nurse Lunsford. Nurse Lunsford was ordered by the physician to send all patients to Valley Baptist Hospital unless the patient had a physician on the hospital's staff or unless it was a "life–death situation."

Upon entering the waiting room, Nurse Lunsford found Mr. Floyd lying on a table complaining of chest pain that had also radiated to his arms. After questioning Mr. Floyd, Nurse Lunsford learned that he had not undertaken any strenuous exercise or eaten anything unusual that day that may have influenced the onset of his symptoms. Despite suspecting "cardiac involvement," Nurse Lunsford did not take Mr. Floyd's vital signs. Nurse Lunsford gave the following instructions to Miss Farrell: take Mr. Floyd to Valley Baptist Hospital; speed there; drive with the automobile's emergency flashers on; and use the automobile's citizen's band radio to call for help on the way to Valley Baptist Hospital. Nurse Lunsford also asked Miss Farrell about her knowledge of cardiopulmonary resuscitation (CPR), because there might be a chance that she may need to use it during transport. Mr. Floyd died five miles from Willacy Hospital on the way to Valley Baptist Hospital.

The Texas Board of Nurse Examiners conducted a hearing on the actions of Nurse Lunsford relating to Mr. Floyd's death. The board found Nurse Lunsford's conduct had been unprofessional and dishonorable and likely to injure patients or the public, and they suspended Nurse Lunsford's Texas RN license for one year. The District Court of Travis County affirmed the board's decision. Nurse Lunsford appealed, citing that she did not owe a duty to Mr. Floyd because a nurse–patient relationship had not been established between the parties. The court of Appeals of Texas, Third District, affirmed the judgment of the District Court (Croke, 2006).

In this case, Nurse Lunsford maintained that she did not have a nurse–patient relationship, because Mr. Floyd hadn't been admitted to the hospital and was not a patient of the staff physician. However, the courts found that the nurse automatically owed a duty to Mr. Floyd through the receipt of her Texas Registered Nurse Licensure and that a nurse–patient relationship existed when she met Mr. Floyd in the hospital waiting room in need of life-threatening emergency care. Dr. Eileen Croke explained the Texas Board of Nurse Examiners Rule 22 in relation to nurse–patient duty. That rule requires an RN

to assess the health status of each patient and institute appropriate nursing actions that might be required to stabilize the patient's condition and/or prevent further complications (Croke, 2006). In this case, the board and the courts found that Nurse Lunsford failed to assess and implement appropriate nursing actions and that she failed to follow the following standards of care:

1. Failure to assess Mr. Floyd's medical status
2. Failure to inform the physician of Mr. Floyd's cardiac condition and potential life–death medical status
3. Failure to institute appropriate nursing actions, such as taking vital signs and placing the patient on an electrocardiogram (ECG) machine, to stabilize Mr. Floyd's medical condition and prevent further complications and, ultimately, his demise

In Dr. Croke's analysis of this case, she notes that Nurse Lunsford should have been able to reasonably foresee the potential complications related to Mr. Floyd's complaints. The courts look for the foreseeability of consequences in relation to actions taken to determine whether or not the actions taken were the cause of the ultimate events that resulted.

One older case and one hypothetical situation presented here illustrate the existence of foreseeability: a patient who was depressed and had suicidal thoughts voluntarily entered a psychiatric unit. He was assigned a suicide watch and suicide prevention nursing supervision status level according to hospital policy and was not allowed to leave the psychiatric unit without a staff escort. About two weeks after admission, the nurses began to allow the patient to leave the ward unescorted even though policy indicated a physician order was necessary to change the patient's supervision level. The patient committed suicide by jumping out a window (*Abille v. U.S.*, 1980). The patient's survivors were awarded $180,000 in damages based on the negligent acts of the hospital nurses. Suicide was a foreseeable event in this instance.

US courts have established that it is the duty of the hospital and its staff to exercise reasonable care to protect suicidal patients against foreseeable harm. If, on the other hand, foreseeability is absent and a patient commits suicide, there is no breach of duty. In a hypothetical example, it is not foreseeable that a patient who is diagnosed with cancer, for instance, will commit suicide as a result of the diagnosis and therefore special suicide precautions would not be necessary or one of the standards of care for such a patient, unless of course the patient complained of suicidal feelings to one of the healthcare team members.

Proximate causation must exist between the deviation of the duty and the resulting injury. In Nurse Lunsford's case, her failure to follow the standards of care of properly assessing Mr. Floyd—performing vital signs and giving him an ECG—was the cause-in-fact of the injury; her conduct was so closely connected with the result—Mr. Floyd's demise—that the law was justified in imposing liability (Croke, 2006).

Examples of Sources of Nursing Standards

Table 15-2 illustrates some of the sources of nursing standards that constitute the resources for establishing the specific duty of nurses in various work settings. These resources should be familiar to the practicing nurse and the nurse leader because they provide a daily guideline or protocol for maintaining the highest standards of practice.

The Most Common Issues in Professional Nursing Malpractice

There's no denying it: the healthcare environment today poses great liability risks for all healthcare providers, including nurses. Increased patient acuity, shorter lengths of stay, advanced technological demands, decreased nurse to patient ratios, increased numbers of unlicensed healthcare personnel, budget cuts, and modified orientation programs for new nurse graduates are all contributing factors.

Interestingly enough, even though the demands of the healthcare industry and the nursing profession today are more varied and more numerous, the nursing acts that constitute malpractice today have remained very similar to those of the past 30 years (Smith-Pittman, 1998; Croke, 2003). Three newer causes of action for malpractice that have resulted from shortened length of stay, reduced nurse to patient ratio, and increased technological complexity are improper delegation, early discharge, and improper use of equipment. However, the most common categories of allegations against nurses have not changed drastically and can be summarized as follows:

- Failure to properly assess (make careful and full observations) of the patient's condition

Table 15-2 Examples of Nursing Standards of Care

Nursing Practice Settings	External Sources of Professional Nursing Standards	Governmental Sources of Regulatory Nursing Practice Standards	Internal Sources of Organizational Nursing Standards
Medical/Surgical Acute Care	American Nurses Association (2004), *Nursing: Scope and Standards of Practice.* www.nursingworld.org American Nurses Association (2003), *Nursing's Social Policy Statement.* www.nursingworld.org American Nurses Association (2001), *Code of Ethics for Nurses With Interpretive Statements.* www.nursingworld.org/ Nursing theoretical and clinical literature (text-books and peer-reviewed nursing magazines)	State Nurse Practice Act The Joint Commission www.jcaho.org Medicare and Medicaid www.medicare.gov Occupational Safety and Health Administration (OSHA) www.osha.gov Centers for Disease Control and Prevention (CDC) www.cdc.gov State infection control (state Departments of Health) Biohazard handling regulations Americans with Disabilities Act (ADA) www.ada.org Health Insurance Porta-bility and Accountability Act of 1996 (HIPAA) www.cms.hhs.gov/hipaa US Department of Health and Human Services Office of Civil Rights www.hhs.gov/ocr/index/html	Policies and procedures of the institution Nurse's job description and related competencies Nursing care plans

continues

Table 15-2 Examples of Nursing Standards of Care—continued

Nursing Practice Settings	External Sources of Professional Nursing Standards	Governmental Sources of Regulatory Nursing Practice Standards	Internal Sources of Organizational Nursing Standards
Perioperative Care	Association of Perioperative Registered Nurses (2008), *Perioperative Standards and Recommended Practices.* www.aorn.org	Same as above American Association for Accreditation of Ambulatory Surgery (AAAASF) www.aaasf.org	Same as above
Pediatric Acute Care	American Nurses Association and Society for Pediatric Nurses (2003), *Family-Centered Care: Putting It Into Action.* www.nursing-world.org	Same as above	Same as above
Perinatal Acute Care	American Nurses Association (2004), *Neonatal Nursing: Scope and Standards of Practice.* www.nursingworld.org	Same as above Emergency Medical Treatment and Active Labor Act (EMTALA)	Same as above
Emergency Care	Emergency Nurses Association (1999), *Scope of Practice.* www.ena.org	Same as above	Same as above
Community Nursing Care/Ambulatory Care	American Nurses Association (2007), *Public Health Nursing Scope and Standards of Practice.* www.nursingworld.org American Public Health Association (APHA), Public Health Nursing Section. www.apha.org	Same as above Accreditation Association for Ambulatory Health Care (AAAHC) www.aaahc.org	Same as above

continues

Table 15-2 Examples of Nursing Standards of Care—continued

Nursing Practice Settings	External Sources of Professional Nursing Standards	Governmental Sources of Regulatory Nursing Practice Standards	Internal Sources of Organizational Nursing Standards
Psychiatric Nursing	American Nurses Association and American Psychiatric Nurses Association (2007), *Psychiatric-Mental Health: Scope and Standards of Practice.* www.nursingworld.org	Same as above State mental health codes	Same as above

---

- Failure to monitor the patient's condition (failure to provide ongoing observations with frequency determined by the patient's acuity level and the related standard of care)
- Failure to document changes in the patient's condition, and/or failure to document concisely, completely, and in a timely manner
- Failure to intervene with appropriate nursing actions, or failure to follow standards of care
- Failure to report alterations in the patient's condition to the appropriate person in a timely manner (Mayberry & Croke, 1996)

Case Examples of the Most Common Issues in Malpractice

The major focus of this chapter is on legal and regulatory issues facing the nurse leader, which refers to the charge nurse, nurse manager, and unit manager. However, to be fully accomplished in any of these positions and especially to supervise nurses providing direct patient care, a nurse leader must be a fully accomplished clinician and provider of direct care. So, the first legal issue and regulatory considerations analysis focuses on direct care in a number of clinical areas and then focuses on those legal and regulatory considerations that face today's nursing leaders.

Failure to Properly Assess (Make Careful and Full Observations) of the Patient's Condition

In *Collins v. Westlake Community Hospital* (Ill. 1974), the jury determined that the nurse's failure to appropriately observe and document progressive circulatory impairment caused by the patient's (plaintiff, in this case) leg cast resulted in the amputation of the patient's leg. The physician had written an order for the nurse to watch the condition of the toes. Expert testimony at trial established that routine nursing care required monitoring the circulation of seriously injured patients as frequently as every 15 minutes, and at least every two hours, without a physician's order.

The nurse testified at trial that she had checked the circulation in the plaintiff's leg every hour throughout the night shift, as is consistent with the standard of care. However, the nurse failed to record any of her observations until 6 A.M. the next day, at which time the medical records merely reflected a note concerning the condition of the plaintiff's toes and a telephone call placed to the attending.

The court rejected the nurse's testimony and stressed the fact that the nurse's notes for the crucial 7-hour period when the patient's condition became critical failed to show that the nurse observed the patient's circulation at any time while she was on duty. The court noted that absent a record, the jury could properly assume that no observations were made during the critical period (Northrop & Kelly, 1987).

This case illustrates the fact that in court the result of the failure to regularly document the status of the patient's condition equates to no observations performed.

Failure to Monitor the Patient's Condition (Provide Ongoing Observations With Frequency Determined by the Patient's Acuity Level and the Related Standard of Care)

The 1993 issue of the *Professional Liability Newsletter* describes a 1989 failure-to-monitor case involving a nurse assigned to care for an acutely ill respiratory patient during the hospital's night shift. Although the nurse just completed a nurs-

ing program and had passed the state nursing licensing examination, the nurse was inexperienced. Chart entries revealed a patient with progressive respiratory difficulties who received a narcotic and a sedative medication during the nurse's shift. There was no evidence in the chart that the nurse had taken the patient's vital signs (Rubsamen, 1993).

The patient was initially seen in the emergency room on Thanksgiving night around 10:30 P.M. by an emergency physician who felt that the patient should be hospitalized. An ear, nose, and throat (ENT) physician was called and responded immediately. The ENT MD performed a history and a physical examination, noting complaints from the patient of having had a sore throat for three days. But that night the sore throat was "extremely severe" and swallowing was difficult. The patient was very obese, but the doctor noted that the patient "did not appear acutely ill" (Rubsamen, 1993, p. 3). The patient was admitted for hydration, with orders for a number of medications. The orders gave no instruction to the nurse that the doctor should be called if the patient developed respiratory distress.

The patient arrived on the unit at 12:30 A.M.; the nurse made chart entries, such as "labored respiration," "difficult respiration," "patient sitting up in bed," and "breathing audible from the hallway" (Rubsamen, 1993, p. 3). Even though these entries were made, no references to the patient's vital signs were found in the patient's record. A supervisor and another nurse were in the hospital, but there was no entry that they had seen the patient until just before the respiratory arrest.

The record showed that at 12:45 A.M. the patient was given Halcion (triazolam); by 2 A.M. he was having a problem breathing; at 4:20 A.M.

Demerol (meperidine) was administered, and 30 minutes later the patient was drowsy and exhibiting signs of apnea. The code team found him unconscious when they were called at 5 A.M. (Rubsamen, 1993).

A neurologist examined the patient the day following the respiratory arrest and diagnosed the patient as having "profound hypoxic encephalopathy" (Rubsamen, 1993, p. 3). The patient never recovered and has remained in a semicomatose state.

Upon review of the chart, it was noted that the nurse established no contact with the emergency physician on duty, who could have gotten to the patient faster than the Ear, Nose, and Throat (ENT) specialist who had admitted and was caring for the patient but was not at the hospital at the time. The nurse chose to leave a message for the ENT physician and await a response to the call.

Throughout the court's analysis of this case, the focus was on the nurse's failure to monitor the patient's changing status at different times, failure to provide complete documentation of vital signs, and failure to administer medication properly. The hospital's liability in the case was that of having placed an inexperienced nurse in charge of an acutely ill patient and not providing the appropriate level of supervision. The patient received a $2.6 million settlement with the majority assessed against the hospital (Mayberry & Croke, 1996).

This case illustrates a number of important issues, but key to the breakdown in performance here was the placement of an inexperienced nurse in a leadership/solo position on an acute medical floor. It is most prudent to prepare new nurses for the many challenges of caring for the acutely ill patient and starting the new nurse on the day shift with a preceptor "buddy" nurse assignment for the first few months. A preceptor orientation period allows the new nurse the opportunity to learn how to prioritize care and systematically assess and monitor patients in a supportive environment. Preceptor orientations may take more staff resources initially, but the supportive preparation of the new nurse will save the hospital's budget in the long run by reducing risks of patient injuries and by the provision of competent safe patient care.

Failure to Document Changes in the Patient's Condition, and/or Failure to Document Concisely, Completely, and in a Timely Manner

In *Pellerin v. Humedicenters* (1997), the plaintiff alleged that the emergency department (ED) nurse administered an injection of Demerol (meperidine) and Vistaril (hydroxyzine pamoate) in a substandard manner, causing a lump at the injection site and continuous pain, which was later diagnosed by a neurologist as a cutaneous gluteal neuropathy. How the injury actually occurred could not be proven at trial. Medical experts gave conflicting testimony regarding the cause of the patient's nerve injury (either the hydroxyzine pamoate or the needle could have caused it). Nurse experts opined that the failure to document the site and mode of injection fell short of the standard of care. At trial, the defendant testified that her customary practice of giving an intramuscular injection met the standard of care. The jury found in favor of the plaintiff and awarded more than $90,000 in damages (Croke, 2003).

Properly charting any nursing interventions is essential even if you routinely perform those interventions in the same manner every time.

The patient's medical record has many functions, chief among them is to communicate patient information among providers. Also important is the record's function as a legal document of the care received by the patient. If an incident is brought to court, the time that lapses can be as long as five to eight years and memories fade. The only current document of the event is the patient's record. Concise, timely, and complete documentation of the nursing process—assessment and nursing diagnosis, nursing care plan, nursing interventions, implementation and evaluation of planned interventions, and the patient's response—are critical elements for successful documentation.

Dr. Croke points out that failure to document physicians' verbal orders that constitute a change from those noted in the chart and failure to document information received from telephone conversations with physicians, including time, content of communication between nurse and physician, and actions taken, can result in a malpractice lawsuit.

Failure to Intervene With Appropriate Nursing Actions or Failure to Follow Standards of Care

In *Alef v. Alta Bates Hospital*, a labor and delivery nurse failed to properly perform Doppler monitoring. The nurse listened to the fetal heart rate after every contraction for 15 seconds and multiplied the results by 4. This technique did not encompass the entire contraction; therefore, late decelerations were missed. The infant suffered severe brain damage because the fetal distress went undetected.

Similarly, in *Uhr v. Lutheran General Hospital*, a 13-year-old patient died during surgery to remove a cyst from her femur because the nurse failed to properly weigh the sponges. The amount of blood loss went undetected until the patient went into cardiac arrest and died (Smith-Pittman, 1998).

Both examples of failure to follow the standard of care for specific procedures are failures in following the steps necessary to correctly perform a fetal monitoring procedure and to appropriately monitor blood loss following surgery. The importance of a consistent, methodical, systematic approach to nursing care cannot be underestimated, and taking shortcuts frequently result in negative—sometimes life-threatening—outcomes.

Failure to Report Alterations in the Patient's Condition to the Appropriate Person in a Timely Manner

The 1988 case *Koeniquer v. Eckrich* involved the death of a patient as a result of sepsis, which was alleged to have developed when she was discharged with a fever 11 days after urinary tract surgery. The decedent's daughter brought a cause of action against two physicians and the Dakota Midland Hospital, alleging deviation from the appropriate standards of care for a patient in postoperative urology.

The decedent's surgery was performed on January 5, 1983. Her temperature fluctuated during her postoperative hospital stay and was recorded as 100.2°F on January 16 at 8:15 A.M., after the treating physician had completed rounds. The patient was discharged at 10:45 A.M. on the same day. She was readmitted to the hospital on January 19 with a diagnosis of sepsis. On January 21, she was transferred to the

University of Minnesota Hospital and on March 6 died of multiple organ failure.

The plaintiff's expert witness stated that the nurses failed to adequately monitor the patient's changing condition and provide acceptable postoperative care. The nurses responded that they had reported the patient's elevated temperature and the condition of the incision and drainage from it to the physician on the day of discharge but had failed to document such a report; the expert also maintained that allowing the patient to be discharged with an elevated temperature and failing to provide the patient with discharge instructions about monitoring her temperature were examples of failing to act as patient advocate.

Although the hospital argued that the decision to discharge was a medical one, the hospital's director of nursing stated in her deposition that sometimes it is the nurse's responsibility to question the physician's order, especially when there has been a significant change in the patient's condition. The director also confirmed the expert's assertions that the nurse has a responsibility to independently evaluate the patient's condition, to bring her concerns to the physician, and to appeal to other authorities if the nurse believes the physician's decision is wrong.

The court accepted the hospital's argument that it is a physician's decision to discharge a patient and, therefore, that the hospital was an inappropriate respondent to the suit. The state supreme court, however, ruled there was expert testimony in the record showing that hospital nurses had a duty to attempt to delay the patient's discharge because of her changing symptoms that day, yet there was no evidence in the record that any nurse questioned or disagreed with the physician's decision to discharge her. The court held that nurses have a duty to ques-

tion a physician's order if they think it is in the patient's best interest to do so and to delay discharge if they believe discharge deviates from acceptable standards of care (Croke, 2003).

The nurses involved in this case neglected their role as advocates for their patient.

Nursing Specialties and the Most Common Deviations From the Expected Standard of Care

It is extremely important to be familiar with the most common areas of risk of improper care to develop preventive systems to prepare yourself and the healthcare team from failing to meet the necessary standards of care in these reoccurring situations. Contained here are many of the most common incidences of high risk for deviation in maintaining the standards of care. There are, of course, many other areas of practice where nurses and doctors can deviate from the established standards of care. This list is by no means all inclusive but is given here as an example of the most common areas of risk for a nurse.

In acute care medical/surgical units, the three most common causes of patient injuries are medication errors, falls, and burns. In perioperative nursing, mistaken identity of the patient and of the surgical site, failure to remove foreign objects, and inadequate postoperative assessment and intervention constitute common areas of breakdown in quality of care. In emergency care, the common areas of risk are inadequate triage, failure to properly assess, and delay in calling a physician. In pediatric care, common areas of deviation from the standard of care are abandonment, medication errors, failure to detect signs and symptoms of dehydration and electrolyte imbalance, failure to protect from burns, improper restraints, and failure to monitor and maintain equipment. Northrop and Kelly (1987) emphasize that the potential for disaster from these and other seemingly less significant errors is greater in the pediatric setting than in the adult setting. In some instances, the same nursing error that would not result in any damage to an adult will be life threatening to an infant or child (Northrop & Kelly, 1987).

In psychiatric nursing care, some of the most common areas for deviation from the standard of care concern the following: the right to treatment, informed consent, right to refuse treatment, privacy and confidentiality, duty to protect and to warn, right to a safe environment, and appropriate discharge procedures.

In perinatal nursing, the common areas of litigation that have continued to be significant over the past 20 years are use of oxytocin, hyperstimulation of uterine activity, fetal heart rate (FHR) pattern interpretation, timely emergent cesarean birth, fundal pressure, shoulder dystocia, operative vaginal birth, neonatal resuscitation, iatrogenic prematurity, and multiple gestation. Other newer areas of risk have developed as a result of new trends in clinical care and more recent recommendations from professional associations and regulatory agencies, such as telephone triage, the Emergency Medical Treatment and Active Labor Act (EMTALA), elective induction of labor, and vaginal birth after cesarean birth (VBAC) (Simpson & Knox, 2003). The article by Dr. Kathleen Simpson and Dr. Eric Knox is an excellent resource on recommendations to promote patient safety and decrease risk exposure.

In elder care and long-term care, the most frequent areas of litigation include repeated falls, pressure sores, dehydration, weight loss, and serious infections (Wager & Creelman, 2004).

Community nursing risks of litigation today differ a great deal from those of 20 years ago as a result of the shorter lengths of stay for hospitalized patients with acute illnesses. Patients having open heart surgery without complications may be released from the hospital one week post surgery. Community health nurses must be experts in the care of all ages of patients, and medical surgical care at home is common. Therefore, many of the same problems that nurses have in the acute care setting can occur in the home: medication errors, failure to properly assess or monitor, and infectious disease control for the patient and family members.

Nursing Management Practice Regulations and the Most Frequently Cited Deviations From the Standards of Care

More than 30 state boards of nursing have revised the administrative rules and regulations governing nursing practice, codifying the legal accountability of the RN who makes assignments, delegates patient care tasks to other team members, and supervises subordinate staff (Campbell-Heider, Krainovich-Miller, King, Sedhom, & Malinski, 1998). Ohio, in 1996, provided detailed guidelines for safe and lawful registered nurse delegation (Ohio Administrative Code, 1996). Part B of these requirements includes the following:

1. An assessment of the individual who needs nursing care
2. The types of nursing care the individual requires
3. The complexity and frequency of the nursing care needed
4. The stability of the individual who needs nursing care

5. A review of assessments performed by other licensed healthcare professionals
6. The training, ability, and skill of the trained unlicensed person who will be performing the delegated nursing activity
7. The nature of the nursing activity being delegated
8. The availability and accessibility of resources (Ohio Administrative Code, Section 4723-13-05, 1996)

In 2007, the Ohio State Board of Nursing revised these regulations, and the revisions reveal some of the recent challenging issues for nurse managers in the current healthcare working environment. The evidence of the expansion of unlicensed personnel responsibility and, more critically, the nurse's responsibility as the person delegating to unlicensed staff members definitely raise the nurse's risk of potential liability.

4723-13-05 CRITERIA AND STANDARDS FOR A LICENSED NURSE DELEGATING TO AN UNLICENSED PERSON

(A) A registered nurse may delegate a nursing task to an unlicensed person if all the conditions for delegation set forth [in this chapter] are met.

(B) A licensed practical nurse may delegate to an unlicensed person only at the direction of the registered nurse and if all the conditions for delegation set forth in this chapter are met.

(C) Except as otherwise authorized by law or this chapter, a licensed nurse may delegate to an unlicensed person the administration of only the following medications:

  (1) Over-the-counter topical medications to be applied to intact skin for the purpose of improving a skin condition or providing a barrier; and

  (2) Over-the-counter eye drop, ear drop, and suppository medications, foot soak treatments, and enemas.

(D) Prior to delegating a nursing task to an unlicensed person, the delegating nurse shall determine each of the following:

  (1) That the nursing task is within the scope of practice of the delegating nurse as set forth in section 4723.01 of the Revised Code;

  (2) That the nursing task is within the knowledge, skill, and ability of the nurse delegating the nursing task;

  (3) That the nursing task is within the training, ability, and skill of the unlicensed person who will be performing the delegated nursing task;

  (4) That the nursing task is delegable as specified in this rule;

  (5) That appropriate resources and support are available for the performance of the task and management of the outcome;

  (6) That adequate and appropriate supervision by a licensed nurse of the performance of the nursing task is available in accordance with, rule 4723-13-07 of the Administrative Code.

(E) Prior to the delegation of any nursing task, the delegating nurse shall

  (1) Identify;

    (a) The individual on whom the nursing task may be performed; and

    (b) A specific time frame during which the delegated nursing task may be performed.

(2) Complete an evaluation of the conditions that relate to the delegation of the nursing task to be performed, including;

    (a) An evaluation of the individual who needs nursing care;

    (b) The types of nursing care the individual requires;

    (c) The complexity and frequency of the nursing care needed;

    (d) The stability of the individual who needs nursing care; and

    (e) A review of the evaluations performed by other licensed health care professionals.

(3) Identify a nursing task as delegable if all of the following apply:

    (a) The nursing task requires no judgment based on nursing knowledge and expertise on the part of the unlicensed person performing the task;

    (b) The results of the nursing task are reasonably predictable;

    (c) The nursing task can be safely performed according to exact, unchanging directions, with no need to alter the standard procedures for performing the task;

    (d) The performance of the nursing task does not require complex observations or critical decisions be made with respect to the nursing task;

    (e) The nursing task does not require repeated performance of nursing assessments; and

    (f) The consequences of performing the nursing task improperly are minimal and not life-threatening.

(F) The delegating nurse shall be accountable for the decision to delegate nursing tasks to an unlicensed person.

(G) If a licensed nurse determines that an unlicensed person is not correctly performing a delegated nursing task, the licensed nurse shall immediately intervene. (Ohio Administrative Code, 4723 Ohio Board of Nursing Chapter 4723-13 Delegation of Nursing Tasks, 2007).

Check your state board regulations to be aware of the guidelines for your practice area.

Case Studies of Nursing Management Malpractice

Real and hypothetical case studies of deviations from nursing management standards and the realities of the regulatory environment are presented here related to the most frequently documented categories of legal allegations against charge nurses and nurse managers.

The analysis of the cases presented can help nurse leaders avoid similar risks in daily practice. Systematic plans of leadership including promotion of regular competency evaluation, the importance of concise and timely management-oriented documentation, regular in-service education, collaboration, managing patient expectations, and building a cohesive shared philosophy of safe care for the entire healthcare team by charge nurses and nursing managers are also discussed.

Some of the most frequent deviations from nursing management standards are the following:

- Inadequate staffing
- Inappropriate staffing
- Overlooked or failure to recognize environmental hazards

- Lack of, inconsistent, or incompetent supervision
- Improper delegation

Inadequate Staffing and Inappropriate Staffing

In the article "The Professional Nurse and Regulation," Denise Flook describes the following hypothetical situation that actually takes place in American hospitals regularly (2003).

Shirley is working as the charge nurse in the postanesthesia acute care unit (PACU) of a 300-bed community hospital. The nursing supervisor informs her that two regular staff nurses from the afternoon shift have called in sick. This will leave the unit, which is already staffed with agency nurses because of an inability to hire more full-time nurses, short another day. Shirley knows that the surgery schedule is full and that she must stay to help cover the unit. The supervisor states that she will pull a patient care technician (PCT) from the surgical unit to assist. Shirley questions if she can provide a safe level of care to the patients and delegate appropriately to the PCT. Chronically working short, she has been asked to do this many times and considers leaving because she is concerned about "putting her license on the line" (Flook, 2003, p. 160).

Flook notes that many questions arise from this scenario, in particular: When is a nurse's license really in jeopardy? What could be the consequences of a nurse leaving the unit because of a staffing shortage as described? She explains that the real risk to a nurse's license may be in abandoning the patients once the nurse is on duty and has accepted assignment of the patients. Leaving would put the patients further at risk and may be viewed as patient abandonment if no other nurse is available to be assigned the patients. Flook advises notifying the super-

visor or nurse manager of the unit that you have concerns about the staffing as outlined in the facility's policies and procedures. For the immediate shift, though, she advises that the nurse must prioritize the care that must be given and delegate appropriately. Ask the supervisor for assistance in making assignments, prioritizing, and providing care (Flook, 2003). The reasonableness test for a nurse manager applies here. It is the charge nurse's responsibility to ensure that he or she is not negligent in making care assignments or providing care. The charge nurse is responsible for providing care at her or his level of education, training, experience, and competence level, and the charge nurse has an obligation to perform as any reasonable nurse would perform.

It is the facility's legal responsibility to provide adequate staffing. If this situation is regularly repeated, it constitutes unsafe working conditions and the charge nurse must advocate for more appropriate staffing up the ladder of responsibility in the hospital (just as the bedside nurse must be an advocate for patients if a doctor's order is unsafe) for the safety of her staff and the safety of those patients under their care. Nurse–patient ratios are mandated in some states; however, having only one RN and filling the rest of the staff with LPNs and unlicensed assistive personnel (UAPs) may not be the correct skill mix to meet the needs of the patients on that unit. To staff by acuities is much more appropriate (Mahlmeister, 1999).

Overlooked or Failure to Recognize Environmental Hazards

Nancy Burden, in her article titled, "Regulatory Compliance in the Ambulatory Surgery Setting:

A Process Improvement Approach," presents two hypothetical case examples of seemingly minor environmental safety considerations that could result in major patient injuries (2003b).

In the first case, an elderly but alert female patient is in the bathroom in the discharge area and falls, unfortunately fracturing her left hip. The woman's weak call for help is not immediately heard because the nurse has stepped away for a moment to assist another person from a stretcher to a chair. The woman in the bathroom on the floor is unable to move because of pain and the position she is in on the floor. She reaches for the call light only to find that the cord, which by law should be hanging within four inches of the floor, has been wrapped around the railing next to the toilet. The nurse does return to find her, but in the interim the patient has suffered significant anxiety and pain and potential delay in treatment because she had no way to summon help.

Burden points out that if charge nurses and unit managers alert their staff members to potential environmental hazards, no matter how seemingly minor, in the long run this can result in having many "eyes looking for, and correcting" potential future infractions and preventing numerous injurious accidents (Burden, 2003b, p. 180).

The second hypothetical example involves a nurse responding to an overhead page for help from the admissions clerk in the lobby of an ambulatory facility. A "Code Blue" has been called, signifying a potential medical crisis. The nurse, joined by several coworkers and an anesthesiologist, must attend to a person in a full code situation. The team has practiced their individual and collective roles and hastens to put the proper protocols in place. Because of the nature of the event and difficulty moving the large man who has suffered a cardiac arrest, they have initiated resuscitation in the lobby. The code cart arrives. In preparing the equipment, they find that no electric plug is within distance for the defibrillator, so they rely on battery mode. Unfortunately, the charge is not sufficient and the man remains in arrest. They continue CPR until outside assistance arrives with a backup defibrillator. Although the man is successfully resuscitated, the event leaves the team in shock and devastated by the implications of what went wrong (Burden, 2003b).

Burden (2003b) reviews what could have gone wrong:

1. Were the results of the risk management checklist the month before addressed?
2. Did anyone investigate the comment that the defibrillator log did not show documentation of battery operation/discharge during the daily checks?
3. Was a new team member unaware of the proper method of testing the defibrillator?
4. Are there other areas of the facility where a person could require electrical equipment, but where that resource is not available? Consider hallways, parking lots, lobbies, and even staff lounges.

Burden stresses that the reason for any compliance plan, environmental inspection, team survey, or regulatory review is the ultimate safety and protection of patients, visitors, and staff members in the facility and the public at large. Using a process of continuous improvement can help move a facility toward that goal.

Lack of, Inconsistent, or Incompetent Supervision

In the 2005 community hospice case *Allen of Michigan, Inc. v. Deputy Director Division of Em-*

ployment & Training, the appropriateness of the decisions and actions of an on-call case manager for a 24-hour hospice program were questioned.

Beacon Hospice (Beacon) provides around-the-clock compassionate care to terminally ill patients and their families. Beacon promises that none of its patients will "die in pain." Beacon provides its after-hours services through a three-tier, on-call system. Beacon's answering service takes all calls from a toll-free number and refers them to a triage nurse. The triage nurse deals directly with the patient and the patient's family. Under a written policy relating to on-call services, the triage nurse determines whether a home visit is necessary.

On June 24, 2002, Nurse Serapiglia began working as a full-time hospice nurse case manager for Beacon. Her duties included assessing and managing pain and symptoms of patients in nursing homes and in home care, making sure they were comfortable and pain free, and providing emotional support to their families. The "after-hours" supervisor for the on-call nurse is the triage nurse. In the early afternoon of Sunday, January 26, 2003, the client, a family of four from Canton, Massachusetts, called seeking services. The patient's daughter asked the triage nurse, Calnan, for a nurse to come to the home to provide services for her father, who was terminally ill. Nurse Calnan decided that a home visit was necessary. She called the on-call nurse, Serapiglia, who lived approximately one and one half hours travel time away. Nurse Calnan maintained that Nurse Serapiglia was "very reluctant to go out." Instead of visiting, Serapiglia called the family, maintaining that a visit was "not necessary."

Shortly after 10 P.M., the patient's son called Calnan to report that the patient was having increased difficulty breathing and was "unresponsive." He was very angry at Beacon because no nurse had visited. Calnan apologized, informing him that she would get a nurse out immediately. She called Serapiglia, expressing disbelief that Serapiglia had failed to visit the family as requested. She ordered her to go to the home immediately. Serapiglia resisted and responded that she would "call the family in an hour." Serapiglia did not go. She called the patient's son and instructed him how to give the patient morphine. Nurse Serapiglia was terminated. Her application for unemployment benefits was initially denied. The nurse appealed. After a hearing, a review examiner awarded benefits to the nurse. The hospital appealed.

The Court of Appeals of Massachusetts reversed the order of the hearing examiner and ordered that benefits be denied. The court held, among other findings, that the cumulative record showed a pattern of clear insubordination (Tammelleo, 2005).

Improper Delegation

Dr. Laura Mahlmeister (1999) discusses improper delegation in her article titled "Professional Accountability and Legal Liability for the Team Leader and Charge Nurse." She cites an unpublished case example in which the team leader was alleged negligent for failure to properly supervise an LPN in the care and stabilization of a neonate after birth.

This case involves a male infant, whose Apgar scores were 8 and 9 at 1 and 5 minutes, respectively, and who weighed 2,600 gm. at 40 weeks gestation. The mother had an essentially normal prenatal and intrapartum course. The infant was assessed by the RN at 30 minutes of age. Vital signs were within the normal range, but the RN documented that the infant was "extremely jittery." She assigned subsequent care to an LPN, directing her to obtain a heel stick capillary blood sample for glucose testing and to feed the infant 15 to 20 mL of 5% dextrose in water if the test results were "low."

The LPN visually read a glucose strip as a "weak 40 mg/dL" and documented that the findings were reported to the RN. She then fed the infant 15 mL of glucose water. There were no additional entries in the infant's medical record regarding his condition for the next 1 hour 10 minutes. At that time (when the neonate was approximately 2 hours old), the mother, who was encouraged by the LPN to maintain skin-to-skin contact with her infant, called for help. The RN found the infant apneic and cyanotic with a weak apical pulse in the range of 80 to 90 bpm. Cardiopulmonary resuscitation was initiated; the infant's condition stabilized, and he was transported to the NICU. The first capillary blood glucose result obtained in the NICU was "zero." The infant experienced permanent neurologic damage. The expert witness hired by the plaintiff's attorney alleged that the RN had violated the Nursing Practice Act by assigning care of an unstable neonate to the LPN. The RN also was criticized for failing to reassess the infant and the glucose level after the initial feeding.

The RN team leader testified in deposition that she did not recheck the neonate because she believed the LPN was "perfectly competent to manage sick infants. She's worked in this unit longer than I have." The LPN testified that after reporting that the glucose was low and feeding the neonate, she assumed the RN would reevaluate the infant because "LPNs can't be responsible for unstable babies." This case was settled before trial for a substantial, but undisclosed, sum of money. The RN team leader was terminated by her employer (Mahlmeister, 1999).

As noted earlier, the state boards of nursing define the legal duties of the RN for delegation and supervision of subordinate staff. The team leader and/or charge nurse in perinatal and other specialty settings must not only be an expert clinician who has the competence to care for the sickest patients but also must be skilled in delegation, supervision, and evaluation of subordinate team member activities (Mahlmeister, 1999).

Systems That Facilitate the Most Effective Management of Healthcare Personnel

Identifying and understanding inherently unsafe nursing and nursing management practices are the first steps in resolving the problems identified and decreasing the overall risk (Edgett Collins, 2007). How can a nurse manager ensure competent safe practice by his or her staff? Patient safety research is in its infancy, but early findings described by Dr. Suzanne Edgett Collins show that nursing process factors in patient safety failures can be subdivided into four major categories that are operational in almost all patient encounters. In summary, they are as follows:

1. Nurses are routinely presented with diverse and unpredictable patients.
2. Inconsistency in the multiple ways of nursing task performance.
3. Complexity in that there are a large number of steps in the process of completing a nursing task (i.e., consider the multiple ways to change a sterile dressing or insert and secure an IV).
4. Tight coupling, meaning that often there is a sequential dependency and necessary order of steps to complete a nursing task, and if there is a failure in one step, there is a resulting cascade of

failure (i.e., insertion of a Foley catheter).

Edgett Collins's comments lend credence to the development of a systematic approach for performing the skills and procedures necessary for each patient care specialty. This concept is being put to use in different ways, from creating a safety nurse position in specialty areas such as perinatal nursing to developing competencies to match the patient care expectations for a particular unit or patient care specialty.

The Safety Nurse

The perinatal safety nurse (PSN) position was developed as a new role to promote safe care for mothers and babies after a proactive clinical initiative in which an interdisciplinary leadership team from five academic medical centers (Columbia University, Cornell University, Johns Hopkins University, the University of Rochester, and Yale University) identified and adopted evidence-based clinical practices to promote quality and minimize risk of patient harm. This group identified obstetrics as the area of highest insurance claims costs and the highest associated risk of preventable patient harm and injury. Most important, as the result of site reviews of all the participating facilities and analysis of their reports for performance improvement, the group prioritized patient safety projects and implementation strategies. A summary of their priorities and recommendations for obstetrical departments is as follows:

- Evaluation of the safety culture in each obstetrical department
- Promotion of interdisciplinary teamwork
- Development of a nonhierarchical clinical environment through team training programs

- Standardization of key clinical policies and protocols based on current science, standards, and guidelines from professional and regulatory agencies (Brown Will, Hennicke, Jacobs, O'Neill, & Raab, 2006)

Also significant is the fact that they planned to improve the accuracy and timeliness of fetal assessment by promoting a common language for electronic fetal monitoring (EFM), using terminology recommended by the National Institute of Child Health and Human Development Research Workshop (NICHD, 1997) and a shared knowledge base on fetal heart rate (FHR) pattern interpretation and expected interventions for nonreassuring FHR patterns. Measures such as this unify the approach used and decrease the variations that can occur in a department compared to the increased risk of error that can occur when a department does not consistently define the standard of care required of the healthcare team. Ongoing education and national certification in electronic fetal monitoring was the means of substantiating and validating this goal.

This group of safety initiative leaders also recognized that to be successful, day-to-day support for all program components with monitoring and outcomes measurement was necessary. The patient safety nurse role was developed to actualize the findings of the leadership group (Brown Will et al., 2006).

Competency Programs

For those hospitals that have issues with maintaining adequate numbers of nursing personnel, creating a new position may not be financially feasible. Another method for decreasing risk is to tie competency processes to job descriptions, orientation checklists, and performance appraisals. Whether the nursing department is acute care or ambulatory surgery, an effective competency program should encompass skills that relate to each employee's job and the specific patient populations served and should apply to all employees (McLane, 2007).

Careful interviewing and checking of references is fine, but until the nurse manager follows and evaluates the performance of new staff members for weeks and, more realistically, months of day-to-day nursing practice, she or he will not know exactly how someone performs. Positive, consistent, safe patient care outcomes will not be seen in the nursing healthcare team unless managers understand what skill competency set is needed for specific patient care areas and are prepared to test the competency of staff. Newly hired staff members should be tested at the time of hire, and then should be placed on a trajectory to improve upon those skills that they have not mastered; competency assessment enables the nurse manager and new nurses to understand where they are weak and in what areas they need improvement. Regular competency reevaluations should be conducted for all staff members to keep them current and competent.

To be able to move closer to expectations for safe patient care, an effective nurse leader needs to develop guidelines or algorithms for the expected competencies for all positions, linking the competencies with the specific job description and encouraging the newly hired and inexperienced RNs to accomplish those competencies within a set time frame. For example, upon hiring a new nurse, present the new nurse with the expected competencies for the position in a pretest to see where he or she places. Use that information to assist them to master their

weak areas and document the total performance; set goals for learning the competencies they didn't master, and then retest in three months. Then, assign them patients appropriate to their skill set. Schedule a time line for your expectations and methods for the RNs to learn what they need to learn to master the position. In this way, newly hired staff members understand what the position entails, what skills they must master at each level of the position, and in what time frame the mastery must take place.

For the supervising nurse, then, the points of evaluation are clear and the time line within which to achieve them is documented. This overall plan applies to all specialty areas; only the specific tasks to be mastered differ. Nursing competence is supported through several mechanisms and specifically required in both Human Resource and Nursing standards of The Joint Commission. The medical and nursing literature confirms that standardized, uniform, evidence-based quality improvement measures do improve the quality and safety of medical and surgical care; however, those measures must be implemented consistently and with a systematic method that provides oversight, continuing education, consistency, and clear expectations for success. A specific competency program developed for each specialty unit is one way to ensure consistent safe care.

The Joint Commission reported the most frequent root causes for all sentinel events concerned the following two categories: unfamiliar situations in which there was insufficient orientation/ training and miscommunication (The Joint Commission, 2008a). A solid competency program facilitates orientation, and in-service training topics should reinforce those areas that staff members need to improve upon.

Competency expectations should apply to those nurses who float and to agency nurses as well. Assessment of the basic skills of these two groups of nurses will be much easier and delegation of tasks much more appropriate if the nurse leader has assessed their competency score.

Finally, Susanne Conley, Patricia Branowicki, and Diane Hanley (2007) write about a competency and preceptor model for new leaders. They maintain that an orientation program for new nurse managers that combines the components of nurse manager competencies, precepting by the nurse manager's supervisor, and written and classroom resources will ensure that new managers are ready to face the challenges that await them.

The Importance of Understanding and Meeting Patients' Expectations

Healthcare literature has shown over many years that patients are much less likely to bring a cause of action against a physician or nurse if that patient felt the healthcare provider and/or the institution was receptive to his or her individual concerns. An effective nurse leader knows how to meet and exceed patients' expectations. If the nurse manager can effectively share that knowledge with staff so that staff members fully understand how they can contribute to the success of the unit, fewer confrontational situations will arise. An extremely helpful reference for meeting patients' expectations is Susan Keane Baker's book *Managing Patient Expectations: The Art of Finding and Keeping Loyal Patients* (1998). The outpatient concepts and guidance offered by Keane are equally applicable to inpatient care.

How Documentation Can Be the Most Effective for Nurse Managers

Concise, complete, and timely patient care documentation is critical for all providers of care regardless of the discipline or specialty. T. M. Marrelli (1997) maintains that the nurse manager needs a dependable method to provide facts to defend positions, plan for the future, and record the unit's and the department's past. The practice of committing to memory observations about behavior, good or bad, without actual notations is no longer feasible and is not responsible to the staff (Marrelli, 1997).

> *During meetings with the staff in a group or on an individual basis, the discussion should be summarized orally and then the plan of action summarized in writing. Short notes kept on the staff's performance can make evaluation time objective and full of examples, positive and negative, on which manager and staff goals are designed. All that must be noted are (1) the topics of discussion and (2) the outcomes or goals for either or both parties. Then the next meeting will first address the progress or steps being taken to meet the goals. (Marrelli, 1997, p. 60)*

Another advantage of keeping regular notes, especially for a new nurse manager, is that when meeting with staff members who report issues, such as needing more equipment or training, the new manager has specific examples to discuss with his or her manager that may provide specific rationales for organizational improvements.

Keeping continual daily chronicles of pertinent meetings and unit occurrences Marrelli calls management by objectives (MBO). Partnering

MBO with the consistent provision and use of evidenced-based procedural competencies facilitates improved patient care and a healthcare team that not only understands the clinical care objectives but is invested in the vision and philosophy of their department.

Summary

A proactive, clinically experienced, assertive, transparent style of leadership can produce motivated providers of safe patient care. The information presented here can assist new nurse leaders to develop a management philosophy that incorporates preventive measures. In this way, the nurse manager and staff can not only avoid potential mishaps that could result in negative legal ramifications but, most importantly, develop a philosophy that consistently promotes the highest standards of care and excellent bedside and community nursing leadership practice.

QUESTIONS

1. The Centers for Medicare and Medicaid Services (CMS) developed a quality improvement road map. Their goal was to
   a. ensure that every person will have the right care every time
   b. establish guidelines for adequate health care
   c. establish patient rights for those who are insured
   d. establish standards for the uninsured

2. The Centers for Medicare and Medicaid Services (CMS) developed strategies for improving care. The one that will most affect the healthcare system is: "To pay in a way that expresses commitment to supporting providers for doing the right thing—improving quality and avoiding unnecessary costs—rather than directing more resources to less effective care" (Edelman, 2008). This means
   a. hospitals will be funded for quality care
   b. providers of care must adhere to standards of care
   c. healthcare providers will no longer be able to bill for charges associated with the hospital-acquired complication
   d. healthcare providers will no longer be able to bill for select charges that cover preventable surgery

3. Patient X was admitted to a local hospital for surgery and following surgery was placed in a regular medical surgical unit instead of a postanesthesia care unit (PACU). The patient attempted to call (using the call bell and verbally calling as well) for assistance during the night, and when no one came, attempted to get out of bed. Patient X fell to the floor, injuring her shoulder, and was not discovered on the floor by a nurse until

approximately 30 minutes after falling. It was discovered that the unit to which Patient X was assigned was short staffed that evening. This was the third accident that occurred on the unit as a result of short staffing. Which of the following statements is true?

   a. It is the facility's legal responsibility to provide adequate staffing. If this situation is regularly repeated, it constitutes an unsafe condition.

   b. The patient should not have attempted to get out of bed without help and is legally liable for the injuries.

   c. The facility cannot be held responsible, because during a nursing shortage it cannot always be required to provide adequate staff.

   d. Because the hospital took care of the patient following the accident and did not charge for additional care, this is a nonissue.

4. Which of the following statements is true?

   a. The old adage and statement, "If you didn't chart it, it is hasn't been done" is no longer true.

   b. The practice of committing to memory observations about behavior, good or bad, without actual notations in chart is okay if you report it to the nurse manager.

   c. Concise, complete, and timely patient care documentation is critical for all providers of care regardless of the discipline or specialty.

   d. A written report in today's world of technology is not necessary.

5. The goal of nursing regulation via licensing is to

   a. protect the public from harm

   b. standardize care

   c. keep the nurse from being sued

   d. garner revenue

References

Abille v. U.S., 482 F. Supp. 703 (Ca. 1980).

Alef v. Alta Bates Hospital, 5 Cal. 4th 208 (Ca. 1992).

Allen of Michigan, Inc. v. Deputy Director Division of Employment & Training, 833 N.E. 2d 627 (Ma. 2005).

Bates, D., & Gawande, A. (2003). Improving safety with information technology. *New England Journal of Medicine, 348*(25), 2526–2534.

Brook, P. (2007). Program update: Promoting patient safety and preventing medical errors. *Journal of Nursing Law, 11*(3), 124–128.

Brown Will, S., Hennicke, K., Jacobs, L., O'Neill, L., & Raab, C. (2006). The perinatal patient safety nurse: A new role to promote safe care for mothers and babies. *Journal of Obstetric, Gynecologic & Neonatal Nursing, 35*(3), 417–423.

Brownlee, S. (2007). *Overtreated: Why too much medicine is making us sicker and poorer.* New York: Bloomsbury.

Burden, N. (2003a). Agencies and acronyms: A guide to regulatory jargon. *Journal of PeriAnesthesia Nurses, 18*(3), 147–151.

Burden, N. (2003b). Regulatory compliance in the ambulatory surgery setting: A process improvement approach. *Journal of PeriAnesthesia Nursing, 18*(3), 173–181.

Burroughs, R., Dmytrow, B., & Lewis, H. (2007). Trends in nurse practitioner professional liability: An analysis of claims with risk management recommendations. *Journal of Nursing Law, 11*(1), 53–60.

Campbell-Heider, N., Krainovich-Miller, B., King, K. B., Sedhom, L., & Malinski, V. (1998). Empowering staff nurses to participate in the American Nurses Association's call for quality indicators research. *Journal of the New York State Nurses Association, 29*(3/4), 21–27.

Centers for Medicare and Medicaid Services (CMS). (2005). Quality improvement roadmap. Retrieved April 15, 2008, from www.cms.hhs.org

Collins v. Westlake Community Hospital, 312 N.E. 2d 614 (Ill. 1974).

Conley, S., Branowicki, P., & Hanley, D. (2007). Nursing leadership orientation: A competency and preceptor model to facilitate new leader success. *Journal of Nursing Administration, 37*(11), 491–498.

Constantino, R. E. (2003). Legalities of emergency pain management. *Nursing Management, 39*(4), 24–25, 62.

Croke, E. (2003). Nurses negligence and malpractice: An analysis based on more than 250 cases against nurses. *American Journal of Nursing, 103*(9), 54–63.

Croke, E. (2006). Nursing malpractice: Determining liability elements for negligent acts. *Journal of Legal Nurse Consulting, 17*(3), 3–7, 24.

Edelman, S. (2008, April 27). Unsafe hands: Epidemic of errors at NY hospitals. *New York Post.* Retrieved November 17, 2008, from http://www.nypost.com/seven/04272008/news/regionalnews/unsafe_hands_108305.htm

Edgett Collins, S. (2007). Setting a new standard of nursing care: Potential legal implications of patient safety research. *Journal of Nursing Law, 11*(2), 87–92.

Emergency Medical Treatment and Active Labor Act, Statutory Regulations, 42 CFR, pt 489 (1992).

Flook, D. (2003). The professional nurse and regulation. *Journal of PeriAnesthesia Nursing, 18*(3), 160–167.

Guido, G. (1997). *Legal issues in nursing* (2nd ed.). East Norwalk, CT: Appleton & Lange.

Hirsch, H. (1979). Risk management: The physician's role. *Legal Aspects of Medical Practice, 7*(1), 49–51.

Institute for Healthcare Improvement. (2006). Savings accounts [Progress Report]. pp. 1–12. Retrieved May 5, 2008, from http://www.ihi.org

Institute of Medicine (IOM). (1999). *To err is human: Building a safer healthcare system.* Washington, DC: National Academy Press.

Institute of Medicine (IOM). (2001). *Crossing the quality chasm.* Washington, DC: National Academy Press.

The Joint Commission. (2008a). Sentinel event statistics. Retrieved April 28, 2008, from http://www/jointcommission.org

The Joint Commission. (2008b). Current 2007 & 2008 Standard Manuals and Accreditation Process Manuals. Retrieved April 28, 2008, from http://www.jointcommission.org

Keane Baker, S. (1998). *Managing patient expectations: The art of finding and keeping loyal patients.* California: Jossey-Bass.

Koeniquer v. Eckrich, 422 N.W. 2d 600 (South Dakota, 1988).

Lunsford v. Board of Nurse Examiners, 648 SW 2d 391 (Texas Civ. App. 1983).

Luquire, R. (1989). Nurse risk management. *Nursing Management, 20*(10), 56–58.

Mahlmeister, L. (1999). Professional accountability and legal liability for the team leader and charge nurse. *Journal of Obstetrical and Gynecological Nursing, 28*(3), 300–309.

Marrelli, T. M. (1997). *The nurse manager's survival guide: Practical answers for everyday problems* (2nd ed.). St. Louis: Mosby.

Mayberry, A., & Croke, E. (1996). Issues leading to malpractice show little change: A review of the literature. *Journal of Legal Nurse Consulting, 7*(2), 16–19.

McEachen, I., & Keogh, J. (2007). *Nurse management demystified.* New York: McGraw-Hill.

McLane, D. (2007). Tie competency process to performance appraisals. *Same–Day Surgery,* 25–26.

Murchison, I., Nichols, T., & Hanson, R. (1982). *Legal accountability in the nursing process* (2nd ed.). St. Louis: Mosby.

Murray, M., & Huelsmann, G. (2007). Perinatal morbidity and mortality: Root causes and common themes in labor and delivery litigation. *Journal of Legal Nurse Consulting*, *18*(4), 13–18.

National Institute of Child Health and Human Development Research Workshop (NICHD). (1997). Electronic fetal heart rate monitoring: Research guidelines for interpretation. *American Journal of Obstetrics and Gynecology*, *177*(6), 1385–1390.

New York State Department of Health. (2007). Certificate of need. Retrieved February 7, 2008, from http://www.health.state.ny.us/nysdoh/cons/

Northrop, C., & Kelly, M. (1987). *Legal issues in nursing.* St. Louis: Mosby.

Ohio Administrative Code. (2007). 4723 Ohio Board of Nursing. *Law Writer, Ohio Laws and Rules*.

Pellerin v. Humedicenters, Inc. 969 So. 2d 590 (La. App., 1997).

Poteet, G. W. (1983). Risk management and nursing. *Nursing Clinics of North America*, *18*(3), 457–465.

Ridge, R. (2006). Regulatory requirements. *Nursing Management*, *37*(3), 56.

Rubsamen, D. S. (1993). The inexperienced nurse and a $2.6 million settlement. *Professional Liability Newsletter, 23*(10), 3.

Simpson, K. R., & Knox, G. E. (2003). Common areas of litigation related to care during labor and birth. *Journal of Perinatal Neonatal Nursing*, *17*(2), 110–125.

Smith-Pittman, M. H. (1998). Nurses and litigation: 1990–1997. *Journal of Nursing Law*, *5*(2), 7–19.

Stiehl, R. (2004). Quality assurance requirements for contract/agency nurses. *Journal of Nursing Administration*, *6*(3), 69–74.

Tammelleo, A. D. (2005). MA: Hospice nurse fails to visit dying patient: Fired nurse not eligible for U.I. benefits. *Nursing Law's Reagan Report*, *46*(4), 3.

Uhr v. Lutheran General Hospital, 589 N.E. 2d 723 (Ill. 1992).

Wager, R., & Creelman, W. (2004). A new image for long-term care. *Healthcare Financial Management*, *58*(4), 70–74.

Williams, S. C., Schmaltz, S. P., Morton, D. J., Koss, R. G., & Loeb, J. M. (2005). Quality of care in U.S. hospitals as reflected by standardized measures, 2002–2004. *New England Journal of Medicine*, *353*(3), 255–264.

Chapter 16

Data Management and Informatics: Using Information Technology to Support Advancing Nursing Practice

Patricia Eckardt

This chapter is designed as a very brief overview of Information Technology (IT) and its basic nomenclature and useful applications for nursing informatics in action. It underscores the need for nursing informatics education for all nurses. The resources and references offered throughout, and at the close of this chapter, are intended as a primer on nursing informatics (NI) for evidence-based nursing practice.

The explosion of technology in business, education, and day-to-day life created and influenced the use of technology in nursing. The use of technology and particularly informatics has invaded every component of the healthcare delivery system, putting a great demand on the involvement of nursing.

The American Nursing Credentialing Center (ANCC) began administering an informatics nurse certification examination in November 1995 (HIMSS Nursing Informatics Task Force, 2007). In 2004, President G. W. Bush issued an executive order creating the Decade of Health IT. The goal of this order was to establish an electronic health record (EHR) for every American within 10 years. Hynes (2006) outlines the benefits of computerized simulation technology, in terms of education and training of intensive care nurses for emergency preparedness. Rare but high-risk clinical scenarios could be re-created using a computer simulator, thereby providing opportunities for repeated training exposure to the situation in a low-risk environment so that intensive care nurses could develop competence in managing such situations safely. As president-elect of the American Nephrology Nurses Association (ANNA), Sandra Bodin put forth that the single most important thing that nephrology nurses can do to provide safety and improve outcomes for patients is to embrace health IT (Bodin, 2007). As noted by Smithers (2007), advances in microscopic and video equipment, robots, lasers, specialized implants, minimally invasive instrumentation, and electronic hemostatic and dissection devices require a level of technological knowledge and specialization of perioperative nurses that was not necessary when many began their careers. Alexander (2008) investigates the use of electronically integrated data and clinical decision support systems (CDSSs) in nursing homes to alert nursing staff regarding a decline or improvement in residents' conditions (constipation, dehydration, loss of skin integrity, weight loss or weight gain) for early nursing diagnosis and intervention that is not possible via a paper charting format unless there is intensive daily chart review.

From these examples of nurse leadership advances, governmental awareness, and growing research in the field of IT and evidence-based nursing, we can make a tenable assumption that nurses are well aware of the impact of IT within their practice. However, awareness of importance and the provision of the education to utilize nursing informatics are separate domains.

The American Nurses Association (2001) in the *Scope and Standards of Nursing Informatics Practice* defines nursing informatics as follows:

A specialty that integrates nursing science, computer science, and information science to manage and communicate data, information, and knowledge in nursing practice. Nursing informatics facilitates the integration of data, information, and knowledge to support patients, nurses, and other providers in their decision-making in all roles and settings. This support is accomplished through the use of information structures, information processes, and IT. (p. 17)

How does a nurse develop these skills required to utilize IT to the fullest in daily practice settings? What skills and competencies are considered the most fundamental for safe evidence-based nursing practice?

McCannon and O'Neal (2003) conducted a national survey to determine the IT skills nurse administrators consider critical for new nurses entering the workforce. The sample consisted of 2000 randomly selected members of the American Organization of Nurse Executives and found that effective use of e-mail, operating basic Windows applications, and searching databases were considered critical IT skills by the nurse executives. The most critical IT skill recorded in this study involved knowing nursing-specific software, such as bedside charting and computer-activated medication dispensers. Simpson (2006) concurs that for 21st-century nursing, the electronic health record (EHR) and computerized physician order entry (CPOE) are instrumental in the move to evidence-based nursing (EBN). These competencies in nursing informatics involve education outside of the scope of this chapter. The Healthcare Information and Management Systems Society informatics task force members published a historical and practical guide to nursing informatics in March 2007 that is required reading for all nurses who want to be educated regarding nursing informatics.

Overview of IT Applications for Nursing and Basic IT Nomenclature

The first section of this chapter reviews some basic IT terms. Though not requisite knowledge for use of nursing informatics, familiarity with these terms will broaden the nurse leader's body of knowledge regarding IT. This terminology is frequently found in technology publications and product purchase descriptions and will assist in interdisciplinary discussions and decisions. The ANA's *Scope and Standards of Nursing Informatics Practice* (2001) identifies three progressive levels of NI competencies: the beginning nurse, experienced nurse, and informatics nurse specialist. This chapter will be most useful for the beginning NI competencies nurse. However, the experienced and specialist NI nurse may also glean some support of existing knowledge from the latter portions of this chapter.

Following is a list of common IT terminology:

Bytes. Bytes are units of measure regarding data storage, from *binary table*. A byte is the common unit of computer storage and is made up of 8 binary digits (bits). The terms you will hear the most often are from smallest to largest (relative to each other): kilobyte, megabyte, gigabyte. For example, you might hear someone say that their external memory device has "40 gigs." *Gigs* is slang for gigabyte (which means giant in Latin) and is the equivalent of 1,000,000,000 bytes. James Huggins (2008) provides a thorough and easy-to-read explanation of the origins and quantitative values for the prefixes associated with bytes.

Disk drive. Disk drive refers to a general category of ways to store information on a computer. There are typically hard drive storage areas on computers: these are frequently labeled C drive in the computer's electronic folders. There are other forms of disk drives available to store data, such as thumb drives and rewritable CDs.

Hardware. Hardware is the physical components (nuts and bolts) of the computer that execute the commands to run software. The hardware includes the central processing unit (CPU) that performs most of the work for the computer to function. The CPU for many desktop computers is in the "tower." In laptops and notebooks, the CPU is in the notebook or laptop itself. The CPU works hard, and it needs to have a fan always functioning to cool it down. You hear the whir of the fan as you work on your computer. In the common vernacular, hardware also refers to external memory storage devices.

Modem. The modem transmits and decodes signals so that a computer can be used to gain Internet access and share information with other computers via electronic mail, Web browsing, research, and so forth. In your home, the modem is typically the little black or silver box that needs to light up with a series of lights for you to have Internet access.

Operating system (OS). The operating system is the software that manages and shares the resources on your computer. Windows, Mac, and Linux are all types of operating systems.

Personal digital assistant (PDA). A PDA is an electronic device that may contain some functionality of a computer, a cellular phone, a camera, some video games. A personal digital assistant is a useful tool for nurse leaders; we discuss PDAs at length later in this chapter.

Peripherals. Peripherals is an encompassing term for external devices that you need to interface with your main PC. Examples of peripheral devices are scanners and printers.

Program. A program is a set of instructions that tells the computer what tasks to perform. A program can be a video game or a software program (such as voice recognition program or a tax preparation program). *Programs* and *software* are frequently used as interchangeable terms.

Software. All computer programs are software; for example, the CD for Microsoft Office that you buy and install on your computer is considered software. Software is readily created, erased, and modified on a computer. The next section is about software because you will work with a lot of software, and there are many different types to familiarize yourself with.

Availability and Useful Applications for Nurses

There used to exist a much sharper distinction between software and hardware for personal computers. However, as computer technology has progressed and continues to advance, greater numbers of both types are available, with less distinction between them. Below are some software and hardware products that many nurse

leaders are quite familiar with and also some that nurse leaders need to get more familiar with to meet the ever-growing demands of our profession.

Software

Nurse leaders utilize software on a daily basis for a wide range of objectives. Whether a nurse executive in a pharmaceutical company is using free Audacity software (http://audacity.sourceforge.net) to record a voice podcast e-mail attachment (Cassey, 2007b), or a sexual assault nurse examiner (SANE) is using the SAKiTA software located on a secure server to track evidence (Lopez-Bonasso & Smith, 2006), software is being utilized.

When you purchase a PC, basic software suites often include word processing software and a spreadsheet program (which many use as a database). Purchased computers can also be outfitted with professional or business usage suites such as presentation software (creation of slideshows on your PC) and relational database software (software intended to help manage large amounts of data, and then access to sort the data as needed). The best guides on how to use installed software programs come with the program on the Help menu. These Help menus and tutorials that accompany most software are user friendly and up to date, come with interactive examples to practice your new skills, and provide space for typing your direct questions and choosing the most appropriate answer from a selected menu. If the software does not have an extensive included Help or user guide, there are frequently Web sites with user tips, syntax, questions posted to share for free. To access these Web sites, if you do not have the exact address, enter the key search terms for the specific software, for example, "STATA syntax," into the

Search box of a search engine, such as Google, Yahoo!, or Ask.com.

The versions of available software are continually being upgraded. The basic operations in each progressive version of software are not that dissimilar. You do not need to repurchase every update of software as it is released. Many IT experts suggest waiting at least a year or so before purchasing any updates that you may want. Many users who purchased Windows Vista are aware of the potential bugs associated with recently released updates. However, the problems surrounding Windows Vista are not unique. As Goldsborough (2007) points out:

> The open architecture of PCs, with thousands of different companies making computers, software, printers, and older peripherals and software drivers to connect peripherals to computers means there always will be countless incompatibilities. One of the wisest pieces of advice in deciding to upgrade any software, whether it's an all encompassing package such as an operating system or a group of smaller but critical applications such as an office suite, is to wait until the first set of bugs is out before migrating to a major upgrade. (p. 20)

"Patch downloads" are available to users who need to correct identified flaws in their new or upgraded software. Bass (2004) offers many available options for patch downloads on already-installed software, as well as resources to keep users aware of upcoming software availability. Bass references such sites as KbAlertz, Feed Demon, WinBeta, and BugBlog Rss feeds and provides the addresses.

The use of Help menus and free software is utilization of resources without incurring further expense or time allocation. Nurse leaders know the importance of efficient resource uti-

lization. Additional software for specific user needs (e.g., statistical software, flow charting, and graphic software) can also be purchased separately and installed on your computer by simply running the installation CD and following the installation prompts, or downloading the software directly from the server and installing into your program files. These independently bought software products usually come with Help menus and user tutorials. Again, if these are not included, a search of the Internet usually provides free help guides and tutorials. For example, I typed "Mac" "OS" "help" into the Google search bar and got more than 100 "hits"; an especially useful one was Griffiths (2006) "secrets Apple won't tell you" Web pages and tutorials.

WORD PROCESSING SOFTWARE

A very basic function of a computer is the use of its word processing software. Word processing software is invaluable for disseminating and archiving policy and procedures. Since the use of word processing programs has become commonplace in healthcare settings, the flow of patient care information and evidence-based protocols and practice are timely and widely available to all nurses. To update a protocol or procedure is now a simple process, not the time-consuming rewrite and scan of an entire document that was required in most institutions just a decade ago. Philip Suydam, RN, BS, and Ann Suydam, MS, MA, (personal interview, August 12, 2007) noted that word processing programs are a welcome replacement for typewriters, saving hours of editing and rewriting as well as archiving documents for easy retrieval and revision. The data isolation and data silos of yesteryear are thankfully gone. Every nurse leader should have access to word processing software and have a cache of documents at her or his fingertips for everyday usage on operational, tactical, and strategic levels of leadership.

Word processing software usage is analogous to the historic use of the typewriter. However, word processing software text can be rearranged with a few clicks of a mouse, margins and formatting can be preset, and the word processing software program can check your spelling and grammar, as well as provide a thesaurus. The language underlying a point-and-click icon style computer is MS-DOS. Combinations of key strokes can produce "shortcut" commands that you did not intend, for example: pressing the Control key and then the V key is the Paste shortcut command. This is a point to be cognizant of as your fingers fly over keys. Remember: if you do something you did not intend to do in a word processing program, you usually can undo the last few actions by using the Undo command on the Edit menu.

Word processing software, as most software and hardware, has options and peripherals available to increase availability to all users. Stodden and Roberts (2005) researched the application of voice recognition software (VRS) as a compensatory strategy for written language difficulties for secondary education students. The user does not have to type in the word processing software, just speak, and the software does the word processing. The possible applications of such technology are numerous and need to be explored in nursing informatics.

Word processing software can also be used for complex analyses. Cassey (2008) demonstrates using Microsoft Office Word 2003 (which has been updated to Microsoft Office Word 2007) to create a spreadsheet/table template for economic value-added analysis for nurse leaders involved in cost analysis. There is spreadsheet software available for these analyses that has the capacity for large amounts of data and complicated formulas embedded in the cells, and these are discussed in the following section.

Spreadsheet Programs

Spreadsheets are analogous to the paper accountant's ledgers, where additions and subtractions to the budget were recorded as profits and losses. Spreadsheet software programs are electronic ledger sheets. These powerhouse ledgers provide the nurse leader with built-in functions of summing, averaging, calculating rates, and just about any other arithmetic operation that can be performed by hand (without some of the human error usually associated with repeated calculations). Most spreadsheets also have the capacity to graph data, draw tables, create pictures of data for presentations, and create run charts to track metrics over time, unit, hospital, or any variable that is of interest.

In a retrospective study of EMS utilization in the South Bronx, the data were initially analyzed in Microsoft Office Excel, and the published graphs were constructed solely using Excel, not statistical package software (Cho, Eckardt, Kilbury, & Acosta, 2007). Spreadsheets are slightly intimidating at first because they are new. People frequently get comfortable with one type of program and do not want to learn a new program. However, many programs, even non-Microsoft products, are designed for the icons and menus to be familiar to Windows users, easing the transition between software programs.

The work product from a spreadsheet is invaluable to many nurse leaders. From the simple tracking of "Sunshine Club" contributions on a patient care unit, to calculating rates of performance with door to balloon time over months in cardiac catheterization labs, this software is a nurse leader's best asset for organization and productivity. Carter (2000) outlines an easy-to-follow utilization of spreadsheets with Microsoft Excel to create a computer productivity measurement tool (CPMT). "A CPMT can be used for measuring, managing, and simulating nursing labor dollars and hours while providing quality nursing care for a varying hospital patient census. The labor CPMT included four components: (a) assumption sheet, (b) labor table, (c) daily hours worked sheet, and (d) summary sheet. The components of the system were easily accessed through use of tabs at the bottom of each of the four sheets in Microsoft Excel" (p. 237). There are many uses for spreadsheets for the nurse leader in quality measures, finance, and research or census tracking. Relational databases are also available for managing large amounts of data, and these are described in the next section.

DATABASES

Databases are software programs not usually included in the "home edition" suites of software on PCs. Instead, they are included in professional or business suites. These software programs look like spreadsheets when you open them up in the default view. However, databases do not operate like spreadsheets, and they serve a different function. Their purpose is to aggregate large silos of information. For example, databases are used by many emergency departments to track patients and their diagnoses, time of arrival, time of discharge, disposition, length of stay, and associated demographics. Because many emergency departments see in excess of 60,000 patients per year, this is a formidable database in size and detail (Korn & Mansfield, 2008). This database is also a rich source of information for performance improvement measures and quality indicators. Report-

able Department of Health and credentialing agency sentinel events and information can be accessed by querying the database and printing a report in a matter of minutes.

Databases are also helpful in tracking cost of healthcare services as demonstrated in Titler and colleagues' (2008) examination of hospitalization costs of older adults with heart failure. Databases require repeated usage to gain expertise, as well as time spent on studying tutorials and using Help menus. Setting up and experimenting with a fabricated database and dummy data is also a method of gaining exposure to a database software program and its intricacies. Users can hone database skills, make common user errors, and then troubleshoot those same errors at no risk to the repository of an actual information database.

As always, the maintenance of patient privacy is of primary concern when setting up and using an electronic database or electronic source of patient information. The practice of protection of databases and software helps us in maintaining this privacy. Many institutions have corporate minimum standards regarding protecting electronic patient information. These guidelines incorporate, but are not limited to, the Health Insurance Portability and Accountability Act standards (also known as HIPAA regulations) enacted by Congress in 1996. These guidelines can be accessed at multiple Web sites. Some electronic resources regarding these guidelines are listed at the end of the chapter.

PRESENTATION SOFTWARE

The software programs for presentations have had a major impact on everything from hospital unit-based meetings to annual professional conferences. The style, formatting, and ease of content inclusion make presentation software a tool of value for conveying ideas in a less restrictive medium than the traditional published paper or journal article. People have different attributes that influence style of learning. The media aspect of presentation software, with its eye-catching fonts, various backgrounds, programmable animations, and clip art, elevate presentation software to the status of a communication tool that can be adjusted to suit various audiences and their particular learning needs and styles.

Team projects can also easily incorporate presentation software into the team's collective work product, and presentations can be e-mailed to respective team members for added input or saved on an intranet or communal drive for manipulation, editing, and presentation. Most software application work product (files, documents, spreadsheets, presentations) can be uploaded to communal sites or drives for team projects and usage. If an intranet is not available within a work organization, wikispaces can be created for free for the same purpose, or password-protected e-mailing of work product serves the same purpose. "Dipping Your Toes in Wikispace" (2006) offers an excellent introductory tutorial on wikispace creations and usage. No matter your organizational decisions regarding presentation and file sharing, Harrison (2006) provides information on password protecting work product, thereby protecting information privacy.

A few common mistakes made when using presentation software are the inclusion of too much content on each slide and the use of too many slides in a presentation. There are rules of thumb (heuristics) and presentation etiquette available on multiple Web sites; further suggested readings regarding these heuristics are at the end of the chapter. Examples of some of these heuristics are as follows:

- Plan to spend a minimum of a full minute on each slide (so, if you have 30 minutes to do a presentation, you should have a maximum of 30 slides).
- Minimum font size for slides is 36 points for titles and 20 points for body content.
- Slide color schemes with high contrast are suggested for ease of viewing.
- Limit animated transitions between slides and other in-slide animations (fly-ins, waves) to one every other slide because more than that has been observed anecdotally to induce vertigo.

STATISTICAL SOFTWARE PACKAGES

It has been said that one's greatest strength is frequently also one's greatest weakness. This particular forewarning is appropriate when it comes to the application of statistical software packages. The use of personal computer software to perform statistical calculations and equations that were once done only by hand and later by experienced statisticians with punch cards and in syntax on large computers has reduced pages of intricate calculations to a few points and clicks of a mouse. These advancements in technology have made statistical description and inference from data available within seconds for any user.

Unfortunately, all of the power packed into the statistical software packages is not inclusive of an education in applied statistics or quantitative methods. The Help menus, whether available online or included as tutorials, are interactive, thorough, and a must for any user of these products. However, the theory and assumptions underlying many statistical tests cannot be understood by the computer program. The software reads data entered by the user. Hopefully, the user has the education to know whether the data entered are in the correct format and meet assumptions that the program cannot test for, and that the correct analysis is being performed on the data.

For example: the nurse leader who has seen a presentation that includes a comparison of multiple averages (such as the difference in length of stays between four different hospitals in the same system) has been looking most probably at an ANOVA (analysis of variance) comparison. The default on one of the most commonly used statistical software packages is to treat all ANOVA comparisons as a priori unless post hoc tests are specifically requested. The differences in inferential results by these different methods can prove significant for a nurse leader's data.

For the more commonly used t test comparisons, one must make research choices as in Cohn's (2007) research regarding clinical pathways in medical surgical nursing education. Cohn had a directional hypothesis and made a decision based on previous empirical evidence to utilize a one-tailed t test for inferential data analysis. A computer software program can report both a one-tailed and a two-tailed significance level for your data but cannot tell you which to use. That is where subject matter expertise is applied. The takeaway with this caution is akin to the caution used before one drives an automobile: there are minimum standards of competency one is required to meet before operating any machinery. Responsible operators also are aware of their level of skill and experience and take them into consideration when planning which roads to navigate solo and how to handle hazardous conditions.

"Much of classical statistics has developed around data sets that can be represented as rectangular (flat) data files. These files are ordinarily structured so that rows represent individuals, and the columns represent variables. This approach is embodied in all of the traditional computer packages for statistical analysis, and is explicit in packages such as SPSS, which structures data in the form of a spreadsheet" (Rindskopf, 1998, p. 184). So, the setup of the view for data entry in most statistical packages when you open it up will look like a spreadsheet. However, the data files in statistical packages do not operate like spreadsheets and cannot execute functions in cells as a spreadsheet software program can (i.e., these data files cannot sum within cell, multiply cells, etc.). The format is similar for user ease; the application and potential for the product are different. Do not expect a statistical software package to behave like an accounting spreadsheet because you will be frustrated and end up with incorrect results.

In summation, statistical software is an invaluable and unique tool for a nurse leader whether comparing the rate of wound infection between units in a prison hospital or measuring modeling factors that contribute to delay in diagnosis in a community health center. A wise nurse leader just remembers "error in, error out" and does not try to replace knowledge with technology. There are many courses available both online and at institutions regarding basic statistical methods, or you can consult a statistician for help. The American Statistical Association Web site URL is included at the end of the chapter for reference.

For the nonnovice statistically minded nurse leader who wants some expert information regarding approaches to data analysis, a highly recommended book chapter is Dr. David Rindskopf's in *Evaluation for Educational Productivity* (1998, pp. 173–192). Rindskopf (a renowned scholar in applied statistical methods) discusses current issues in statistical methods, design, and data analysis problems faced by evaluators and researchers. The chapter is fittingly entitled "Statistical Methods for Real-World Evaluation." The chapter was written for a book on advances in educational policy; however, statistical methods are tools that can be applied to all sciences, from agriculture to zoology. Rindskopf writes his chapter in a voice that is informative and clear, and he deals with issues common to nursing research such as missing data and exploratory data analysis.

Much of the real-world data in nursing science research require fuzzy sets analysis. Verkuilen (2005) states, "Fuzzy sets involve concepts which are vague, in the sense that it is frequently very difficult to assign objects to exactly defined categories" (p. 462). Data such as these can be thoroughly analyzed statistically, while not violating the theoretical properties of the data using these complex analyses. Advancements in IT have made these types of analyses available to users. For a nontechnical discussion on fuzzy set analysis, the Verkuilen article is excellent. The importance IT has had in advancing the statistical rigor and theoretical altruism available to today's nurse researcher is clear when discussing these quantitative topics.

REFERENCE SOFTWARE AND ELECTRONIC SOURCE USAGE FOR RESEARCH

Whether conducting a literature review for a thesis or dissertation or researching to strengthen one's knowledge regarding a new nursing protocol or standard of care, the Internet offers a wealth of resources. Anderson and Klemm (2008) discuss the possibilities and cautions when utilizing the Internet for research.

Many institutions of higher learning now have electronic library resources (virtual libraries) where a student or faculty member can be at home on their PC, sign on to the university intranet, and access many online journals and articles. The process for an online search shares many of the components of a physical library search. However, there are elements in the process that are unique to an online reference search and that require specific education for complete use of the electronic resources available for research. Simpson (2006) notes that "in a recent study of 3,000 licensed U.S. nurses, eighty-two percent had Internet access somewhere in their facility, but fewer than 50% had a workstation where they could access it easily, such as on patient units or at the nurses' station. Most of those surveyed didn't search Medline (55%), the majority (73%) didn't search CINAHL, and almost 38% believed their colleagues did not use research findings in the practice environment" (p. 13).

Systematic electronic searches are a key to evidence-based nursing research. However, Hoss and Hanson (2008) signal that researchers are discovering significant gaps in practicing nurses' skills in identifying, accessing, retrieving, evaluating, and utilizing published evidence. Chalmers, Hedges, and Cooper (2002) and Glanville (n.d.) provide insightful information regarding a systematic review of electronic resources and the proper methodology and application of electronic searches to research and evidence-based practice. Systematic review requires access to the professional literature (electronic and nonelectronic). Hand searches can be aided by an online search and noting dates of publication limitations and a World Wide Web query for white papers and conference proceedings.

For direct access to excellent electronic information, an appropriate search of key Web sites should be conducted. Cassey (2007c) states:

Most nurses are aware of the American Nurses Association's extensive library of professional nursing Standards of Practice. Those standards guide the art of nursing and create a general framework for applying and integrating the science of nursing into daily nursing practice. Complementary to the nursing standards are the interdisciplinary practice guidelines organized and distributed by the National Guideline Clearinghouse (NGC). The NGC offers an extensive collection of peer-reviewed, current, scientific standards to support clinical decision making in nursing practice. Becoming familiar with these resources is critical to safe and professional nursing practice. (p. 302)

Meta-analysis has also been a growing area of research, in part because of the availability of shared data and research on the Internet and via electronic libraries. The *Cochrane Handbook for Systematic Reviews of Interventions* (Higgins & Green, 2006) is the source for information on nursing and healthcare meta-analyses. The Cochrane Web site offers multiple tutorials in meta-analytic processes, as well as a repository for meta-analyses conducted in the healthcare sciences. For inclusion of dissertations and unpublished sources of research to decrease possible publication bias in evidence-based research, there is also the online dissertation database available in most electronic libraries. The use of electronic resources for any research begins with a basic inquiry into a subject.

To answer some basic questions on how to best utilize electronic resources and databases for basic nurse research, I interviewed Jeff Gutkin, Director of Academic Computing at Wagner College, Staten Island, New York (J. Gutkin, personal communication, July 15, 2007), who offered these solutions regarding inquiry and search words:

- Draw one or two of the most unique words contained in your thesis statement or research question. Start by using them as keywords.
- The database only matches the word you type in to where it is found in a record. Try to think of what word the author would use when writing an article on your topic. An article on nursing might never contain the word "nurse."
- Search for authors by subject, authority, and keyword. Some authors have published many articles on the same subject. By placing that name in an author search, you will get only the articles that author has written. Typing that name in a subject search will list articles written about the author. Putting the name in a keyword search will list articles that mention the author's name.
- Learn how to use Boolean operators or "wildcards." Many databases have the OR, NOT, and AND functions built into their advanced search feature. Using OR returns an article that has one word or another word and will return the highest volume of hits. NOT can exclude articles that contain a certain word; for example, *bipolar type 1, NOT 2* will return only articles about type 1. AND is inclusive and limits the search to an article that contains both words. You can also use quotation marks to limit a search, but you should use them with caution. For example, a search for "nurse–midwives" will return only articles that contain that exact phrase. Each database has its own list of operators and wildcards that it uses and there is usually a help section that contains this information.

Librarians are an excellent resource for acquisition of electronic reference materials, as well as systematic search approaches for subject items including gray or fugitive literature, such as white papers, dissertations, and conference proceedings. Rosenthal (1994) and Rothstein (2008) discuss the importance of gray literature and its inclusion in systematic reviews, especially in light of the ease of electronic literature reviews that may lead to the preclusion of gray literature review. Software is available that tracks and organizes articles, papers, and information retrieved on research subjects. Endnote and Zotero are two examples of bibliography tracking software to organize references for primary research. Comprehensive Meta Analysis (CMA) software is a meta-analytic software package that also organizes references for comparison and effect size computation and data extraction. These products are designed to aid the nurse in research endeavors.

Last, primary research involves theoretical grounding and often the use of a tool to measure a variable. Researchers are aware of the need for a theoretical framework for construct development, as well as a valid and reliable instrument to directly or indirectly measure constructs and variables of interest. Web sites dedicated to compiling nurse research resources and theories often include reliable and valid tools for measurement. These resources are listed at the close of the chapter in the section titled "Internet Resources Available to You."

Hardware

As noted earlier in the earlier chapter, hardware is the internal workings of your computer, the central processing unit. Many peripherals now hold memory, transfer files, and are sold as hardware. The most common of these products are listed below with a brief comment section on each product.

Flash Drives

There are very few nurses still using floppy disks to store electronic files. Since 1995, few PCs come equipped with a standard floppy drive. File storage is now frequently on *flash drives* (also known as *thumb drives* or *jump drives*) for ease of storage and transportation. Flash drives are inexpensive and are compatible with most PCs. If your computer does not initially recognize the flash drive when you plug it in to the USB port, you can install the software for that particular brand of flash drive from the accompanying installation CD or download it from the Internet at the flash drive company Web site.

There are two cautions for external memory devices. The first is *always* back up important files in at least two places: if you have a flash drive for school courses, be certain to also copy those files onto your home computer's C drive on a regular (weekly) basis. If you primarily store your files on the C drive on your home computer, then back up files on an external drive weekly. As mentioned earlier, most recent computers do not come with floppy disk capacity. You need to purchase a peripheral floppy disk device if you have old files you want to access (such as data files that came with old texts). One additional step to ease your access to these files in the future is to save the data from the floppy disks to a rewritable CD, a memory key, or some other form of external memory. If you save data to CDs, make certain that they are rewritable discs; otherwise, once you save your data, you cannot edit or add to the disc. A rewritable CD is labeled CD-R, CD+R, or CD-RW.

Any of these formats may be used as potential patient education tools. Cassey (2007a) outlines two specific IT tools available for patient education where English is not the primary language. Both the Spanish Access to Literature/Uso Directo (SALUD) Web page and Healthy Roads Media have materials available in multiple formats that can be used online and can be downloaded and used offline as well. Healthy Roads has audio (mp3) versions that can be downloaded and transferred to a PDA or iPod for sharing with patients. Both of these options seem a natural and necessary extension for the nurse involved in direct patient teaching (acute care; clinics; home care; community, industrial, or prison population settings). Nurses are innovators in patient advocacy, and ensuring patient access to the most current information available is a skill to add to your cache.

External Memory

Other types of external memory serve the same basic function as a flash drive; they just usually store more gigabytes. For example, I have a 37.2-gigabyte external memory bank that functions as my mini memory and travels with me daily. I have every file on it backed up to my home PC or my university intranet, depending on where I will use the file. I doubt I will ever use 37.2 gigabytes of active files at one time, but if I start storing .jpeg and scanned items in mass quantities, I just may.

Scanned images are utilized in health care for many different purposes. One example described by Simonian (2008) involves the implementation of fax and document imaging technology to electronically communicate medication orders from nursing stations to the pharmacy by Sharp Health Care in San Diego, California, hospitals. The system consists of existing fax machines and document imaging software that captures images of written orders and sends them from nursing stations to a central database server. Pharmacists then retrieve the images and enter

the orders in an electronic medical record system. The central database server in that application was designed to store images that require large amounts of working memory. Handheld devices also have a fair amount of working memory and are being used with increasing frequency by nursing professionals.

PDAs

Personal digital assistants (PDAs) have replaced the four inches of reference books shoved in a nurse's lab coat pockets while in a clinical setting. The personal digital assistant fits neatly in any pocket and holds a wealth of information regarding clinical pathways, medications, and emergency algorithms, and they can also access Internet resources. The speed of these devices retrieves full description of disease sequelae, treatment, risks, medication administration guidelines, and contraindications in seconds. The obstetric (OB) wheel used to plan the Estimated Date of Conception (EDC) and gestational age requires just a few clicks, and voilà, it is calculated!

The best feature of the PDA is that the information is always current. The user can upload newer versions of software for free or at reduced rates. The user does not need to buy a new hard copy drug book annually (remember the cost of that?), just the electronic updates after initial purchase. At Adelphi University in Garden City, New York, the use of PDAs by first-year nursing students in the clinical settings was championed by administration and rolled out by S. Greenfield, an assistant professor in the School of Nursing. Dr. Greenfield found that nursing students who used a nursing student software PDA to answer six medication questions outperformed students who used a nursing textbook as their resource on accuracy ($p = .037$) and speed ($p = .002$) variables (Greenfield, 2007).

I spoke with Dr. Greenfield regarding suggestions on how to begin using a PDA for nurses and nursing students, and common pitfalls and mistakes when using PDAs as resources. Her suggestions on how to begin using a PDA for nurses and nursing students are these: first, remember that to use a PDA you need to have a computer. The data on your PDA is backed up on your computer and many software programs are downloaded and/or updated when you "hot sync" your PDA to the Internet connection of your home computer. Next, think about what you will be using the PDA for and your budget for purchasing the PDA and software. If the PDA is to reference data at the bedside, then you need to ensure that the PDA you choose has enough memory or a slot for a memory card to be able to run the program (software) that you choose. All Web sites for nursing/medical/healthcare software have the memory requirements listed and all PDAs will list the amount of memory they have. Last, all PDAs have one of two operating systems, OS and PC. Each has their own advantages. A good Web site to compare the two is www.mobiletechreview.com (listed in the resources section at the end of the chapter).

Two common pitfalls of using PDAs are spending more money than you need to and not going through the included tutorials (personal communication, July 30, 2007). Koeniger-Donohue (2008) conducted a pilot program in the clinical area utilizing Palm Pilots as references and found qualitative results that support the use of PDAs in the clinical academic setting. The PDA has many applications, with promising areas of application being researched each year. Davies, Stock, and Wehmeyer (2003) found that a PDA, the Pocket Compass, could act as an aid for individuals with intellectual disabilities to increase independent decision making. The applications of PDAs increase

daily, and like all mobile technology they have broad implications for use in remote or access-impaired settings or populations.

Peripherals, Hardware, and Software for Increased Technology Access

Increased access to technology can be achieved via training as Mirza, Anandan, Madnick, and Hammel (2006) demonstrated when they pilot-tested and evaluated an innovative program providing IT access to people with disabilities transitioning out of nursing homes into the community. Their methodology was a participatory approach and included pre- and post-training data collection on the 61 program participants to reflect these broad areas related to the IT training experience: performance; self-efficacy; importance, satisfaction, and control. The results indicated the feasibility, effectiveness, and value of IT access for people with disabilities, particularly those transitioning from institutional life to community living.

Accessibility can also be increased by development and implementation of peripherals, hardware, and software designed to broaden the reach of IT access and application. Software that provides read-aloud texts for the blind (Code Red, 2007), the freeware books described by Van Horn (2007) available to financially burdened populations at such sites as LibriVox (www.librivox.org), and the eye blink–directed hardware available for quadriplegic populations described by Ohno, Mukawa, and Yoshikawa (2002) are all venues that increase user IT availability. This increased accessibility for all populations is a trend driven in part by legislation. But as Brooks (2007) is quick to point out, even though the Disability Discrimination Act of 1995 made accessibility a legal requirement, implementation remains poor. This is yet another area for nurses as patient advocates to raise their voices for change.

Internet Resources Available to You

This section includes a few Internet resources available for further information. This is not an all-inclusive list and is meant as a starting point. Some key concepts to remember are the demonstrated effectiveness of IT in nursing and patient education and research. Magnussen (2008) outlines the inclusion of significant learning principles in the e-learning environment. Ornes and Gassert (2007) describe a baccalaureate (BSN) curriculum evaluation of nursing informatics content. Results could be used to inform faculty about strategies that could strengthen informatics competencies.

As stated earlier in this chapter, new nurses need informatics skills to work efficiently in an environment that increasingly relies on IT to promote patient safety. In addition, a federal order mandates that all Americans have an electronic medical record by 2014. Nursing programs must incorporate informatics content into their current curricula to fully prepare new nurses to competently utilize IT. Examples of the application of this technology curriculum are found in the Nokes and associates (2005) Web-based service learning curriculum for student nurses; Harvey-Teeley's (2007) hybrid learning course outline in a Massachusetts school of nursing; and the proposed Accelerated Career Entry (ACE) Program at Drexel University described by Suplee and Glasgow (2008), which includes a substantial amount of IT-incorporated learning in the curricula, and which has graduated more than 500 nurses since

its inception, with a successful 95–100% National Council Licensure Examination (NCLEX) pass rate.

INTERNET RESOURCES

Nursing associations and organizations
- Boards of Nursing from Allnurses: A Nursing Community for Nurses: http://allnurses.com/boards-of-nursing-info.html
- Healthcare Information and Management Systems Society (HIMSS): http://himss.org/ASP/index.asp

Government Web sites and large databases of interest to nurses
- National Center for Health Statistics: http://www.cdc.gov/nchs/nhis.htm
- Registered Nurse Population: Findings from the 2004 National Sample Survey of Registered Nurses: http://bhpr.hrsa.gov/healthworkforce/rnsurvey04/
- US Department of Health and Human Services: http://aspe.hhs.gov/admnsimp/

Product Help, tutorials, and information
- Audacity, The Free, Cross-Platform Sound Editor: http://audacity.sourceforge.net/
- CollectiveMed.com: http://www.collectivemed.com
- Comprehensive Meta-Analysis: http://www.meta-analysis.com/pages/why_use.html
- EndNote: http://www.endnote.com/
- Epocrates: http://www.epocrates.com
- HIPAA.org: http://www.hipaa.org/
- LibriVox: http://www.librivox.org
- Microsoft Office Online: http://office.microsoft.com/en-us/

- Mobile Tech review: http://www. mobiletechreview.com/tips/palm_vs_ pocketPC.htm
- PDA Cortex: http://www.pdacortex.com
- PEPID: http://www.pepid.com
- Zotero: http://www.zotero.org/

Nursing research and education

- All Nursing Schools: http://www. allnursingschools.com/?src=trl_ans
- Cardinal Stritch University Library: http://library.stritch.edu/research/ subjects/nursingtheorists/overview.htm
- CINAHL: http://www.cinahl.com
- Clayton State University Department of Nursing: http://healthsci.clayton.edu/ eichelberger/nursing.htm
- The Cochrane Collaboration: http:// www.cochrane.org/
- Computer Retrieval of Information on Scientific Projects (CRISP): http://crisp. cit.nih.gov/
- NurseScribe: http://www.enursescribe. com/nurse_theorists.htm
- University of San Diego, Hahn School of Nursing and Health Science: http:// www.sandiego.edu/academics/nursing/ theory

Statistics

- American Statistical Association: http:// www.amstat.org/index.cfm?fuseaction= main
- David M Lane HyperStat: http:// davidmlane.com/hyperstat/
- Judea Pearl home page: http://bayes. cs.ucla.edu/jp_home.html
- Notes on MCMC (Markov Chain Monte Carlo) methods: http://www.stats.ox. ac.uk/~reinert/mcmc/mcmc07.html

and http://www.stats.ox.ac.uk/~reinert/ mcmc/practical07.pdf

- R Project for Statistical Computing: http://www.r-project.org/
- Spiegelhalter book: http://www. amazon.com/Bayesian-Approaches-Health-Care-Evaluation-Statistics/ dp/0471499757
- Spiegelhalter article: "Incorporating Bayesian Ideas into Health-Care Evaluation": http://projecteuclid.org/ DPubS/Repository/1.0/Disseminate? view=body&id=pdfview_1&handle= euclid.ss/1089808280

Summary

This brief chapter is an introduction to the IT definitions, tools, and resources that are available to nurse leaders today to shape health care tomorrow. The purpose of this chapter is to discuss some of the applications of IT by nurse leaders today and in the healthcare environment and to list some excellent further resources for nurse leaders and IT. Hospitals now devote about 7% of their operating budgets to clinical, business, and patient-outreach IT applications (Joch, 2008).

Jenkins, Hewitt, and Bakken (2006) note, "Nurses must be prepared to participate in the evolving National Health Information Infrastructure and the changes that will consequently occur in health care practice and documentation. Informatics technologies will be used to develop EHRs with integrated decision support features that will likely lead to enhanced health care quality and safety" (p. 141). Nursing informatics will help to better serve patient populations. Use this chapter's resources as a starting or continuation point in the development of your nursing informatics competence.

QUESTIONS

1. Which of the following is true about databases?
   a. Databases are used exactly like spreadsheets and serve the same function.
   b. Databases are used by emergency departments to track patient information.
   c. Databases cannot be accessed using a PC.
   d. Databases are on all laptop computers.

2. The American Nursing Credentialing Center (ANCC)
   a. has not yet endorsed the use of technology in nursing
   b. has written many programs to guide nurses in the use of technology
   c. has begun administering an informatics nurse certification exam
   d. does not approve of use of patient information databases

3. A modem is
   a. not necessary for most computer use
   b. a piece of hardware that transmits and decodes signals so that a computer can be used to connect to the Internet
   c. outmoded and most computers no longer need a modem to access the Internet
   d. used for word processing

4. Most nursing programs have incorporated computer technology into their programs, because
   a. new nurses need informatics skills to work efficiently in an environment that increasingly relies on IT to promote patient safety
   b. a federal order mandates that all Americans have an electronic medical record by 2014
   c. nursing programs must incorporate informatics content into their current curricula to fully prepare new nurses to competently utilize IT
   d. All of the above

5. The increased use of technology to maintain patient information has created the need to be diligent about
   a. maintaining patient privacy because it is of primary concern when using an electronic database or electronic source of patient information
   b. accuracy in data collection
   c. input of confidential materials
   d. which computer program is being utilized because the wrong program can interfere with collection of accurate data

Recommended Reading

Cooper, H. (1998). *Synthesizing research: A guide for literature reviews* (3rd ed.). Thousand Oaks, CA: Sage.

Hannah, K. J., Ball, M. J., & Edwards, K. J. (1999). *Introduction to nursing informatics* (2nd ed.). New York: Springer-Verlag.

Petticrew, M., & Roberts, H. (2005). *Systematic reviews in the social sciences: A practical guide.* Oxford, UK: Wiley-Blackwell.

Smith, J. (2000). *Health management information systems: A handbook for decision makers.* Buckingham, UK: Open University Press.

Thede, L. Q. (2003). *Informatics and nursing: Opportunities and challenges* (2nd ed.). Philadelphia: Lippincott Williams & Wilkins.

References

Alexander, G. (2008, February). Analysis of an integrated clinical decision support system in nursing home clinical information systems. *Journal of Gerontological Nursing, 34*(2), 15–20.

American Nurses Association. (2001). *Scope and standards of nursing informatics practice.* Washington, DC: Author.

Anderson, A., & Klemm, P. (2008). The Internet: Friend or foe when providing patient education? *Clinical Journal of Oncology Nursing, 12*(1), 55–63.

Bass, S. (2004). 11 easy ways to keep a PC up-to-date. *PC World, 22*(10), 55.

Bodin, S. (2007). President-elect message. Evidence and nursing informatics to improve safety and outcomes. *Nephrology Nursing Journal, 34*(2), 135–136.

Brooks, G. (2007, June 8). Making websites accessible to all. Retrieved April 27, 2008, from http://www.nma.co.uk/home/articles/Brooks/june2007_8.html

Carter, M. (2000, September). Use of a nursing labor computer productivity measurement tool. *Nursing Economics, 18*(5), 237–242.

Cassey, M. (2007a, May). Information systems and technology. Building a case for using technology: Health literacy and patient education. *Nursing Economics, 25*(3), 186–188.

Cassey, M. (2007b, July). Information systems and technology. Using technology to let your voice be heard. *Nursing Economics, 25*(4), 230–232.

Cassey, M. (2007c, September). Information systems and technology. Incorporating the National Guideline Clearinghouse into evidence-based nursing practice. *Nursing Economics, 25*(5), 302–303.

Cassey, M. (2008, January–February). Information systems and technology. Using a spreadsheet/table template for economic value added analysis. *Nursing Economics, 26*(1), 61–63.

Chalmers, I., Hedges, L. V., & Cooper, H. M. (2002). A brief history of research synthesis. *Evaluation and the Health Professions, 25*(1), 12–37.

Cho, E., Eckardt, P., Kilbury, L., & Acosta, J. (2007, January) Is EMS over- or under-utilized in the South Bronx: A retrospective view. *New York Medical Journal, 2*(1), 16–20.

Code red: Is Braille losing its touch? (2007, October 26). *Weekly Reader News—Senior.*

Cohn, E. (2007). Eastern Nursing Research Society, building bridges between academia and service: Using clinical pathways as a teaching tool in medical-surgical nursing. Poster. Providence, Rhode Island, April 14, 2007.

Davies, D., Stock, S., & Wehmeyer, M. (2003, Winter). A palmtop computer-based intelligent aid for individuals with intellectual disabilities to increase independent decision making. *Research & Practice for Persons with Severe Disabilities, 28*(4), 182–193.

Dipping your toes in wiki-space. (2006). *Associations Now.* Retrieved April 2, 2008, from MasterFILE Premier database.

Glanville, J. (n.d.). *Identification of research.* York, UK: Center for Research and Dissemination.

Goldsborough, R. (2007, August 13). Software upgrades not without pitfalls. *New Orleans CityBusiness, 28*(3), 20–22. Retrieved February 22, 2008, from MasterFILE Premier database.

Greenfield, S. (2007, March). Medication error reduction and the use of PDA technology. *Journal of Nursing Education, 46*(3), 127–131.

Griffiths, R. (2006). Mac OS X hints. *Macworld, 23*(7), 80–82. Retrieved April 22, 2008, from Academic Search Premier database.

Harrison, W. (2006). Passwords and passion. *IEEE Software, 23*(4), 5–7.

Harvey-Teeley, K. (2007). Educational innovations. Designing hybrid Web-based courses for accelerated nursing students. *Journal of Nursing Education, 46*(9), 417–422.

Healthcare Information and Management Systems Society (HIMSS) Nursing Informatics Task Force. (2007, March). An emerging giant: Nursing informatics. *Nursing Management, 38*(3), 38–42.

Higgins, J. P. T., & Green, S., (Eds.). Cochrane handbook for systematic reviews of interventions 4.2.6 (updated September 2006). Retrieved February 6, 2008, from http://www.cochrane.org/resources/handbook/hbook.htm

Hoss, B., & Hanson, D. (2008). Evaluating the evidence: Web sites. *AORN Journal, 87*(1), 124–141.

Huggins, J. (2008, March 27). Where did kilo, mega, giga and all those other prefixes come from? Retrieved April 14, 2008, from http://www.jamesshuggins.com/h/tek1/prefixes.htm

Hynes, P. (2006, Winter). Reflections on critical care emergency preparedness: The necessity of planned education and leadership training for nurses. *Dynamics, 17*(4), 19–22.

Jenkins, M., Hewitt, C., & Bakken, S. (2006). Women's health nursing in the context of the National Health Information Infrastructure. *JOGNN: Journal of Obstetric, Gynecologic, & Neonatal Nursing, 35*(1), 141–150.

Joch, A. (2008). IT at a crossroads (cover story). *H&HN: Hospitals & Health Networks, 82*(2), 45–50.

Koeniger-Donohue, R. (2008). Handheld computers in nursing education: A PDA pilot project. *Journal of Nursing Education, 47*(2), 74–77.

Korn, R., & Mansfield, M. (2008). ED overcrowding: An assessment tool to monitor ED registered nurse workload that accounts for admitted patients residing in the emergency department. *Journal of Emergency Nursing, 34*(5), 441–446.

Lopez-Bonasso, D., & Smith, T. (2006, Summer). Sexual assault kit tracking application (SAKiTA): Technology at work in West Virginia. *Journal of Forensic Nursing, 2*(2), 92–95.

Magnussen, L. (2008). Applying the principles of significant learning in the e-learning environment. *Journal of Nursing Education, 47*(2), 82–86.

McCannon, M., & O'Neal, P. (2003). Results of a national survey indicating IT skills needed by nurses at time of entry into the work force. *Journal of Nursing Education, 42*(8), 337–340.

Mirza, M., Anandan, N., Madnick, F., & Hammel, J. (2006). A participatory program evaluation of a systems change program to improve access to information technology by people with disabilities. *Disability & Rehabilitation, 28*(19), 1185–1199.

Nokes, K., Nickitas, D., Keida, R., & Neville, S. (2005). Does service-learning increase cultural competency, critical thinking, and civic engagement? *Journal of Nursing Education, 44*(2), 65–70.

Ohno, T., Mukawa , N., & Yoshikawa, A. (2002). FreeGaze: A gaze tracking system for everyday gaze interaction. *Proceedings of the 2002 Symposium on Eye Tracking Research and Applications*. New Orleans, Louisiana.

Ornes, L., & Gassert, C. (2007). Computer competencies in a BSN program. *Journal of Nursing Education, 46*(2), 75–78.

Rindskopf, D. (1998). Statistical methods for real-world evaluation. In A. J. Reynolds & H. J. Walberg (Eds.), *Evaluation for educational productivity* (pp. 173–192). Greenwich, CT: JAI Press.

Rosenthal, M. C. (1994). The fugitive literature. In H. Cooper & L. V. Hedges (Eds.), *The handbook of research synthesis*. New York: Russell Sage Foundation.

Rothstein, H. (2008). Publication bias as a threat to the validity of meta-analytic results. *Journal of Experimental Criminology, 4*(1), 61–81.

Simonian, A. (2008). Medication order communication using fax and document-imaging technologies. *American Journal of Health-System Pharmacy, 65*(6), 570–573.

Simpson, R. (2006, June). Information technology. Automation: The vanguard of EBN. *Nursing Management, 37*(6), 13–14.

Smithers, J. (2007). Rationales for developing a perioperative Web-based resource: Informatics in action. *AORN Journal, 86*(2), 239–248.

Stodden, R., & Roberts, K. (2005). The use of voice recognition software as a compensatory strategy for postsecondary education students receiving services under the category of learning disabled. *Journal of Vocational Rehabilitation, 22*(1), 49–64.

Suplee, P., & Glasgow, M. (2008). Curriculum innovation in an accelerated BSN program: The ACE Model. *International Journal of Nursing Education Scholarship, 5*(1), 1–13.

Titler, M., Jensen, G., Dochterman, J., Xie, X., Kanak, M., Reed, D., et al. (2008). Cost of hospital care for older adults with heart failure: Medical, pharmaceutical, and nursing costs. *Health Services Research, 43*(2), 635–655.

Van Horn, R. (2007). Online books and audio books. *Phi Delta Kappan, 89*(2), 154–155.

Verkuilen, J. (2005). Assigning membership in a fuzzy set analysis. *Sociological Methods & Research, 33*(4), 462–496.

Unit Four

Caring for Nurses

Chapter 17

Caring for the Nurses Who Provide Patient Care

Bonnie Ewing and
Marie Hayden-
Miles

OUTLINE

Nurses today are challenged to provide leadership within a healthcare system that is becoming increasingly complex. High patient acuity, sophisticated technology, the shifting of healthcare delivery from the hospital to community settings, and a nursing shortage demand effective leadership practices to guide nurses who are stressed and burdened in chaotic systems. To be able to provide an optimal level of care to patients, nurses need to have a sense that their leaders care about them and appreciate the work they do. Nursing leaders, therefore, must be guided by a set of core values and principles that communicate caring to others. In addition, they need to assist nurses by developing safe work environments that promote health and well-being. Wesorick (2002) states, "The legacy of leadership will be determined by the ability to co-create the best places to practice and receive care" (p. 18).

Caring: The Core of Leadership

Caring, a core value of the nursing profession, has been examined extensively by nursing theorists and researchers. Nightingale (1859) wrote "nursing's most important work is caring" and

Leininger (1984) describes caring as "the essence of nursing." Nursing has traditionally been concerned with caring as a principle for nursing action (Cronin & Harrison, 1988). Leininger (1988) views caring as the central and unifying domain for the body of knowledge and practices that are nursing relationships. Nursing leaders such as Watson (2006) and Nyberg (1998) claim that caring is not only about patients but that caring exists within us and needs to be conveyed to individuals who care for patients.

Models of Caring

Nyberg (1998), who developed a Model of Caring Administration, states that caring is foundational. In Nyberg's model, nursing administrators communicate caring as both an ethic and a philosophy. Caring relates not only to patients, but it is also the life approach of nurses. Caring individuals can make the work environment more pleasant. Having a sense of compassion and empathy imparts concern, thereby enhancing trusting relationships. Watson (2000) also describes caring as foundational, but goes further, calling caring the moral foundation of the profession and central to the profession's roles and responsibilities. She argues that caring-healing leadership "may be the primary source of nursing's survival in this 21st century" (p. 6).

So important is caring leadership that several nursing authors (Watson, 2006; Kerfoot, 1997; Boykin & Schoenhofer, 2001) consider it a moral imperative. Kerfoot (1997) describes a community of caring as "the greatest gift a leader can give" (p. 50). Understanding that the world is filled with uncertainty, leaders must adopt practices and strategies that are open to the changes and nuances existing in the surrounding culture

(Porter-O'Grady & Malloch, 2003). Change in the 21st century requires that leaders address workplace relationships (Wesorick, 2002). The American Association of Critical Care Nurses (2004) considers a professionally and psychologically sound work environment essential to improving patient safety, staff retention, and recruitment. Such an environment is empowering and respectful of all staff.

It is important that nursing leaders not only enact caring practices but also relate to nurses in a way that communicates their inherent worth and dignity. Unpublished research by Hayden-Miles and Ewing (2007) indicates that even small acts can sustain nurses through difficult times, as revealed by one nurse: "Everyday one of the nurse administrators would come by and thank us for doing this 'important work.' It really made a difference. I found myself looking forward to her visits." Research by Ray, Turkel, and Marino (2002) supports visibility as an important part of leadership practice: "One administrator felt that being visible and modeling caring was a core value and made time to make rounds on a consistent basis" (p. 12).

Individuals who feel cared for are better able to provide care to patients; therefore, leaders must find ways to make caring visible and tangible. Creating a culture of care need not be expensive. Simple gestures can demonstrate caring. For example, soliciting input and involving people in decision making, when appropriate, give individuals a sense that their opinions are respected. Being considerate and sensitive to the fact that people have obligations and responsibilities outside of the work environment helps them feel valued. Fostering a respectful environment in which others are treated as valued colleagues, and who are attended to as people, supports their spirits, freeing them to be better nurses. "Authentic leaders bring love, hope, relationship-centered principles and inspiration to the workplace everyday" (Kerfoot, 2006, p. 595).

Leaders may struggle to find a balance between creating caring environments and their responsibility to contain costs. However, some researchers argue that caring has economic value. "Although caring and economics may seem paradoxical, contemporary health care concerns emphasize the importance of understanding caring in terms of cost" (Turkel, 2001, p. 81). Research by Parsons and Cornett (2005) demonstrates that harmonious work environments increase retention. A reduced turnover saves the cost of recruiting and orienting new employees. Felgen (2003) argues that caring is a resource and is most valuable when it permeates the organization. "When caring exists in every fiber of the fabric of their work environment, nurses feel cared for and relevant, empowered to do what they do best . . . care for others" (p. 214). Caring, respectful leadership practices can reduce costs by increasing patient satisfaction, improving patient outcomes, and maintaining a healthier work environment for staff.

Caring Leadership Practices

By utilizing caring practices, leaders can facilitate and support the movement toward healthy workplace standards (Kerfoot, 2006; AACN, 2004). Leaders need to understand how best to function to create workplaces that are healthier. Their style, manner, and way of relating to people can have a major impact on the way others feel about their ability to function and perform. Nyberg (1998) states that by developing attributes such as a commitment to a caring relationship, self-worth, prioritization, and openness, the leader can influence others and bring out

their potential. "Caring is an ethic that affects all life relationships. It is a way of relating to people that involves special skills of openness and responsiveness to the needs of others" (p. 36). The following practices embody caring concepts that can be utilized by leaders to promote healthy work cultures that will ultimately affect how individuals and groups perform.

Integrity, Trust, and Respect

Imparting values will give others the knowledge that the leader has integrity. In a comparative descriptive study of nurse executives and women leaders, Carroll (2005) found that personal integrity, including ethical standards, trustworthiness, and credibility, received the highest level of importance for both groups. Trust is an essential component of relationships that may take time to develop with people. Individuals want to trust that their leaders are competent, will safeguard confidences, and will not harm them (Rowley, 2007). Leaders who establish trusting relationships can develop enduring relationships with shared purpose. If leaders are open and honest in their relationships, they establish connections that build commitment. Rogers (2005) emphasizes that effective strategies for building and maintaining trusting relationships between nurse managers and staff are ability, benevolence, and integrity identified by Mayer, Davis, and Shoorman (1995).

Ability is maintaining competency within a domain so that others will trust in the expertise of the leader. A leader who is benevolent is concerned and caring about employees. Integrity requires functioning with principles, being honest with staff, and demonstrating openly values and beliefs by articulating them and acting in ways consistent with the values stated. Respect is at the core of developing relationships that are healing for caregivers in relation to one another and to patients, the recipients of their care. Respect is a way of life that needs constant support and nurturing. It is essential to know when disrespect occurs and with whom. Sustaining respectful relationships requires creating infrastructures to support and initiate healing relationships in which the caregivers and recipients of care can be engaged (Malloch & Porter-O'Grady, 2005).

Inspirational Dialogue

Listening and hearing what another is trying to say and the hidden messages conveyed through nonverbal cues enhance communication. Clarifying what is being said and acknowledging understanding shows that the leader is interested in knowing what others feel and think (Boyatzis & McKee, 2005). Within systems that are rapidly changing, articulating the signs of change and using inspiring language are vital for others to understand the value of the change that might be occurring (Malloch & Porter-O'Grady, 2005). Empathetic leaders foster an inclusive approach with others that helps them to feel that their leaders care. When people discuss what they feel, they uncover causes of problems. Shared language surfaces that emanates from powerful feelings, resulting in moving people from talk to action. People become involved in identifying problems, issues, hopes, and aspirations and create a shared language about the current reality. This ultimately releases energy to move their common goals forward (Boyatzis & McKee, 2005).

Professional Style

People are magnetized by leaders and imitate their behaviors; therefore, the more caring, professional, and positive the leader, the more people will respond positively (George, 2003). The leader's style is a behavioral signature that lets others know how the leader functions and what the leader values (Rowley, 2007). Professional nursing leaders model values and beliefs through their actions and practices. They are authentic leaders who desire to serve others and to empower them to make a difference in the lives of their patients. They work hard to overcome their own shortcomings and lead with purpose, value, and meaning. Refusing to compromise principles, they let others know where they stand by setting boundaries.

The professional nursing leader recognizes that leadership is a lifetime of professional and personal growth. The behaviors of the professional leader illuminate the foundational beliefs and values of the nursing profession. For example, nursing educators who are caring and compassionate toward their students show them how to be caring toward their patients. The leader can affect how others think, reason, and interact. Emotions spread from expressive people; therefore, the leader is in a prime position to affect the behavior of others. Professional leaders are concerned about other people's ways of doing things but recognize that others' ideas may or may not be more important than their own. Assertive leaders are able to agree or disagree and be comfortable about giving and receiving honest feedback even if it is unpopular.

A professional leader needs to be self-aware by recognizing feelings about one's self in relation to others. Knowing one's own feelings frees the leader to have a better ability to assess and read how others relate and perform. Boyatzis and McKee (2005) state that when leaders are mindful of who they are, they understand their own responses in relation to others. They are then able to maintain self-control to manage the stresses and dynamics inherent in leadership. Resonating with one's self can create resonance with others. Reflection, contemplation, and internal explorations are ways to attend to the self that help the leader learn how to attend consciously to other people and the surrounding culture.

Engagement

Individuals require attention to their needs and problems, and it is the responsibility of the leader to show interest in others so that they will perform. By spending time with employees, the leader learns about them and the ways that they work. Learning about people by evaluating their performance, the leader can help them adapt to new changes, especially if they are threatened by the chaos that change can create. Leaders who care will help others to understand the importance of their work as it relates to the whole of what is happening.

Helping people who operate within the context of established ways to unlearn and undo what has been done for years is a challenge. In such cases, the leader is required to lend clarity and psychological support. By being aware of forces and drives, the leader can assist others to create goals, objectives, and project outcomes (Malloch & Porter-O'Grady, 2005). Subjective satisfaction enhances the well-being of individuals and groups. A desire for setting goals, achieving them, and finding meaning and fulfillment in achievement is essential to experiencing a sense of well-being. Through praise and encouragement, healthcare leaders can work to promote and encourage performance. Outcomes of self-efficacy include vitality, feelings of accomplishment, and social well-being (Leddy, 2006).

Team Building

One of the essential skills of a nursing leader is team building. Building successful teams is critical to healthcare organizations because a high level of teamwork leads to increased work satisfaction and reduced burnout among nurses (Rafferty, Ball, & Aiken, 2001). How leaders gather team members together can contribute to the success or failure of the team. The leader who brings passion and enthusiasm for nursing calls out the best in the team. Creating a team with diverse perspectives and intellect and helping the members carve out time to cultivate thinking and the exploration of multiple perspectives help ensure that creative solutions are devised to assist the patients for whom they care. Like team members, leaders, too, must create an environment in which diversity of opinion is encouraged and negative feedback is accepted.

Helping the team to understand how important it is for nurses to know and connect with each other so that they can work together to resolve problems is essential. Inviting members to introduce themselves and tell how much they know and what kinds of experiences they are bringing to the team invites collaboration and a respect for diversity of intellect and perspective. An important aspect of team building is how we attend to the work environment, that is, how team members work together to create fair and respectful communities. Listening to each other helps team members connect with and understand each other, thereby building community between and among them. Fostering relationships and partnerships not only helps to eliminate isolation and competitiveness but also helps staff feel they have someone to turn to for assistance (Kalisch & Begeny, 2005).

Leaders need to be seen as partners who can be relied on to help team members through unfamiliar or difficult situations, addressing questions and concerns and sustaining them through the everyday stresses of working as nurses.

Shared Visions

A shared vision means to have a common purpose. It is the way that people come together and share feelings and thoughts about what they believe their ideals are. Leaders need to find their voices within to know how they can connect others to their ideal vision of the organization (Goleman, Boyatzis, & McKee, 2002). If a leader has a sense of hope, envisioning the future with others is possible, but the key is to have a clear mental picture of the future that is inspiring.

The idea of creating together is exciting for the leader as well as a group of individuals who establish a common purpose. People who feel a collective excitement are attuned to the organization and with one another in a manner creating resonance that builds organizational harmony. When the leader works with individuals on exciting projects and takes less credit, more good ideas arise. Working on projects together often results in more ideas that emanate from the original (Porter-O'Grady & Malloch, 2003). The leader's sense of self in relation to a future has an impact upon cognitive flexibility, willingness to seek variety, and persistence. Positive emotions affect how effectively individuals think, reason, and interact with others. Meaning and purpose often follow positive images of the future that powerfully drive the behavior of the leader and, in turn, the activities of those with whom the leader works. By sharing the vision together, organizational goals can be achieved with meaning and purpose.

Caring for Nurses

Nursing leaders in education and practice need to examine more closely how nurses care for their own selves and how this affects the care of their patients. Performance demands, heavy workloads, and work relationships, as well as personal issues, can create enormous stress.

In 1990, with the passing of a resolution on nursing education by the National League for Nursing, a curriculum revolution began. The curriculum revolution was not about what was taught but about how it was taught. Caring, as a core value in nursing curricula, was a major theme of the curriculum revolution (Tanner, 1999). This revolution supported a change in faculty–student relationships and faculty–faculty relationships to enhance caring practices. Nursing students learn best when they are in trusting relationships with their instructors and see them as partners and co-learners in the educational process (Hayden-Miles, 2002).

Research by Knowlden (1991) indicates that nurse caring is knowledge constructed from personal experiences in nursing education and practice. That is, one learns caring by experiencing caring practices. This can occur only when the climate of the school is supportive of these practices (Beck, 2001). Many healthcare institutions are beginning to understand the importance of showing their concern for their employees by including wellness activities in the workplace (Pender, Murdaugh, & Parsons, 2006). The promotion of health and well-being involves enhancing quality of life. Quality of life is multidimensional and includes health, emotional concerns, environmental factors, and lifestyle (Leddy, 2006). These components of our overall sense of well-being are related to stress and how we cope.

Self-care, which includes physical, emotional, spiritual, and intellectual dimensions, affects how nurses respond to patients and colleagues (Sherwood, 2003) and is therefore essential. Wellness centers can be established both in the workplace environment and in nursing schools to promote health and well-being in keeping with the national initiative of *Healthy People 2010* (US Department of Health and Human Services, 2001). This initiative strives to prevent illness and disease by empowering people to become more responsible for their own health and well-being.

From an ecological perspective (Tiedje, 2001), well-being can be promoted by physical and emotional environments. Places that evoke tranquil and pleasurable experiences can be effective in reducing stress. Creating an environment that promotes professional and personal satisfaction and that emphasizes the importance of a positive state of well-being helps individuals to develop, grow, and learn more productively. Stress reduction rooms can provide an atmosphere where people can go to relax and meditate. Such rooms are being established for people to seek a respite (Klainberg, Ewing, & Ryan, In press). Soothing sounds and an atmosphere of soothing colors provide a way to escape and reduce stress.

Negative behaviors such as overeating and alcohol abuse can be substituted with positive experiences that will result in a healthier lifestyle, provided individuals receive the appropriate guidance. Nutrition programs are being included in some workplace settings, giving employees more opportunity to select healthier foods. Exercise programs to promote fitness and yoga are suggested to improve overall health. Nurses are recognizing the importance of touch therapies such as massage, reiki, and reflexology as important to promoting relaxation, while music can reduce physiologic stress, pain, and anxiety (Guzzetta, 2005).

Various forms of counseling include mentors, friends, faculty, and spiritual advisors. Individuals who need counseling should be referred appropriately by leaders who are sensitive and understanding to their special needs, problems, and issues. Committing to helping each other is a major step to addressing the concerns that affect the well-being of nurses and ultimately patients. If nurses do not care for themselves and each other, their own quality of life will worsen.

A caring leader offers to be a mentor for individuals who need guidance. The leader–mentor assumes the role of developing another individual by providing guidance, support, and training to a junior person or protégé (Stone, 2004). Mentoring is essential for people assuming new positions, such as new graduates, as they attempt to adjust to highly stressful environments. New nurses need not only role models to follow but also to have a person in whom they can confide and trust to discuss their reactions to a new workplace.

Organizational cultures are becoming increasingly diverse, and leaders must be conscious of racial differences, ethnic bias, sexual sensitivity, classism, and religious orientation (Schein, 2004; Walters, 2004). Identifying multicultural barriers such as stereotypes is crucial to prevent conflicts and oppressive behavior. Each generation has a different way of responding in the job setting. Knowing about the generations and their differences can impart understanding and create opportunities for others to share their knowledge and work together (Hu, Herrik, & Hodgin, 2004). Efforts can be made creatively within healthcare settings and campuses to provide nurses and nursing students with opportunities to understand the importance of self-care and the promotion of health and well-being. For example, The Good Work Project (2008) is a multisite effort to identify individuals and institutions that exemplify work that is excellent in quality, socially responsible, and meaningful to its practitioners. It determines how best to increase the incidence of good work in our society. This project explores variables that have sustained nurses (new and experienced) in attempts to perform good work in today's rapidly changing, complex environments. The influences of role models and mentors prove to be invaluable to their professional careers.

A supportive work environment that sustains nurses includes teamwork, cohesiveness, shared values, and expressions of gratitude. Creating a positive culture by supporting nurses and valuing them improves quality of care, morale, and successful recruitment and retention (Miller, 2006). Student nurses need to be taught the value of addressing health and well-being on the college campus. Wellness programs and virtual health and wellness centers can provide places for nursing students to destress and access information for health care (Ewing, Ryan, & Zarco, 2007). Seasoned nurses and nursing educators must help students to understand the significance of caring for themselves by encouraging them to seek excellence in their own health care. Students also need to be taught how to stand up for their needs and request those things that are important to their lives, such as good nutrition and excellent counseling services.

Summary

Changes in health care will affect the future development of the nursing profession in ways that are unknown. The nursing shortage, retirement, and shifts in the population will result in enormous changes that will affect nursing education and practice. Nursing professionals will need to readjust from traditional methods and develop new models of leadership to meet the challenges of a fast-paced, changing, and complex world. New leaders must be resilient and capable of adjusting quickly to contextual changes affected by economics and political systems. Knowing and understanding the culture of systems, forces, and drives enhance the leader's ability to perform, function, and provide guidance to change. With understanding that life is uncertain and filled with surprises, leaders need to be flexible. Maintaining a sense of hope and optimism promotes a sense that shared visions can become possible. By developing authentic, flexible, and emotionally sensitive practices, caring leaders are able to share visions and achieve goals together to promote health and well-being for patients and the nursing profession.

QUESTIONS

1. In Nyberg's model of caring, nursing administrators communicate caring as
   a. something that is required to get work done
   b. an ethic and a philosophy
   c. both appropriate and necessary
   d. None of the above
2. Nyberg believes that caring
   a. relates only to how we treat our patients
   b. is closely related to the technical skills we possess

   c. exists within us and needs to be conveyed to individuals who care for patients

   d. can interfere with the quality of care a nurse gives a patient, if the nurse cares too much

3. According to Watson, healing leadership and caring are believed to be
   a. unimportant as compared with skills and techniques
   b. foundational to nursing
   c. important for one's belief in patient care
   d. part of the code of ethics

4. A professional leader needs to be self-aware because
   a. knowing his or her own feelings allows the leader to be able to assess others
   b. it gives the leader a sense of how to manage the stress of leadership
   c. knowing his or her feelings allows the leader to respond in relationship to others
   d. All of the above

5. A shared vision means to have a common purpose. A good leader will express this by
   a. controlling the environment to prevent staff from providing poor care to patients
   b. helping the staff feel a collective excitement about what they are doing and the creativity related to their work
   c. letting individuals establish their own purpose in relationship to their work
   d. discouraging one single purpose for the group and encouraging total individuality

References

American Association of Critical Care Nurses (AACN). (2004). *AACN's healthwork environment initiative backgrounder.* Retrieved December 1, 2008, from www.aacn.org/WD/Practice/Docs/HWEBBBack grounder.pdf

Beck, C. T. (2001). Caring within nursing education: A metasynthesis. *Journal of Nursing Education, 40*(3), 101–109.

Boyatzis, R., & McKee, A. (2005). *Resonant leadership.* Boston: Harvard Business School Press.

Boykin, A., & Schoenhofer, S. (2001). The role of nursing leadership in creating caring environments in health care delivery systems. *Nursing Administration Quarterly, 25*(3), 1–7.

Carroll, T. L. (2005). Leadership skills and attributes of women and nurse executives: Challenges for the 21st century. *Journal of Nursing Administration Quarterly, 29*(2), 146–153.

Cronin, S., & Harrison, B. (1988). Importance of nurse caring behaviours as perceived by patients after a myocardial infarction. *Heart and Lung, 17*(4), 374–380.

Ewing, B., Ryan, M., & Zarco, E. (2007). A campus wellness program: Accepting the challenge. *Journal of the New York State Nurses Association, 38*(1), 13–16.

Felgen, J. (2003). Caring core value, currency, and commodity…is it time to get tough about "soft"? *Nursing Administration Quarterly, 27*(3), 208–214.

George, B. (2003). *Authentic leadership: Rediscovering the secrets to creating lasting value.* San Francisco: Jossey-Bass.

Goleman, D., Boyatzis, R., & McKee, A. (2002). *Primal leadership: Learning to lead with emotional intelligence.* Boston: Harvard Business School Press.

The Good Work Project. (2008). Retrieved December 30, 2008, from http://www.goodworkproject.org

Guzzetta, C. E. (2005). Music therapy: Hearing the melody of the soul. In B. M. Dossey, L. Keegan, & C. E. Guzzetta (Eds.), *Holistic nursing: A handbook for practice* (4th ed., pp. 619–624). Sudbury, MA: Jones and Bartlett.

Hayden-Miles, M. (2002). Humor in clinical nursing education. *Journal of Nursing Education, 41*(9), 420–424.

Hayden-Miles, M., & Ewing, B. (2007, March). *The meaning of being a novice nurse.* Paper presented at 3rd Annual Leadership Conference: Research and Education: The Gateway to Leadership, Adelphi University.

Hu, J., Herrik, C., & Hodgin, K. (2004). Managing the multigenerational team. *Healthcare Manager, 23*(4), 334–340.

Kalisch, B. J., & Begeny, S. M. (2005). Improving nursing unit teamwork. *Journal of Nursing Administration, 35*(12), 550–556.

Kerfoot, K. (1997). Leadership: The courage to care. *Nursing Economics, 15*(1), 50–51.

Kerfoot, K. (2006). Authentic leadership. *Dermatology Nursing, 18*(6), 595–596.

Klainberg, M., Ewing, B., & Ryan, M. (In press). Stress reduction on a college campus. *Journal of the New York State Nurses Association.*

Knowlden, V. (1991). Nurse caring as constructed knowledge. In R. McNeil & R. Watts (Eds.), *Caring and nursing: Explorations in feminist perspectives* (pp. 201–208). New York: National League for Nursing Press.

Leddy, S. K. (2006). *Health promotion: Mobilizing strengths to enhance health, wellness, and well-being.* Philadelphia: F. A. Davis.

Leininger, M. (1984). *The essence of nursing and health.* Thorofare, NJ: Slack.

Leininger, M. (1988). Leininger's theory of nursing: Cultural care, diversity and universality. *Nursing Science Quarterly, 1*(4), 175–181.

Malloch, K., & Porter-O'Grady, T. (2005). *The quantum leader: Applications for the new world of work.* Sudbury, MA: Jones and Bartlett.

Mayer, R. C., Davis, J. H., & Shoorman, F. D. (1995). An integration model of organizational trust. *Academic Management Review, 20*(3), 709–734.

Miller, J. F. (2006). Opportunities and obstacles for good work in nursing. *Nursing Ethics, 13*(5), 471–487.

Nightingale, F. (1859). *Notes on nursing.* New York: Dover.

Nyberg, J. J. (1998). *A caring approach in nursing administration.* Boulder, CO: University Press of Colorado.

Parsons, M. L., & Cornett, P. (2005). The voice of staff nurses in creating a healthy workplace. *International Journal for Human Caring, 9*(2), 70.

Pender, N. J., Murdaugh, C. L., & Parsons, M. A. (2006). *Health promotion in nursing practice* (5th ed.). Upper Saddle River, NJ: Pearson Prentice Hall.

Porter-O'Grady, T. (1997). Quantum mechanics and the future of healthcare leadership. *Journal of Nursing Administration, 27*(1), 15–20.

Porter-O'Grady, T., & Malloch, K. (2003). *Quantum leadership: A textbook of new leadership.* Sudbury, MA: Jones and Bartlett.

Rafferty, A. M., Ball, J., & Aiken, L. H. (2001). Are teamwork and professional autonomy compatible, and do they result in improved hospital care? *Quality in Health Care, 10*(4), 32–36.

Ray, M. A., Turkel, M. C., & Marino, F. (2002). The transformative process for nursing in workforce redevelopment. *Nursing Administration Quarterly, 26*(2), 1–14.

Rogers, L. G. (2005). Leadership development: Why trust matters: The nurse manager–staff nurse relationship. *Journal of Nursing Administration, 35*(10), 421–423.

Rowley, A. (2007). *Leadership therapy: Inside the mind of Microsoft.* New York: Palgrave Macmillan.

Schein, E. (2004). *Organizational culture and leadership* (3rd ed.). New York: Wiley.

Sherwood, G. (2003). Leadership for a healthy work environment: Caring for the human spirit. *Nurse Leader, 1*(5), 36–40.

Stone, F. (2004). *The mentoring advantage: Creating the next generation of leaders.* Chicago: Dearborn Trade Publishing.

Tanner, C. (1999). Caring as a value in nursing education. *Nursing Outlook, 38*(2), 70–72.

Tiedje, L. B. (2001). Caring for the family in health and illness. In K. S. Lundy & S. Janes (Eds.), *Community health nursing: Caring for the public's health* (pp. 710–721). Sudbury, MA: Jones and Bartlett.

Turkel, M. C. (2001). Struggling to find a balance between caring and economics. *Nursing Administration Quarterly, 26*(1), 67–82.

US Department of Health and Human Services. (2001). *Healthy people 2010*. McLean, VA: International Medical Publishing.

Walters, V. L. (2004). Cultivate corporate culture and diversity. *Nursing Management*, *35*(1), 36–37, 50.

Watson, J. (2006). Caring theory as an ethical guide to administrative and clinical practices. *JONA's Healthcare Law, Ethics, and Regulation*, *3*(8), 87–93.

Wesorick, B. (2002). 21st century leadership challenge: Creating and sustaining healthy, healing work cultures and integrated service at the point of care. *Nursing Administration Quarterly*, *26*(5), 18–32.

Chapter 18

Creating a Culture of Care for the Maturing Nurse

Stephen Paul
Holzemer

OUTLINE

This chapter is intended to assist the novice nurse in forming collaborative relationships in a changing and challenging workforce environment. Not unlike the general population, the people who do the work of nursing are aging. Maturing nurses can be viewed as a significant part of the core of today's nursing profession. The average age of registered nurses (RNs) has increased to 46.8 years in 2004, and of these RNs, 41% were 50 years of age or older (US Department of Health and Human Services, 2007). This is an increase of 33% from 2000. Only 8% of RNs were under the age of 30 in 2004 compared to 25% in 1980 (US Department of Health and Human Services, 2007).

The profession of nursing, until recently, often focused on the care and needs of novice nurses. Nursing is now challenged to shift its gaze to the core of the profession—older (maturing) nurses—as they struggle to maintain their position in the workforce (Buerhaus, Staiger, & Auerbach, 2000, 2009; Hoover, 2007). Another phenomenon has occurred to increase the aging workforce in nursing: as a result of a shift in the economy and a population that is living longer, many are entering the nursing workforce as a change of career or a second career and contribute to the growth in numbers of mature nurses.

Of great concern to the nursing profession and, more importantly, a cause of a possible threat to the public's health is the loss of experienced nurses from the workforce. This is real from a local as well as global perspective. The value of the nurse—demonstrating wisdom unfolding from age and experience—is receiving national attention (Keenan, 2003; Letvak, 2003) and influencing national health policy (Mason, Leavitt, & Chaffee, 2007; Milstead, 2008).

Mature nurses embody the core of professional wisdom developed from their expertise as nurses as well as other lived experiences (Hatcher, 2006). Many of the people who do the work of nursing are aging and, like the rest of the population, can be expected to experience personal health-related challenges as they age. The nursing shortage, compounded by the potential loss of the wise-mature nurse, is the catalyst for examining an approach to create and protect a culture of caring for nursing (and other health professions). The relationship between maturity and professional wisdom is evident in nurses working in the profession as a career over time. Cumulative experience and education provide the nurse with knowledge of how to meet the needs of clients in the healthcare delivery system from a comprehensive perspective. In addition, the mature nurse who is new to the profession may bring professional wisdom from previous work and life experience (McLean & Anema, 2004).

Maturity and Professional Wisdom

From a global perspective, the integrity of many professions and trades is at risk from the loss of their aging members. The graying of the world's population provides an opportunity to rethink the meaning of the potential loss of the richest talent pool in many disciplines (Manpower, 2008). Some professions are slow to reinvent competitive strategies to retain their skilled workforce, while others experience shrinking pools of personnel entering their workforce. The result is a dearth of skilled professionals to perform and oversee the work on which society depends. Government regulation of nursing practice becomes increasingly complex as the nursing shortage expands (Loversidge, 2008).

Examination of the phenomenon of the maturing of the nursing workforce is not related to any form of discrimination against people who are aging. Avoiding ageism in the discussion of the maturing nursing workforce should be a paramount consideration. The concepts of aging and maturing used in this discussion are viewed as adjuncts in comprehending the process of moving nursing and other health-related professions to full professional potential. The potential of creating a reality where all age cohorts of nurses participate fully in the process of their mission—maintaining the public's health—is a concern for the whole profession (Cohen, 2006; Rosenfeld, 2007).

Retaining older, mature nurses in the workforce is not, in itself, a solution to the overall nursing shortage. Assisting older nurses to "hang on" or "work a few more years" seemingly will only stall the crisis at hand—not enough nurses committed to the work of nursing. The nursing profession, at times, does not seem to meet the needs of at least some of the experienced nurses considering retirement from the profession. Nursing does not have a well-articulated plan for creating and protecting a culture of care to keep mature nurses in the workforce until they are ready to leave it. Leadership is emerging, however, among nurse executives in magnet institutions and nurse executives who use the philosophy of nurturing the workforce to keep it productive (Mensik, 2007; Ulrich, Buerhaus, Donelan, Norman, & Dittus, 2007).

The Mature Nurse as Care Provider, Educator, Researcher

Each state Nurse Practice Act and the ethical principles of the *Code of Ethics for Nurses* (American Nurses Association, 2001) provide guidance on how the nursing workforce can protect the public. The maturing nurse must be able to physically and emotionally accomplish the art and science of nursing, at the bedside, in the classroom, and in the research environment. Threats to providing comprehensive nursing care in these settings may surface from problems in the nurses' physical and/or psychosocial integrity (Krowchuk & Letvak, 2005; Kovner, Brewer, Cheng, & Djukic, 2007).

Although experienced nurses are not unsafe to practice solely because of their age, increasing attention is being given to the meaning of nurse competency and safety for all practitioners (Bolton & Moritz, 2007; Henneman & Gawlinski, 2004). Increasing attention is being focused on environments that promote safety for the provider and recipient of care (National Council of State Boards of Nursing, 2005) before these environments drive nurses from the profession (Bingham, 2002).

Physical and Psychosocial Integrity of the Mature Nurse

Nurses experience physical and psychosocial health challenges throughout their professional lives. These mirror the physical and psychosocial health challenges to integrity of all aging persons (Bennett & Flaherty-Robb, 2003). Of particular concern are health challenges that occur in professions and occupations where stress and other work variables may promote or support addictive behaviors and make reporting them difficult (Badzek, Mitchell, Marra, & Bower, 1998; Beckstead, 2002). Addictions to alcohol and other nonprescribed drugs or misuse of these and prescribed medications are concerns that need to be illuminated. Addiction to food, sexual behavior, and computer use and debilitating conditions such as anxiety and depression escort many nurses into retirement, voluntary or mandated. A systematic plan on how to better support nurses using a supportive and confidential approach needs to be developed. Nursing's attempts to address the need for a hope-based, recovery-focused approach to care for nurses has been under consideration for decades (Jefferson & Ensor, 1982; McGee, 2000; Menzies & Taca, 2008).

The psychosocial integrity of the mature nurse may be less understood in part because of diagnostic stigma. Major threats to psychosocial integrity of the aging population, and therefore the mature nurse, include anxiety, depression, addiction, and other mental illnesses. It is thought that nurses are approximately at the same risk for these illnesses as the general population (Handley & Ward-Smith, 2005; Kenna & Lewis, 2008; Trinkoff & Storr, 1998). Nurses may, however, underreport or deny these problems because of concerns with seeking treatment while maintaining employment (Kenna & Lewis, 2008). It is anticipated that the threats to psychosocial integrity of the mature nurse may be better understood by the increase in research by nurses in the area (Stevenson & Sommers, 2005; Walton-Moss & Campbell, 2002).

Use of technology with intent to improve the physical and psychosocial environment of work has been documented and implemented (Bolton & Moritz, 2007). The need to promote the physical integrity of the mature nurse is evident in the development of ergonomically positive changes in the physical nature of how nursing care is provided. Implementation of "lift teams" and providing nurses with flexible schedules (consecutive hours and days worked) are maximizing the contribution of nurses wanting to remain part of the healthcare team. Addressing physical problems at the work site can maximize the contribution of mature nurses who experience conditions and diseases associated with aging (Hatcher, 2006).

Taking Action: Application of the Alliance for Health Model to Support the Physical and Psychosocial Integrity of the Mature Nurse

Nurses can demonstrate self-advocacy by actively creating a later-in-career scenario that maximizes potential and minimizes nonsupportive employment situations. Nurses can participate in the critical assessment activities that should be strategic in keeping them viable in the workforce. The Alliance for Health model, originally created for general community assessment (Holzemer & Arnold, 1998), can be applied by nurses to support their self-advocacy efforts as they mature. Use of the Alliance for Health model provides insight into creating and protecting a culture of caring for nursing (and other health disciplines).

The Alliance for Health model provides structure to assess five important areas of concern that may be helpful for nurses to consider as they direct their employment future. The areas of concern are: (1) community-based needs, (2) systems of care management, (3) influences on resource allocation decisions, (4) validation of services by the client, and (5) expertise of the interdisciplinary team. Each of the five areas of concern is discussed in this chapter as it relates to the mature nurse population. Figure 18-1 provides a representation of the components of the model. The Alliance for Health model provides a structure for all nurses working in a nursing and/or (other) healthcare system to assess the needs of nurses in the workforce. The language of the model is adapted to this specific goal of creating and protecting a culture of caring for the maturing nurse.

Figure 18-1 Alliance for Health Model—Creating and Protecting a Culture of Care for All Nurses

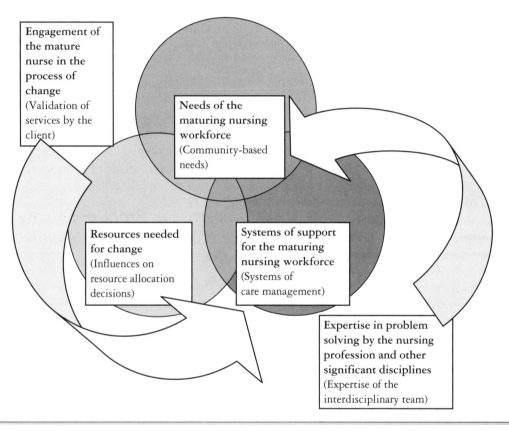

Source: Author

Needs of the Maturing Nursing Workforce (Community-Based Needs)

The community-based needs component focuses on the needs of the mature nurse. As previously identified, the mature nurse has needs for physiologic and psychosocial integrity. Nurses need to share their particular needs (physical and psychosocial) and be willing to participate in exploring ways, such as by adapting the work environment, that will better meet their needs. Younger nurses can play a strategic role in this process by supporting their peers and improving the work environment for their peers, and themselves, as they mature.

Systems of Support for the Maturing Nursing Workforce (Systems of Care Management)

Systems of care management include the systems in place to support the mature nurse and the development of a culture of caring. These could include formal educational and support service programs for retention of nurses in the workforce and for the reentry of nurses returning to the workforce. The various needs identified by all nurses working in the process of creating systems of support need to be evaluated for effectiveness. To date, systems of support for nurses have been identified and reflect ergonomic, financial (current and retirement compensation), educational, and other physical and psychosocial needs (Cohen, 2006; Keenan, 2003).

Resources Needed for Change (Influences on Resource Allocation Decisions)

Nurses need to influence resource allocation decisions, which include those that provide the resources needed for creating and protecting a culture of care. The cost to the institution and the community of losing the mature and wise nurse has been studied (Hatcher, 2006; Keenan, 2003). Institutions need to invest in nursing's future today for the mature nurse and tomorrow for the next generation of nurses just entering the workforce. Resources are needed to evaluate and support the competence of nurses and keep the nursing workforce from eroding to levels unsafe to provide necessary care to the public (National Council of State Boards of Nursing, 2005).

Engagement of the Mature Nurse in the Process of Change (Validation of Services by the Client)

The mature nurse needs to validate services provided to create and protect a culture of care. Maturing or aging nurses need to learn to value realistic employment options and, for some, accept limitations in their scope of work. As with all nurses, these nurses cannot be expected to work in environments that are not supportive of meeting their needs. Collective action is needed by nurses to secure a safe environment in which to work (Spetz, 2008).

Expertise in Problem Solving by the Nursing Profession and Other Significant Disciplines (Expertise of the Interdisciplinary Team)

The interdisciplinary team in this situation is made up of administrators, human resource professionals, mature nurses, and others who possess the expertise to create and protect a culture of care. Mature and age-sympathetic nurses and other providers need to bring their lived experience to the table to participate in resolving the current workforce dilemma.

Solutions to the Challenge of Creating and Protecting a Culture of Caring

Exploring a solution to the challenge of creating and protecting a culture of caring should be grounded in the principles of project management. A formal project management approach provides the opportunity to secure the essential human and material resources for success. A project management venue commits the experts in nursing, medicine, human resource management, and corporate administration to a process of change fostering accountability. Project management explicates the relationship between the time necessary to achieve outcomes with the necessary fiscal resources to complete the project. Project management secures administrative support by connecting projects to the goals and philosophy of the sponsoring institution (Meredith & Mantel, 2006).

There are five components in this proposed solution to the challenge of creating and protecting a culture of caring for the nursing profession. This approach extends beyond a focus on the current group of maturing nurses in that the fundamental change creates a support network for all nurses. The components are: (1) establishing institutional support for and commitment to creating and protecting a culture of caring (for all nurses), (2) creating and protecting role redesign for the institution and the community, (3) implementing requisite aesthetic and environmental changes needed to increase productivity, (4) stabilizing nurses in work and recruiting and reorienting nurses returning to work, and (5) fostering the ongoing relationship between nurses and a program to monitor the creation and protection of a culture of care for nurses. Figure 18-2 provides a visual representation of these components.

Institutional Support and Commitment to Create and Protect a Culture of Caring

Institutional support and commitment to create and protect a culture of caring are critical to this process. Without institutional support and

commitment, no change is likely to occur. There are five aspects of institutional support and commitment (see Figure 18-3):

- Recognizing a skill set—emotional and physical fitness for work
- Aesthetics and quality of the work environment
- Human resource practices
- Collegial support within and outside of the institution
- Vision and action by the nurse executive team

Each is discussed in the following subsections.

RECOGNIZING A SKILL SET: EMOTIONAL AND PHYSICAL FITNESS FOR WORK

Currently used performance evaluations identify the skill set needed by nurses in their work. Nurses should be able to identify how changes in the emotional and physical expectations of their work might be improved. Nurses should be engaged in the conversation about how technology, for example, might improve their ability to engage in the ongoing safe practice of nursing, including finding a niche of less taxing emotional and physical work, if that is necessary.

AESTHETICS AND QUALITY OF THE WORK ENVIRONMENT

Asking nurses to express concerns with the aesthetics and quality of the work environment may provide insight into making the work experience more productive. Standard ergonomic improvements as well as specific (and prudent) changes in the work environment for individuals or groups of nurses need consideration.

HUMAN RESOURCE PRACTICES

Making modifications in work requirements to assist the mature nurse in completing required

Figure 18-2 Exploring a Solution to the Challenge of Creating and Protecting a Culture of Caring

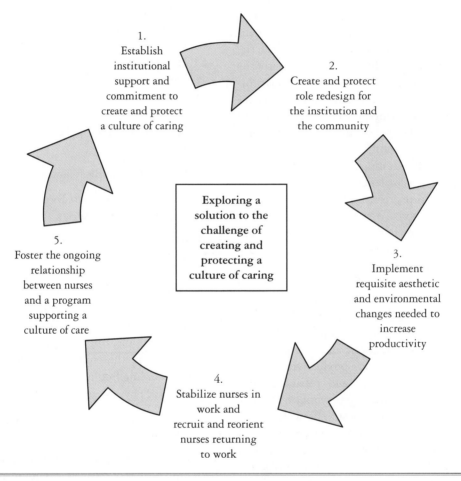

1.
Establish
institutional
support and
commitment to
create and protect
a culture of caring

2.
Create and protect
role redesign for
the institution and
the community

**Exploring a
solution to the
challenge of
creating and
protecting a
culture of caring**

5.
Foster the ongoing
relationship
between nurses
and a program
supporting a
culture of care

3.
Implement
requisite aesthetic
and environmental
changes needed to
increase
productivity

4.
Stabilize nurses in
work and
recruit and reorient
nurses returning
to work

Source: Author

activities should be discussed. Variations in total work hours or consecutive days worked may be components in innovative work solutions. Release time or day care for aging relatives, for example, along with day care for children, are age-appropriate solutions. Human resource policies and procedures need to be evaluated for how they meet the needs of maturing nurses.

These include improvement of the use of technology to create a work environment that reduces unnecessary physical demands.

COLLEGIAL SUPPORT WITHIN AND OUTSIDE OF THE INSTITUTION

The potential for shifting employment responsibilities may allow for the mature nurse to

Figure 18-3 Institutional Support to Create and Protect a Culture of Caring for All Nurses

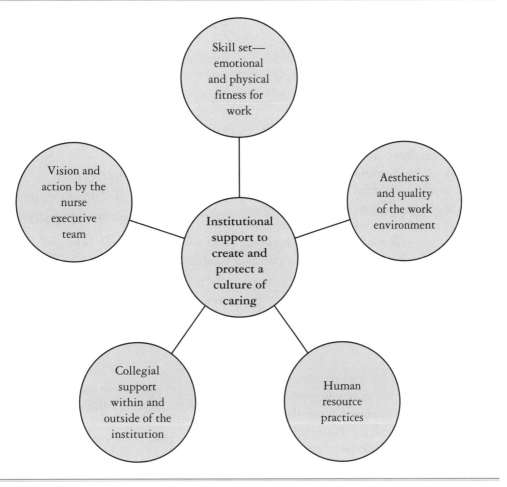

Source: Author

move into more teaching, mentoring, and coaching-focused roles and responsibilities. Because these roles are so critical to the functioning of the nursing department, relationships with schools of nursing could be established or broadened to augment the credentialing of these nurses for a change in their practice. Certification and degree programs on site can assist with the process of legitimizing role change among nurses involved in role redesign.

VISION AND ACTION BY THE NURSE EXECUTIVE TEAM

The ongoing vision and action by the nurse executive team, in one or a group of cooperating institutions, is paramount in developing and sustaining institutional support and commitment to create and protect a culture of caring. The nurse executive team needs to play a central role in securing a preferred future for the nursing profession at work.

Creating and Protecting Role Redesign for the Institution and the Community

Creating and protecting role redesign for the institution and the community move the activity of meeting the needs of mature nurses into the long-range goals of the institution. Preparing for role redesign supports a natural evolution of maximizing the potential of nurses. The crisis response of "finding a place for nurses to work" is replaced by the grooming of nurses for the best fit between their needs and the needs of the organization.

Implementing Requisite Aesthetic and Environmental Changes Needed to Increase Productivity

Implementing requisite aesthetic and environmental changes needed to increase productivity can hardly be argued to be a nonessential component of change. As previously identified, involving nurses in the development and monitoring of the benefits of aesthetic and environmental changes is critical. Certainly, the maturing workforce has special needs previously not identified because of the increasing numbers of nurses in this category.

Stabilizing Nurses in Work and Recruiting and Reorienting Nurses Returning to Work

Improving the work experience of nurses currently working and the activities of recruiting and reorienting nurses returning to work require special attention. Demonstrating institutional commitment to meeting the needs of the mature nurse working and returning to work can be supported by a broad educational plan. Lessons learned from work redesign for the employed nurse can be applied to the nurse returning to work. A comprehensive plan might improve the retention of returning nurses, fostering a dedication to the institution that is willing to develop the expertise of the nurses working in the institution.

Fostering the Ongoing Relationship Between Nurses and a Program to Monitor the Creation and Protection of a Culture of Caring for Nurses

The ongoing fostering of the relationship between nurses and a program to monitor the creation and protection of a culture of caring for nurses can have important consequences for stabilizing the nursing workforce. Ongoing and future problems could be more quickly identified and resolved by using the personnel and material resources at hand. A systematic search for new, previously untapped resources could eliminate the "crisis approach" often used in meeting nursing's employment needs.

Summary

Wisdom in the nursing profession can be maintained, in part, by creating and protecting a culture of caring for the maturing nurse. This culture of caring, to succeed, must be constructed by all nurses and other participants in healthcare delivery. Special needs of the mature nurse care provider, educator, and researcher need to be identified and embraced to create and protect a culture of caring for the discipline. Special concerns for the physical and psychosocial integrity of the mature nurse, including those holding stigma and involving less than compassionate understanding, need to be examined in detail.

The use of the Alliance for Health model provides one method to direct assessment in five areas. These areas of concern, including community-based needs, systems of care management, influences on resource allocation decisions, validation of services by the client, and expertise of the interdisciplinary team, may be helpful for nurses to consider as they direct their future. The Alliance for Health model identifies issues that impact the problems of improving the work experience of the mature nurse.

Institutions that wish to engage in the process of problem solving as it relates to the work experience of the mature nurse need to make the decision to formalize the problem-solving process using the principles of project management. Project management ties intended outcomes to a time line and financial plan to maximize success, while directly relating problems to corporate goals and philosophy.

Components of creating one solution for addressing this dilemma include establishing institutional support and commitment to create and protect a culture of caring (for all nurses), creating and protecting role redesign, implementing requisite aesthetic and environmental changes, stabilizing nurses in work and recruiting and reorienting nurses returning to work, and fostering the ongoing relationship between nurses and a program to monitor the creation and protection of a culture of caring for nurses. Using a broad problem-solving approach involving key players and centering the project in the nurse executive team provides hope for meeting the needs of the mature nurse remaining in the workforce.

QUESTIONS

1. A trend in nursing that reflects that of society is that
   a. maturing nurses are not viewed as a part of today's nursing profession
   b. the general population is aging and working nurses are aging
   c. maturing nurses have no role in today's high-tech profession
   d. we revere the younger population and nurses reflect this

2. To utilize the input of maturing nurses, the profession should
   a. create and protect a culture of caring and support for the maturing nurse
   b. upon a nurse's retirement, interview the nurses for his or her expertise
   c. provide each maturing nurse someone with whom to consult
   d. test the maturing nurse for competency

3. Maturing nurses should be included as part of an interdisciplinary team to
   a. use their lived experiences and history to help in resolving current workforce dilemmas
   b. maintain leadership of the team

   c. delegate workload to the team

   d. provide their lived experiences as a basis for care, using advanced technology

4. The maturing nursing population provides an important role in health care today. Loss of the mature nurse would create a void. Therefore, institutions should

   a. create an environment of caring and support for the mature nurse, which will benefit future generations of nurses entering the workforce

   b. include a financial bonus for older nurses who remain in the workforce

   c. decrease hiring new nurses and invest in the mature nurse workforce

   d. create an environment in which the new nurses are hired to work with mature nurses and pick up most of their workload

5. The nurse manager of an orthopedic unit is aware that many of the nurses working on the unit are maturing. Patients on the unit often need lifting, and their care requires enormous amounts of physical hardiness and endurance. Which of the following solutions, which will affect the maturing nurses as well as all the nurses on the unit, will best solve the problem?

   a. The nurse manager requests that older nurses be transferred to a less strenuous floor in the hospital and hires all young nurses to provide care for the patients in this unit.

   b. The nurse manager requests funds from the institution to implement a "lift team" that will work with all nurses to help with the physical care they need to provide to patients.

   c. The nurse manager provides assistance to all maturing nurses in the provision of care.

   d. The nurse manager requires maturing nurses to care only for nonstrenuous cases.

References

American Nurses Association. (2001). *Code of ethics for nurses with interpretive statements*. Washington, DC: Author.

Badzek, L. A., Mitchell, K., Marra, S. E., & Bower, M. M. (1998). Administrative ethics and confidentiality/privacy issues. *Online Journal of Issues in Nursing*. Retrieved December 22, 2008, from http://www.nursingworld.org/MainMenuCategories/ANAMarketplace/ANAPeriodicals/OJIN/TableofContents/Vol31998/No3Dec1998/PrivacyIssues.aspx

Beckstead, J. W. (2002). Modeling attitudinal antecedents of nurses' decisions to report impaired colleagues. *Western Journal of Nursing Research*, *24*(5), 537–551.

Bennett, J. A., & Flaherty-Robb, M. K. (2003). Issues affecting the health of older citizens: The challenge. *Online Journal of Issues in Nursing*. Retrieved December 4, 2008, from http://www.ncbi.nlm.nih.gov/pubmed/12795628

Bingham, R. (2002). Leaving nursing. *Health Affairs*, *21*(1), 211–217.

Bolton, L. B., & Moritz, P. (2007). Using technology to mitigate the nursing shortage. In D. J. Mason, J. K. Leavitt, & M. W. Chaffee (Eds.), *Policy and politics in nursing and health care* (5th ed., pp. 540–549). St. Louis: Saunders.

Buerhaus, P. I., Staiger, D. O., & Auerbach, D. I. (2000). Implications of an aging registered nurse workforce. *Journal of the American Medical Association.* Retrieved April 16, 2008, from http://jama. ama-assn.org/cgi/content/full/283/22/2948

Buerhaus, P. I., Staiger, D. O., & Auerbach, D. I. (2009). *The future of the nursing workforce in the United States: Data, trends, and implications.* Sudbury, MA: Jones and Bartlett.

Cohen, J. D. (2006). The aging nursing workforce: How to retain experienced nurses. *Journal of Healthcare Management, 51*(4), 233–245.

Handley, S. M., & Ward-Smith, P. (2005). Alcohol misuse, abuse, and addiction in young and middle adulthood. *Annual Review of Nursing Research, 23,* 213–244.

Hatcher, B. (Ed.). (2006). *Wisdom at work: The importance of the older and experienced nurse in the workforce.* Princeton, NJ: Robert Wood Johnson Foundation.

Henneman, E. A., & Gawlinski, A. (2004). A "near-miss" model for describing the nurse's role in the recovery of medical errors. *Journal of Professional Nursing, 20*(3), 196–201.

Holzemer, S. P., & Arnold, J. (1998). Alliance for health: A model for community health assessment. In M. Klainberg, S. Holzemer, M. Leonard, & J. Arnold (Eds.), *Community health nursing: An alliance for health* (pp. 79–93). New York: McGraw-Hill.

Hoover, K. W. (2007). The nursing workforce: Supply and demand. In D. J. Mason, J. K. Leavitt, & M. W. Chaffee (Eds.), *Policy and politics in nursing and health care* (5th ed., pp. 509–518). St. Louis: Saunders.

Jefferson, L. V., & Ensor, B. E. (1982). Help for the helper: Confronting a chemically-impaired colleague. *American Journal of Nursing, 82*(4), 573–577.

Keenan, P. (2003, April). *The nursing workforce shortage: Causes, consequences, proposed solutions.* New York: Commonwealth Fund.

Kenna, G. A., & Lewis, D. C. (2008). Risk factors for alcohol and other drug use by healthcare professionals. *Substance Abuse Treatment, Prevention, and Policy, 3*(3). Retrieved May 6, 2008, from http://www.substanceabusepolicy.com/content/3/1/3

Kovner, C. T., Brewer, C. S., Cheng, Y., & Djukic, M. (2007). Work attitudes of older RNs. *Policy, Politics, & Nursing Practice, 8*(2), 107–119.

Krowchuk, H. V., & Letvak, S. A. (2005). Second opinion: Should a staff nurse's age be a consideration in making patient and shift assignments? *American Journal of Maternal/Child Nursing, 30*(2), 84.

Letvak, S. (2003). The experience of being an older staff nurse. *Western Journal of Nursing Research, 25*(1), 45–56.

Loversidge, J. M. (2008). Government regulation: Parallel and powerful. In J. A. Milstead (Ed.), *Health policy and politics: A nurse's guide.* Sudbury, MA: Jones and Bartlett.

Manpower, Inc. (2008). *Confronting the talent crunch: 2008.* Milwaukee, WI: Author.

Mason, D. J., Leavitt, J. K., & Chaffee, M. W. (Eds.). (2007). *Policy and politics in nursing and health care* (5th ed.). St. Louis, MO: Saunders.

McGee, E. M. (2000). Alcoholics Anonymous and nursing: Lessons in holism and spiritual care. *Journal of Holistic Nursing, 18*(1), 11–26.

McLean, T., & Anema, M. (2004). Reduce the nursing shortage: Help inactive nurses return to work. *Journal of Continuing Education in Nursing, 35*(4), 211–215.

Mensik, J. S. (2007). The essentials of magnetism for home health. *Journal of Nursing Administration, 37*(5), 230–234.

Menzies, P., & Taca, A. C. (2008). New hope for treating addictions in health care professionals. *Missouri Medicine, 105*(1), 25–26.

Meredith, J. R., & Mantel, S. J. (2006). *Project management: A managerial approach* (6th ed.). Hoboken, NJ: Wiley.

Milstead, J. A. (Ed.). (2008). *Health policy and politics: A nurse's guide.* Sudbury, MA: Jones and Bartlett.

National Council of State Boards of Nursing. (2005). Continued competence concept paper: Meeting the ongoing challenge of continued competence. Chicago: Author.

Rosenfeld, P. (2007). Workplace practices for retaining older hospital nurses: Implications from a study of nurses with eldercare responsibilities. *Policy, Politics, & Nursing Practice, 8*(2), 120–129.

Spetz, J. (2008). Nurse satisfaction and the implementation of minimum nurse staffing regulations. *Policy, Politics, & Nursing Practice, 9*(1), 15–21.

Stevenson, J. S., & Sommers, M. S. (2005). The case for alcohol research as a focus of study by nurse researchers. *Annual Review of Nursing Research, 23,* 3–26.

Trinkoff, A. M., & Storr, C. L. (1998). Substance use among nurses: Differences between specialties. *American Journal of Public Health, 88*(4), 581–585.

Ulrich, B. T., Buerhaus, P. I., Donelan, K., Norman, L., & Dittus, R. (2007). Magnet status and registered nurse views of the work environment and nursing as a career. *Journal of Nursing Administration*, *37*(5), 212–220.

US Department of Health and Human Services. (2007, February 20). Nursing workforce expands as average age of RNs increases, HRSA survey finds. HRSA News. Retrieved July 16, 2008, from http://newsroom.hrsa.gov/releases/2007/nursing-survey.htm

Walton-Moss, B. J., & Campbell, J. C. (2002). Intimate partner violence: Implications for nursing. *Online Journal of Issues in Nursing*, *7*(1). Retrieved December 22, 2008, from http://www.nursingworld.org/MainMenuCategories/ANAMarketplace/ANA Periodicals/OJIN/TableofContents/Volume72002/No1Jan2002/IntimatePartnerViolence.aspx

Spiritual Leadership in Nursing: Leading With "Spirit" in a Changing Healthcare Environment

Sharon R. Kowalchuk

OUTLINE

From the beginning in Nightingale's time, nurses and nursing theorists have been discussing the creation of an environment in which healing occurs. An environment in which the nurse cares for the unique human being: body, mind, emotion, and spirit (Erickson, Tomlin, & Swain, 1983)—the whole person who is unique and greater than the sum of his parts (Rogers,

1980). This whole person is a coherent being who continually strives to make sense of his world (Riehl-Sisca & Roy, 1980). Nurses recognize the power within the patient to enable higher levels of consciousness (Neuman, 1982). According to Watson (2005), this valued person is cared for, respected, nurtured, understood, and assisted toward health through unity and harmony in the mind, body, and soul (Marriner-Tomey, 1989).

Nursing theories have evolved to describe what we as nurses do as caring persons for others. Yet, we have not given as much attention to the "caring for" our followers and ourselves as healthcare leaders. Do we see nurses in the same way we describe our patients? Do we give the same sacred care to each individual nurse and team member? Do we honor the uniqueness of each co-worker? Do we care for, respect, and enable each other to reach a higher level of consciousness? Do we turn to the other person to find out who he or she is as a unique individual in *mind*, *body*, and *spirit*?

Why Do Nurses Avoid Addressing the "Spirit" in Each Other?

As a discipline, nursing has roots in spiritual and religious institutions. In our quest to define nursing as a profession and separate nursing from traditional religious caregiver roles, we have deemphasized the spiritual realm, that is, until recently. A more obvious reason is the level of discomfort most people feel talking about things of the spirit. *Spirit* has a religious connotation and not a scientific one. Perhaps we fear that spirituality may be viewed by others as weakness, not strength, as a leadership trait. In Joint Commission recommendations, the one

common area of weakness consistently identified is "spiritual assessment." This is one of the deficiencies most difficult to correct and one of the assessment skills most difficult to teach. Many confuse the term *spiritual* with religion or view it as too personal to discuss or to put into words on an assessment.

Addressing This "Spirit" as Leaders in Nursing

Nurse leaders need to begin by defining the terms *religion*, *spirituality*, and *spirit*. *Religion* and *spirituality* can be synonymous in some people's minds and different in others' perception. The difference is in the eye of the beholder. Usually, *religion* is understood to refer to the more formalized institutions of faith, whereas *spirituality* denotes a way of being, an attitude toward life. Hence, some who regard themselves as spiritual may not align themselves with any particular form of religion. In a broader sense, spirituality is more personal, less dogmatic, and more encompassing than the faiths of established religions (Visser, 2005).

Spirituality refers to a search for meaning that transcends material well-being and focuses on basic, deep-rooted human values and a relationship with a universal source of power or divinity. Spirituality can be defined as the expression of the active and vital connection to an invisible force, power, or core value deep within the self; this definition of spirituality opens the concept to all individuals in the workplace.

What Defines the Spiritual Leader?

The spiritual leader has a deep sense of purpose and respect for the receivers of care and for the individuals who contribute to this caregiving paradigm. This leader looks to establish for self and followers meaning and value in the work to be done. The leader nourishes the spirit, creativity, and connection to that which is sacred in each person.

The spiritual leader is visionary and has the ability to *see* the invisible, "the spirit," in each individual and utilize this powerful force to build group cohesion and accomplish organizational goals. This leader is not new but newly recognized in the business literature and referred to as a "spiritual" or core values leader. Other descriptors are *visionary*, *edgewalker*, *bridge-builder* (Neal, 2006).

Have You Met a Spiritual Nurse Leader?

In nursing, we have all at one time met this type of leader. Usually, the leader was a head nurse who had a deep sense of respect for each employee. This nurse treated all fairly and as unique human beings. Most of all, this nurse leader had a deep respect for the patient, commitment to the patient's care, and a clearly communicated vision of how that care was to be rendered. This nurse was decisive and addressed with immediacy any deviation from her vision. We rallied around this nurse as a team and came to take on this nurse leader's values. This nurse leader influenced us. Why? Because this nurse lead by example, demonstrated results, and believed in developing us as people and showed respect for our personhood (Maxwell & Dornan, 1997).

Spirituality operates in several realms:

1. *Cognitive*: A person's search for meaning, purpose, truth
2. *Emotional*: Feelings of love, hope, connectedness, inner peace, comfort, support

3. *Behavioral*: How we manifest our beliefs and inner spiritual state through relationships, connections with others, our community, nature, and a greater power (Anandarajah & Hight, 2001)

Spiritual leaders recognize and respond to these cognitive, emotional, and behavioral expressions. They risk entering another's world, risk allowing another into theirs, are fully present in the moment, and have a deep sense of meaning and valuing clearly established.

One such nursing leader today is Marie Anker. In Box 19-1 you can read how Marie's humble background, her growth and development in nursing, and her eventual leadership of a multi-hospital system illustrate the journey of a spiritual leader.

Today's Healthcare Workplace Demands a New Style of Leadership

Top-down leadership comes naturally to most people and is congruent with the medical model and the structure of healthcare organizations in general. This is the model used by most leaders in healthcare organizations today. In this model, abuses of authority over delegation, lack of listening, dictatorial decision making, inability to let go or give credit where credit is due, and withholding of information occur. This style is no longer able to motivate workers toward greater productivity.

Recent changes in the global climate, terrorism, lack of job security, and distrust of the organization have forced workers to look inside rather than outside for the answers. Workers want to know that what they are doing has *value and meaning*. Businesses trying to compete have been forced to look for new ways to enhance

---

Box 19-1 A Memoir

Marie Anker

My grandparents were immigrants from very different cultures, backgrounds, and experiences. My father's parents arrived through Ellis Island as young adults with their respective families from Avellino and San Benvenuto, Italy, in the early 1900s. They met and married in the United States. My grandma shared that her family had wanted her to have an arranged marriage, as was done for her other older siblings. She resisted and married the man she chose at the tender age of 18.

Ben and Teresa eventually raised five children, four sons and a daughter. They were very family oriented. My recollections of visits as a child included everyone gathered around the dining room table, enjoying a five-course meal and lively, loud discussion related to daily life, politics, work, and current events. Grandchildren ran and played, and the men in the family provided music with their mandolins.

Devoted, loving, and caring, my grandparents lived to enjoy 11 grandchildren and 49 years of marriage. My grandfather believed in education and was very hard working, having mastered a variety of trades to provide for his family.

My mother's mother wanted to come to America as a young girl. Born in Germany, Mary was one of six siblings. To honor her request, her oldest sister, Matilde, was sent to accompany her. They were sponsored by an uncle in New Jersey. Reportedly, Mary was young and adventurous. Tilla, her older sister, was serious, loyal, and not interested in leaving her family or her homeland. Living in New York City during the war was very difficult with family at home. She first returned to Germany to see her family at age 74.

Mary and Ludwig met and married in New York. My grandmother Mary lived in Brooklyn and had two children. Ludwig, her husband, was a sailor before arriving in New York. He had sailed with Count Van Luckner in his teen years. In New York City, he worked as a painter. In 1930, he fell from a scaffold while working on an apartment building on 86th Street in Manhattan. Having no medical insurance, he did not seek medical care and died a few days later from a fractured skull at the age of 34. At the time, my mom was two years old and her brother an infant.

My mom was raised by her aunt and uncle. They moved between Brooklyn, Queens, and the Bronx, where she attended Walton High School. One night after the end of World War II, she was at a dance in Brooklyn with her friends, and she met my dad. When he left, he wrote her phone number on a matchbook. She never expected to hear from him, but he surprised her when he called and asked her for a date. They were married within the year and moved to the Bronx. Because my mom was not Catholic, they were not permitted to marry in the church. Their ceremony was held in the rectory.

My dad loved learning; he had an extensive vocabulary. As the oldest of five, he did not complete Evader Childs High School, because he worked with his father in their butcher store during the Depression. Working hard, they bartered services with customers, providing meat for a teacher's family in return for English lessons for the children. Work in the butcher business was physically taxing with long hours in cold refrigerators. When he was home, he would rest or we would visit his parents or go for a ride in the country.

Education was an important family value. My parents sacrificed to have all of their children attend Catholic elementary school. It happened to be in an Italian area in the Bronx. It wasn't until years later that I realized that the reason we were treated differently by many of our classmates was our blended heritage. Most of the students were solely Italian.

At the age of 13, I met Father Soraci. He was an Italian priest assigned to Santa Maria. In life, certain people stand out in the development of who we become. I am thankful to him for his support, guidance, and direction. I joined the Junior Sodality of Our Lady and began to volunteer. My first experience was at Providence Rest Home in the Bronx. Every week, I would walk there from Westchester Square. As a volunteer, I would read to the seniors or help transport them to and from the dining room. This experience piqued my interest in service.

In eighth grade, I was accepted into Cardinal Spellman High School. At the time, it was a new archdiocesan program that provided tuition support for the students who were accepted. As an average student, I remember the eighth-grade class president challenging me as to how I was accepted and

she wasn't. Grammar school was a very painful interpersonal experience.

You could get lost at Spellman. Although coed, the boys were on one side of the building and the girls on the other side. The school was very competitive. The scholastic requirements were rigid. Regents exams were required with each course, and it was expected that you would pass the course as well as the Regents. I graduated with an academic and a Regents' diploma. Speaking with my counselor prior to graduation, I shared that I was interested in nursing. She informed me that I would never be accepted into a nursing program.

At home, my dad did not want me to become a nurse. Whatever his experience was during the war, he did not think highly of the work of nurses. So, what did I do? During Easter vacation, I discovered that Westchester Square Hospital offered a nurse aide training program, so I applied, was accepted, attended, and completed the program. The hospital was around the corner from my house, so I was able to work weekends, summers, and days off. That was the best experience of all. I was able to work under the supervision of the deputy director and the RNs on the various units. By working with a variety of patients and staff, I was able to expand my knowledge and skills and build confidence in my interpersonal interactions with everyone I came in contact with.

Upon graduation from high school, I applied for various nursing programs. I shared with my dad that, even as an unlicensed driver at the time, I planned to buy a car and drive to Rockland County every day to attend school. You can imagine his response. So, when I was accepted to Westchester School of Nursing in Valhalla, my parents supported my application. The entire tuition was less than $400 for the three years. This included books, uniforms, and housing. Finances were tight, because I had three siblings still at home in elementary and high school.

I worked hard and enjoyed my nursing education at Westchester. As a diploma school, we were expected to become knowledgeable and perform all clinical nursing skills prior to graduation. Our records were meticulously maintained by the director, who was aware of the number of hours spent by each individual student on each clinical competency.

Upon graduation, I returned to the Bronx and accepted an offer of employment at Einstein Hospital. Serendipitously, I began studying at Lehman College in the evening for credits toward my BSN. I married during this time and accepted a new position in a methadone inpatient detox unit. This position had a flexible schedule, which allowed me to continue my education. In the 1970s, Pace was one of the only educational programs that offered flexibility for working RNs, allowing them to advance their education. Classes were offered in the evenings and on weekends. In 1977, my friend Betsy and I completed our BSNs. A few years earlier, I initiated employment at Jacobi Medical Center. Having three years of RN experience, Ms. Kaufman assigned me to the Surgical ICU Burn Unit. I will always remember the patients served and this experience; it was rewarding, competency building, and challenging.

Having completed my BSN, I could still feel school in my blood when Pace initiated

a master's program. Having a supportive husband and family, I continued my studies in the evening and completed a master's degree in nursing administration and education in 1984. I was fortunate to have excellent professors and mentors. Jean Kijek (Program Director), Joan Moore (Nursing Research), Carolyn Chambers Clarke (Wellness Model), and Lori Sudal (VP Nursing and mentor) were RNs who made a major contribution to my professional development and for whom I will be eternally grateful.

Over the 18 years at Jacobi, I, like many others, was able to advance within the system based upon my additional education and clinical and administrative experience. Joining the private sector in 1993, initially in a small Westchester community hospital and later in a tertiary care facility in the Bronx, served to expand my knowledge and skills related to systems, health care, quality, and nursing services. In addition, I was able to find time to complete a postmaster's certificate in HIV/AIDS nursing and become an adjunct professor in nursing for the College of New Rochelle, first in the undergraduate and then in the RN to BSN program. In 2002, while assisting an RN during her BSN community nursing placement at Jacobi, I learned about the posting for an Assistant Vice President (AVP) for Nursing for the New York City Health and Hospitals Corporation. After a lengthy process, I was appointed as AVP in the spring of 2003.

Working at New York City Health and Hospitals Corporation (HHC) is both exciting and demanding. As a nurse, you need to be compassionate about the work and the commitment to the mission of the organization. Our goal over the years has not altered: to provide care to everyone who enters our doors regardless of their ability to pay. In this municipal hospital system, opportunities for growth and professional advancement abound. Education is encouraged.

This position has allowed me to be the voice of nursing for the corporation. In col- laboration with the senior leadership— focused upon patient and healthcare delivery, safety, and quality—the nursing agenda is built to ensure the provision of high-quality nursing services throughout the corporation.

What an honor for the granddaughter of immigrants.

human potential. One answer has been a new flat or side-by-side organizational style with participatory management and servant leaders who are effective and active listeners. Operating within this type of structure, companies such as Kyocera, Keyspan, The Body Shop, Xerox, and numerous others have begun to develop a spiri- tual connection in the workplace.

"Business is essentially a human enterprise facing all the challenges of the human relation- ship. Engaging in these relationships in a fair, loving, caring and compassionate way is the essence of spirituality"(Visser, 2005). Nursing leaders—not business leaders—should be at the forefront of this new model. Our business *is* car- ing. In our work, we are continually identifying the patient's human spirit to offer hope. Our work is inherently stressful and requires us to find meaning in suffering. The nature of most of our work is teamwork. Teams function best when they hold the same values.

What About Diversity?

Thirty years ago, we would not have needed to discuss diversity of values. We all worked within a 10-mile radius of where we were born and raised and were of similar ethnic, cultural, reli- gious, and social groups. Our patients were from the same community as ours. We did not even know the word *diversity* existed. We all spoke the same language. Working with the diversity we encounter today, we must put respect and valu- ing as top-priority behaviors in the work envi- ronment. As team members we must ask, "What are the core values we all agree upon?"

In his research on a global code of ethics for the 21st century, Kidder (1994) found that despite diversity, men and women around the world hold in common eight core values: love, truth, fairness, freedom, unity, tolerance, responsibility, and respect for life. As nurses, we do agree upon these core values. They are all in our code of ethics for nurses. The spiritual nurse leader begins here, by helping the group identify the values they all hold in common—not their differences. One of the most potent group experiences occurs when a work group realizes that, despite their diversity, they hold in common the same core values.

Encountering a Spiritual Leader

Great leaders inspire us to go places we would never go on our own, and to attempt things we never thought we had in us.

—Finzel, *Top Ten Mistakes Leaders Make*

One of the earliest role models in my career was a head nurse on the children's psychiatric unit of a large city hospital. The hospital had a famous reputation, but the employees and leaders were uncaring, lazy, and unmotivated. Upon arrival to this unit, a different atmosphere was noted. A stunning black woman in her 30s with blonde hair, designer clothing, dripping with jewelry, sporting fake green nails and high heels greeted me at the door to the children's ward for my first day of transfer. The unit had a reputation of being different; staff from units in the hospital spoke of the head nurse as being "different and stuck up" with unrealistic expectations of her staff.

Well, she certainly looked different from the other head nurses. Her orientation to the unit was caring and crystal clear. She defined the culture and her staff expectations: "We treat these children with care and respect. They are all here, because they have been harmed in some way by those they loved or trusted. We never restrain them or medicate them—only in dire emergencies." In her tenure of 16 years, that had occurred twice. Was I clear? Could I practice within these parameters? These were visionary ideas, not the common practices of the time or of the greater hospital culture.

As a young graduate nurse, I was willing and eager to give it a try. My question was how she got these older resistant workers to follow her lead. I watched her closely. She led by example. She was a role model with the patients. She was present on the unit just enough to see that her philosophy was carried out. She saw her job as nurturing and caring about her staff. She made it a career to really know what made each staff member respond: what their life was about, what concerned and motivated each of them. When one worker was hurting or having a bad day or had a personal need, the others took up the slack. She never had to direct that; it was the culture, the expectation.

People hated to float in or out of the unit. The culture was so divergent from the main cul-

ture of the institution. Supervisors, doctors, the unit chief, and the researchers all deferred to this head nurse's values. Workers did things well outside of their specified job descriptions. She used praise whenever she found an opportunity and sparingly, quietly, and confidentially would identify things you might have done differently. She never identified these things as mistakes, only opportunities to look at what we might have done differently. Her positive attitude never waivered. It was always neutral and non-judgmental. She treated and respected all of us for the unique human beings we were. She identified, utilized, and developed all of our talents because she saw and appreciated the human spirit in each of us. She never aspired to greater positions in nursing. She is still there in the same position she has held since her graduation. I did not know at the time that she was my first spiritual leader in nursing.

Becoming a Spiritual Nursing Leader

Leaders have a unique mission. They need a clear and compelling vision with their own mission statement. They establish measurable goals and success criteria. A spiritual leader looks to establish for self and followers meaning and value in the work, the process, and conditions under which the work is done.

One famous leader in nursing, Martha Rogers, was my lecturer in the first semester of graduate school. She did not depend on anyone else to communicate her message, her theory, or her beliefs. She taught the introductory course to make sure the message was communicated with her spiritual intent. The Dean of Nursing at New York University (NYU) still teaches the freshman seminar course. She wants students to know what she believes and stands for in nursing. She wants to mold them. Great leaders in nursing do not delegate the task of orientation to followers. They make sure they are an active part of the orientation of each new employee or student and that their values are imparted clearly and directly.

The second person of significance in my career was an assistant director of nursing at a large research institution. She set a high standard of care and high expectations for all of us. When she identified something you were good at, you were on a committee or teaching it to others. She took a professional interest in each of us. She may not have known us personally, but she readily identified our professional strengths and utilized them to motivate each of us. She established for staff belief in the value and meaning of the work. When the process or conditions of the work were less than ideal, she listened to the workers and took the steps needed to improve conditions. She identified and valued each person's contribution to getting the job done and gave the person the authority and respect needed to get it done. I learned the key principle of delegation: after you have delegated it to the right person, get out of the way or he will not believe that you believe he can do it. She believed in and expected the best in others. She was not blind to conflict or slips from standards, and when they occurred she addressed each in a clear and positive mode. She helped us to identify meaning and value in our work, our patients, and each other. She led us in questioning processes and conditions that were not optimal and gave us the encouragement and support needed to improve them.

These were the models that I developed from. In the subsequent years, my career took me to other institutions and areas of responsibility in supervision, staff development, administration, and education. I drew upon these experiences and role models. I used their management style, never being able to articulate it clearly. The more I read about management theory, the more I was sure these managers were not adequately described by any of them. Their management behaviors are the foundations of what I believe *is* spiritual leadership: (1) a belief in your own mission in life and nursing, (2) a positive belief about the intentions of others, (3) a clear identification of the core values in your life and work from which you operate, (4) identification of the risks you are willing to take, (5) a plan for how you will build the bridges needed to get the work done, and (6) implementing the structure and the plan needed for the team to accomplish the goal.

The spiritual leader believes it can be done. The spiritual leader is an *implementer*. The team will tell you how to get it done if you listen carefully. Once you put your idea into words and define the project with enthusiasm, others will come forward to be on the team.

Spiritual leadership starts with a self-audit. Ask yourself the following questions:

1. What is my mission statement?
2. What do I believe about others?
3. What are my beliefs about the intentions of others?
4. What are my core values in life and work?
5. What risks am I willing to take?
6. How can I build bridges between workers, departments, management, patients, and staff?

Spiritual leaders develop their team by using the following techniques:

1. Being effective listeners
2. Being fully present in the moment

3. Clearly communicating the project and issues
4. Facilitating change and creative approaches
5. Properly delegating and following up
6. Practicing and modeling healthy conflict resolution

Productivity and Staff Retention

The reason for a surging interest in a new type of nursing management and leadership is the dwindling nursing workforce. We cannot educate nurses fast enough to keep up with the pace of those leaving or retiring. The organizations and leaders ahead of the curve will be those who retain the precious resources they have and cultivate those coming up in the ranks.

Organizational Development or Appreciative Inquiry? What Does This Have to Do With Spiritual Leadership?

The field of business and management has been operating for some time with the model of organizational development. With this model, one examines the organization in terms of what is wrong and what systems, processes, procedures, and people need to change. One then sets out to find change agents to spearhead the changes that will need to take place.

The organizational development field began with a conception of the worker as a physical being, moved to understanding the worker as an emotional being, and evolved to appreciating the worker as an intellectual being. We are now on the cusp of understanding that employees are also spiritual beings, and that when we tap into

that spiritual energy we are able to provide a sense of meaning and fulfillment for the workers and a higher level of commitment and creativity in accomplishing organizational goals: body, mind, emotion, and spirit (Neal, 2006).

If this is so, how do we tap into all four energies, and particularly into the spiritual energy, when we are attempting to improve the delivery of care, the team, or the entire organization? Appreciative inquiry is one method designed to do just that.

Appreciative inquiry looks at what is right, special, unique, and positive. What gives employees a sense of esteem about what they do? It requires a tapping into each employee's uniqueness of spirit, who they are, and what they bring from the other areas of their life (Stavros & Torres, 2005).

Action in the Field

Spiritual leadership requires a recognition and response to the multifaceted expressions of spirituality encountered in our co-workers and patients each day. Forward-thinking organizations are trying to tap into this unexplored human potential to enhance customer service and productivity. In healthcare organizations, the Healthcare Chaplaincy, Inc. (HCI), services have stepped in with their award titled "The Whole Life Award." This award is given to the staff member who, in their care for others, demonstrates respect for human beings as whole persons; practices healthcare with an appreciation for the interrelated functions of body, mind, and spirit in illness and in healing; models teamwork; and embodies in personal and professional life a substantial degree of wholeness in striving for a balance of physical, mental, and spiritual well-being.

The Spiritual Leader Is a Values Coach

The spiritual leader first aligns her values with the organization's values. The spiritual leader recognizes the importance of contribution and welcomes all levels of employees in the team and the project. The spiritual leader shares the organization's values and translates them into rational terms that make sense and bring meaning to the work and the part each is playing in the achievement of the goal.

One Person Can Make a Difference: An Outline for Change

Several years ago the chief executive officer (CEO) of a health system wanted to change the entire system and its organization. He approached staff development for a plan of how the staff would be trained to meet the demands of the new job descriptions. This was a tremendous undertaking for two educators. We had a choice. We could take on the task and lead the change with enthusiasm and motivate others to do the same, or we could resist. Resistance would probably bring about more stress and demands. It was a turning point. We both had to decide whether this change was in alignment with our core values. We knew it was unpopular. What were the risks? To move it forward we needed to be committed. Once committed to the idea, we developed a transition plan and enlisted support from the executive team; we were ready to lead the organizational change. In two weeks, we evolved from a department of nursing staff developers to an organization-wide training and development department. Over the next five years, this transition plan became the foundation utilized to bring about system-wide alignment of mission and core values.

What Type of Leadership Is Required During the Process of Rapid Organizational Change?

For many years as a staff nurse, teacher, supervisor, and educator, I heard the staff refer to administration as "they." *They* think I am invisible; *they* do not care; *they* do not know what I do. On the other hand, administration referred to staff with comments such as *"They* do not want to work hard; *they* can do it; it is no big deal; *they'll* just have to handle it." On both sides of the table, these people were *invisible* to each other. Administration was hiding behind policies, directives, and memos, referring to themselves as "the executive staff" instead of by name. Workers hid behind union contracts and union representatives. I saw invisibility and blindness to each other's values and worth as the main issues.

What Did the Workers and Organizational Leaders Really Want?

Administration wanted the goals of the organization accomplished with compassion and caring toward the patients. The employees wanted their work of caring to be visible to "the executive staff." The employees knew that what they shared with patients was invisible, yet of great value in the patient's healing process. They did not believe this *invisible* group of executives saw any value in what they offered patients. This seemed to be a common theme throughout my career, no matter which organization I was working in.

As the leader of education across a vast system, my charge was to develop one organizational culture from the many. I began by spending much time in each organization, listening first and teaching second. What did any of these organizational cultures hold in common? What could be said to be held in common by all of the members of the larger system? My work began as I listened intently and spent time with staff in each organization. I found common themes. Each region and each organization's chant was *We are invisible to them*. I needed to transform a group of parts into a whole.

I began by building bridges between the two groups, sharing the values of each group with the other. I looked for one person in each group to show some willingness to see the other side. Through dialoguing about core values and our common mission, each organization began to value the contributions made by the others to the larger system and toward enhancing their organization. It was a slow process with many hours spent on education and sometimes coerced collaboration, but the system began to work together.

What happened next was not predictable. The CEO asked me to an executive team meeting and then charged each of us to write up our ideas on spiritual leadership in behavioral health. I had not thought of any of the things we were doing as spiritual: mission driven and caring, yes, but not spiritual. As we left the meeting, the CEO asked for our ideas to develop his written summary and plan. Others in the meeting made it clear to me that they had no intention of putting anything in writing about spirituality. As I walked back to my office, the theme of visibility and invisibility rang out in my head.

What I wrote follows:

NOTES ON SPIRITUAL LEADERSHIP

1. How does it fit into the strategic plan?
2. How will it address improving the quality of patient care?
3. How will it help us to integrate the mission and values into our daily work?
4. How can we come up with a program theme and name that is tied to our goals?
5. How do we make the invisible, "the spirit," in each of us visible in our daily work to create an environment of caring?

After another meeting with the executives and board, a new position was created for a mission and spiritual leader for the staff. This person, Sister Karen Helfenstein, a veteran nurse, administrator, educator, and spiritual leader, became my other half, my guide in the process. Together, we put into words and programs what was needed to unite the staff behind the mission despite their geographic location.

In the beginning of the process, we were not identified as organizational leaders and our role and mission were not spelled out. We had each identified values that were important to us and to the organization. We both believed in the mission and in the value of each person within the organization. We set out with these as guiding principles and along the way tried to make the values come alive in the staff we encountered each day.

Sister Karen identified many resources as well as values leaders in the process. One person who greatly influenced our work together was Judi Neal. She opened her work, her heart, and her home to us and was a guide and inspiration to us in the process. Mostly, she made real to us all the things we thought were only invisible. Judi told her life story and how her consciousness of her personal values grew. She spoke of deep-down knowledge of what she needed to do because of who she was. Risks, results, growth, pain, suffering, and new life were all along her spiritual path. She shared new terms and definitions such as *spiritually grounded*—when one holds values sacred, acts according to those values with discipline and faithfulness, and pays attention to what comes next. One must be alert to personal epiphanies/revelations learned only by values. Values are our North Star on the spiritual journey (Neal, 2006).

Margaret Wheatley's book *Turning to One Another* (2002) provided a terrific starting point and foundation for group work with the staff. Sister Karen faithfully ran groups with whatever staff were interested in each and every hospital and outpatient service in the entire system. Staff were reluctant and cautious at first. Once in the group, they shared incredibly personal and sensitive observations and windows to their soul and spirit and their real motivations for the work they were doing with patients.

Beginning Steps in the Process of Encouraging Spiritual Expression

The beginning steps in encouraging spiritual expression should be taken in offering small, nonthreatening, informal group meetings where staff do not feel the need to respond but instead listen and reflect on a reading or a quote, or something universal and nonspecific to the group. Initially, these groups are formed on a voluntary basis.

Conducting Informal Meetings

During the implementation process, we used informal meetings to share and reinforce core values. Sister Karen began the sessions with an outside reading from Wheatley's book *Turning to One Another*. Following are great group conversation starters:

- What do I believe about others?
- What is my faith in the future?
- When have I experienced good listening?
- What is my unique contribution to the whole?
- When do I experience sacred?

We utilized the organization's own defined core values for group work. Here are some examples for group work sessions. These were also used as a reorientation of staff after six months of employment to reinforce core organizational values and enhance retention:

CORE VALUE: RESPECT

- What is your own experience with respect?
- When was the first time in your life experience that you can remember feeling respected? How did that feel? How was respect communicated to you?
- Think of an experience you have had where you felt disrespected. How did that feel? What were the elements?
- Have you felt respected? By whom? How?
- Have you felt disrespected? How? By whom and/or in what way?
- Have you been able to communicate respect? How? And to whom?

CORE VALUE: FAIRNESS

- Have you seen honesty among co-workers?
- Do you feel you are dealt with fairly?

- Are you free to bring forth issues to your co-workers in an honest and constructive manner?
- What about to your manager?
- Do you see the fairness in action in our dealings with patients? With each other?

CORE VALUE: COMPASSION

- Have you witnessed compassion?
- When?
- Have you been compassionate?

Following are the beginning steps in the spiritual organizational awareness process:

1. Define what core values are important to your organization and the work you do.
2. Interview for these values.
3. Orient to these values. During the orientation, select out those who do not fit.
4. Build a team of employees whose values are congruent with the mission and purpose of the organization.

Impacting the Change Process in the Organization

Change in the organization is a process that begins with the leader's alignment of his or her values with the core values of the organization. The leader then assesses what key factors, issues, processes, attitudes, or beliefs are having the most negative impact on his or her team and what visibles and invisibles he or she needs to change.

Make an Assessment

The leader begins the assessment by taking note of the most obvious forces and influences in the organization; the leader then turns his or her full attention to uncovering those forces and influences that are less visible, but usually the most powerful forces preventing change. The leader should begin to:

- Map the invisible workplace. Look at the ways things really get done—often these go unnoticed or are invisible; assess these first before assuming how to change the work environment.
- Identify invisible anchors that may keep the group from changing.
- Benchmark the attitudes and values of employees at the outset.
- Use data from employee surveys.
- Benchmark quality with existing quality assessment (QA) indicators.
- Benchmark customer satisfaction with existing indicators.
- Restate and emphasize the standards and values.
- Determine whether any gaps exist between the espoused values of the organization and those of the employee in the prehire, orientation, and evaluation processes.

Planning

Look at the overall issues in the organization or on your team. Prioritize what processes, if implemented, could best impact the spiritual culture of the organization or team. Significant items to focus on might be to:

- Change the selection process. Interview for values congruent with the new organization.
- Encourage mentoring and coaching of new employees and leaders by those who exemplify the values and standards you want to embed.

- Appoint positive energy and core values persons to key committees.
- Move negative employees to less visible responsibilities, positions where they have less influence on the group.

Implementation

Launch recognition efforts that are consistent with the mission and the idea of making the "spirit" more visible to others as a caring service organization:

- Reinforce values-guided behaviors and attitudes reflected in everyday work.
- Share insights into the "invisible" ways things get done. (Each department or employee can come up with two examples.)
- Share ways each department feels invisible to another department and/or management.
- Ask individuals to share behaviors of others that make them feel invisible in their daily work. (Later this can be used as a takeoff for customer/patient service changes.)
- Ask each department to come up with ideas for visibility. (They can submit a quote, drawing, photograph, etc. that speaks to who they are.)
- Create a sacred space for reflection (a break room, meditation room, or chapel).

Outcomes

The business literature has come alive with spiritually based leadership examples and terminology. It is the new buzzword associated with improving the bottom line. "Spirituality is essential to health, trust, creativity, commitment, ethical behavior, and productivity. Spirituality tends to ground us in a greater good beyond the self, helps us value other people and creates in us more depth and sensitivity" (Miller, 1999).

Spirituality in the workplace is the practice of reflection and celebration that reminds colleagues of the meaning of life and the dignity of our work. A series of structures can be created by the individual leader or the organization to give colleagues opportunities to realize sacredness in everyday encounters. Spirituality deepens our awareness of our own experiences of the mystery of life and invites us to reflect on the significance of those experiences. It builds community in the workplace and respect for each other's beliefs and traditions. The visible outcome is improved staff retention and customer satisfaction. The invisible is a deep respect for the whole person, body, mind, and spirit, visible through demonstrated respect in each human encounter.

Margaret Benefiel's book *Soul at Work: Spiritual Leadership in Organizations* (2005) uses the term "soulful leadership" to demonstrate how the spiritual centeredness of leaders translates into the way employees and customers are treated. Benefiel reminds us that even if the keys to nurture a soulful organization are missing in the place we work, we can still have an impact on our sphere of influence. As leaders, we can be positive and proactive in nurturing the culture around us.

Your self-audit is something that needs continual attention. What you believe about the intention of others is also a strong determinant of your effectiveness as a spiritual leader. Do you believe, as Harry Truman did, that "when we understand the other fellow's viewpoint—understand what he is trying to do—nine out of ten times he is trying to do it right"?

The spiritual leader, according to Benefiel: (1) brings her soul to work, (2) finds ways to sustain that soul inside and outside of work and in the midst of the workplace, and (3) brings that spiritually grounded presence into her sphere of influence, being responsible to cultivate her own spiritual health as well as recognizing the spiritual nature and needs of co-workers (Benefiel, 2005).

According to Walt Disney, "There are three kinds of people in the world. There are the well poisoners, who discourage others, stomp on their creativity and tell them they can't do. There are the lawn mowers. People who have good intentions, but are self-absorbed, who mow their own lawns, but never help others. And there are life enhancers. This last category contains people who reach out to enrich the lives of others, who lift them up and inspire them" (Maxwell & Dornan, 1997, p. 55).

As nurse leaders, I believe we want to be life enhancers. As we move into the next era, we have to develop these spiritual leadership skills to retain our staff and sustain ourselves. I ask you to reflect upon the nursing leaders that have motivated and inspired you. What can you do to bring their spiritual leadership example to your team?

Summary

Spirituality helps to maintain the organizational system. This chapter discusses methods of being a supportive spiritual team leader. By using scenarios and examples, this chapter explores the methodology of providing team leadership.

QUESTIONS

1. The spiritual leader who is working as a coach does which of the following?
   a. first, aligns her values with the organizational values
   b. adjusts the values of the organization to meet the needs of the employees
   c. chooses leadership from the employees and has them set values
   d. assigns roles to each of the employers and staff

2. To address The Joint Commission recommendations concerning assessment of patient spirituality, nursing education should include
   a. traditional and nontraditional religion as part of nursing education
   b. a spiritual assessment as part of the nursing assessment of the client
   c. self assessment of one's own spiritual beliefs and values
   d. All of the above

3. The concern about including spiritualism in health care is that some consider
   a. one's spirituality as too personal to discuss or to put into words on an assessment
   b. religion and spirituality the same and as such not appropriate to be part of a health-care assessment

c. the healthcare focus as treating only the body

d. All of the above

4. People often confuse *spirituality* with *religion*. Spirituality is defined as a

a. formal religion

b. way of being, an attitude toward life

c. realm totally exclusive of religion

d. way of meeting one's need to help others

5. The spiritual nurse leader in helping a group to identify their commonalities would

a. first identify their differences

b. utilize the nursing code of ethics as a representation of the commonality they hold in their core values

c. have the group explore their cultural diversity

d. have the group agree on all their values

References

Anandarajah, G., & Hight, E. (2001). Spirituality and medical practice: Using the HOPE questions as a practical tool for spiritual assessment. *American Family Physician, 63*(1), 81–89.

Benefiel, M. (2005). *Soul at work: Spiritual leadership in organizations.* New York: Seabury Books.

Erickson, H., Tomlin, E., & Swain, M. (1983). *Modeling and role modeling: A theory and paradigm for nursing.* Englewood Cliffs, NJ: Prentice Hall.

Finzel, H. (2000). *Top ten mistakes leaders make.* Colorado Springs, CO: Cook Communication Ministries.

Kidder, R. M. (1994). *Shared values for a troubled world: Conversations with men and women of conscience.* San Francisco: Jossey-Bass.

Marriner-Tomey, A. (1989). *Nursing theorists and their work.* St. Louis: Mosby.

Maxwell, J., & Dornan, J. (1997). *Becoming a person of influence.* Nashville: Thomas Nelson.

Miller, W. C. (1999). *Flash of brilliance: Inspiring creativity where you work.* New York: Basic Books.

Neal, J. (2006). *Edgewalkers: People and organizations that take risks, build bridges and break new ground.* Westport, CT: Praeger.

Neuman, B. (1982). *The Neuman system model: Application to nursing education and practice.* Norwalk, CT: Appleton-Century-Crofts.

Riehl-Sisca, J. P., & Roy, C. (1980). *Conceptual models for nursing practice* (2nd ed.). New York: Appleton-Century-Crofts.

Rogers, M. E. (1980). A science of unitary man. In J. P. Riehl-Sisca & C. Roy (Eds.) *Conceptual models for nursing practice* (2nd ed., pp. 329–337). New York: Appleton-Century-Crofts.

Stavros, J., & Torres, C. (2005). *Dynamic relationships: Unleashing the power of appreciative inquiry in daily living.* Chagrin Falls, OH: Taos Publishing.

Visser, W. (2005). Spirituality in the workplace: Interview for a special issue, *Effective Executive.* Retrieved March 27, 2007, from http://www.waynevisser.com/articles.htm

Watson, J. (2005) *Caring science as sacred science.* Philadelphia: F. A. Davis.

Wheatley, M. J. (2002). *Turning to one another: Simple conversations to return hope to the future.* San Francisco: Berrett-Koehler.

Additional Resources

Spirituality and Practice:
http://www.spiritualityandpractice.com

International Center for Spirit at Work:
http://www.spiritatwork.org

Centre for Spirituality at Work:
http://www.spiritualityatwork.org

Index